Here are your

2000 World Book Health & Medical Annual Cross-Reference Tabs

For insertion in your WORLD BOOK set

The Cross-Reference Tab System is designed to help link THE WORLD BOOK HEALTH & MEDICAL ANNUAL's major articles to related WORLD BOOK articles. When you later look up a topic in your WORLD BOOK and find a Tab by the article, you will know that one of your HEALTH & MEDICAL ANNUALS has newer or more detailed information.

How to use these Tabs

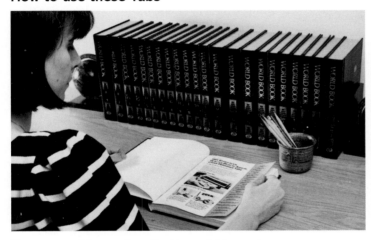

First, remove this page from THE HEALTH & MEDICAL ANNUAL.

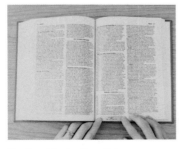

Begin with the first Tab, **ADOLESCENT.** Take the *A* volume of your WORLD BOOK set and find the **ADOLESCENT** article. Moisten the **ADOLESCENT** tab and affix it to that page by the article.

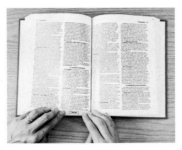

Glue all the other Tabs in the appropriate volumes.

THE WORLD BOOK

HEALTH & MEDICAL ANNUAL

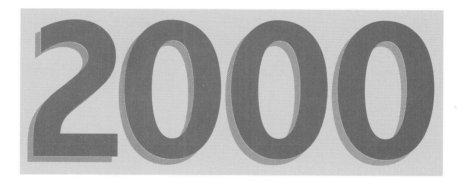

2000

World Book, Inc.
a Scott Fetzer company
Chicago

www.worldbook.com

THE YEAR'S MAJOR HEALTH STORIES

New brain cells

Various studies in 1998 and 1999 add to evidence that, contrary to long-held beliefs, new brain cells can form in adult brains. In the Health Updates section, see BRAIN AND NERVOUS SYSTEM.

From reports of a record drop in AIDS deaths to the promise of new drugs to treat arthritis, it was an eventful year in medicine. On these two pages are stories that editors selected as among the year's most important, memorable, or promising, along with information about where to find them in the book.

The Editors

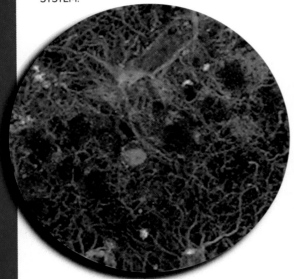

A new treatment for obesity

The FDA in April 1999 approved the use of orlistat as a treatment for obesity. In the Health Updates section, see WEIGHT CONTROL.

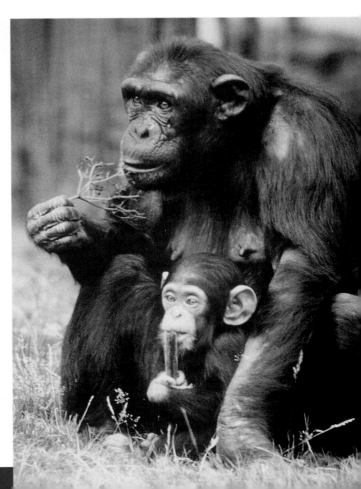

Chimps linked to AIDS virus

In January 1999, researchers identified a subspecies of chimpanzees in Africa as the source of the AIDS-like virus that evolved into human HIV. In the Health Updates section, see AIDS.

World Book, Inc.
525 W. Monroe
Chicago, IL 60661

ISBN 0-7166-1150-3
ISSN 0890-4480
Library of Congress Catalog Card Number: 87-648075
Printed in the United States of America

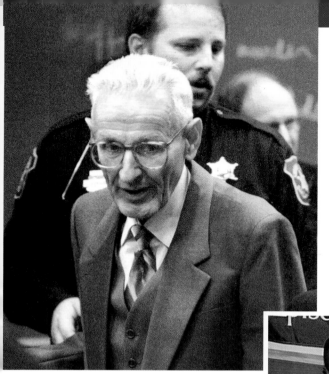

Kevorkian convicted of murder

A Michigan judge in March 1999 convicted Jack Kevorkian of second-degree murder. The retired pathologist had been charged with assisting in the suicide of a terminally ill man. In the Health Updates section, see MEDICAL ETHICS.

Surgeons perform hand transplant

Surgeons in September 1998 performed the first successful hand transplant. In the Health Updates section, see SURGERY.

World's first octuplets

A woman in Texas gave birth in December 1998 to the world's first known surviving set of octuplets. In the Health Updates Section, see HEALTH CARE ISSUES.

Drop in AIDS deaths

The number of deaths from AIDS fell by 47 percent in 1997, causing health officials in 1998 to remove the disease from the U.S. government's list of 10 leading causes of death. In the Health Updates section, see AIDS.

FDA approves "super aspirins"

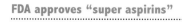

The FDA in 1998 and 1999 approved four new drugs to treat arthritis. In the Health Updates section, see DRUGS.

CONTENTS

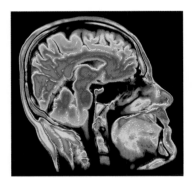

See page 22.

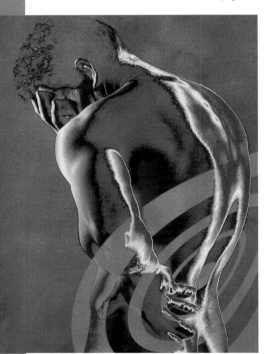

See page 62.

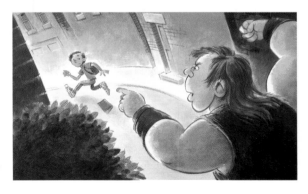

See page 130.

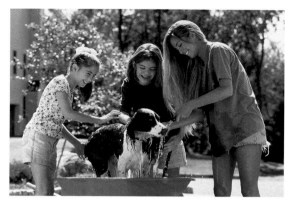

See page 156.

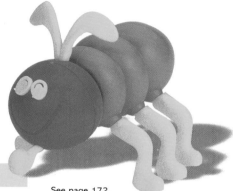

See page 172.

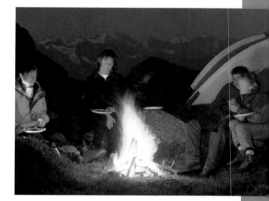

See page 196.

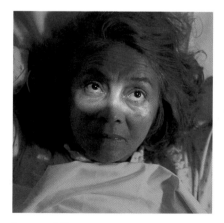

See page 213.

STAFF

IMPORTANT NOTE: The information contained in this publication is not intended as a substitute for the medical advice of physicians or other medical or health-care professionals. Always consult a physician or other appropriate health-care professional on any matters related to health and particularly regarding symptoms that may require diagnosis or medical attention.

EDITORIAL ADVISORY BOARD

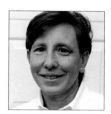

Jan Ellen Berger is Medical Director of Managed Care for the Pediatric Faculty Foundation at Children's Memorial Hospital. She received the B.A. degree in 1979 from Skidmore College, the M.D. degree in 1982 from Loyola Stritch Medical School, and a Master's degree in Jurisprudence and Health Law in 1989 from Loyola University. She is the chairperson of the National Committee on Medical Liability for American Academy of Pediatrics, ,a member of the Advisory Committee of Academic Primary Care at Children's Memorial Hospital, and a member of the managed care subcommittee of the American Medical Association Specialty Society Medical Liability Project.

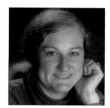

Nadine C. Bruce, M.D., is Director of MetroHealth Medical Associates and Residency Clinics at MetroHealth Medical Center in Cleveland, Associate Professor of Medicine at Case Western Reserve University School of Medicine, and Medical Director of the Kethley House in Cleveland. She received the B.S. degree in 1964 from the College of St. Francis and the M.D. degree in 1970 from the University of Illinois at Chicago. She is board-certified in both Internal Medicine and Geriatrics. Dr. Bruce is a Master of the American College of Physicians and former Governor of the College.

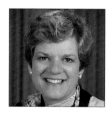

Linda Hawes Clever, M.D., is Chair of the Department of Occupational Health at California Pacific Medical Center and Clinical Professor of Medicine at the University of California at San Francisco. She received the A.B. degree in 1962 and the M.D. degree in 1965, both from Stanford University. Dr. Clever served on both the Board of Governors of the American College of Physicians and its Board of Regents. She was Editor of the *Western Journal of Medicine* between 1990 and 1998. She is a member of the Institute of Medicine of the National Academy of Sciences and the Board of Scientific Counselors of the National Institute of Occupational Safety and Health.

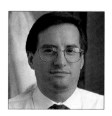

Mark W. Stolar, M.D., is an Associate Professor of Clinical Medicine at Northwestern University Medical School. Dr. Stolar received the B.A. degree from Northwestern University in 1975 and the M.D. degree from the University of Illinois in 1979. He is board certified in both internal medicine and endocrinology. He is on the board of the Endocrine Fellows Foundation and is a member of the American College of Physicians, the Endocrine Society, and the American Diabetes Association.

CONTRIBUTORS

Auerbach, Vivian, Ph.D.
Neuropsychologist and Adjunct
Associate Professor,
Emory University.
[Medical and Safety Alerts: *Teen
Suicide: A Growing Concern*]

Baker, Suzanne M., B.A., M.A.
Director of Development Research,
University of Chicago.
[Health Updates and Resources:
Surgery]

Balk, Robert A., M.D.
Director of Pulmonary and Critical
Care Medicine,
Rush-Presbyterian-St. Luke's
Medical Center.
[Health Updates and Resources:
Respiratory System]

Barone, Jeanine, M.S.
Nutritionist, Exercise Physiologist,
Sports Medicine, and Nutrition
Editor,
*University of California at Berkeley
Wellness Letter.*
[Health Updates and Resources:
Nutrition and Food]

Birnbaum, Gary, M.D.
Co-Director of Multiple Sclerosis
Center,
Minneapolis Clinic of Neurology.
[Health Updates and Resources:
Brain and Nervous System]

Bushie, Laura D., M.A., Ph.D.
Research Biologist and Free-Lance
Medical Writer.
[Spotlight on Medicine: *The Aging
Population; Medicine in the 21st
Century;* Health Updates and Re-
sources: *Cancer; Sexually Transmit-
ted Diseases; Skin; Stroke*]

Connaughton, Dennis, B.A.
Free-lance Medical Writer.
[A Healthy You: *Can You Hear
What I'm Saying*]

Courtouise, Jeffrey W., M.D.
Medical Historian.
[Spotlight on Medicine: *Medical
Advances of the 20th Century*]

Crawford, Michael H., M.D.
Chief, Division of Cardiology,
University of New Mexico
Health Sciences Center.
[Health Updates and Resources:
Heart and Blood Vessels]

Despres, Renee, Ph.D.
Free-lance Writer.
[Medical and Safety Alerts: *The
Great (and Safe) Outdoors;* Health
Updates and Resources: *Exercise
and Fitness; Glands and Hormones;
Mental Health*]

Friedman, Emily, B.A.
Health Policy Analyst.
[Health Updates and Resources:
Health Care Issues]

Gerber, Glenn S., M.D.
Associate Professor,
Department of Surgery,
University of Chicago.
[Health Updates and Resources:
Urology]

Gillespie, Gregory M., B.A.
Free-lance Writer.
[Consumer Health: *Controlling the
Costs of Pet Health Care*]

Hales, Dianne, B.A., M.S.
Free-lance Writer.
[A Healthy Family: *Bullying: A
Silent Nightmare in the Schoolyard*]

Hussar, Daniel A., M.S., Ph.D.
Remington Professor of Pharmacy,
Philadelphia College of Pharmacy
University of the Sciences.
[Health Updates and Resources:
Drugs]

Kass, Philip H., D.V.M., M.P.V.M.,
M.S., Ph.D.
Associate Professor of
Epidemiology,
University of California at Davis.
[Health Updates and Resources:
Veterinary Medicine]

Levine, Carol, M.A.
Director,
Families and Health Care Project,
United Hospital Fund.
[Health Updates and Resources:
Medical Ethics]

Lewis, David, C., M.D.
Professor of Medicine and
Community Health,
Brown University.
[Health Updates and Resources:
*Alcohol and Drug Abuse;
Smoking*]

Livingston, Pamela, B.A.
Free-lance Medical Writer.
[A Healthy Family: *Treating and
Preventing Childhood Obesity*]

Love, Lauren, B.A., M.F.A.
Free-lance Writer.
[Consumer Health: *Home Exercise
Equipment*; Health Updates and Re-
sources: *Birth Control; Weight Con-
trol*]

Luebbers, Lorna, B.S., C.M.T.
Free-lance Writer
[Consumer Health: *Selecting Safe
Toys*; Health Updates and Re-
sources: *Digestive System*]

Maugh, Thomas H., II, Ph.D.
Science Writer,
Los Angeles Times.
[Health Updates and Resources:
Environmental Health]

McInerney, Joseph D.,
B.S., M.A., M.S.
Director, Foundation for Genetic
Education and Counseling.
[Health Updates and Resources:
Genetic Medicine]

Minotti, Dominick A., M.D.,
Allergist,
Northwest Asthma and Allergy
Center.
[Health Updates and Resources:
Allergies and Asthma]

Moore, Margaret E.,
A.M.L.S., M.P.H.
Head, User Services Department,
Health Sciences Library,
University of North Carolina at
Chapel Hill.
[Health Updates and Resources:
Books of Health and Medicine]

Pisetsky, David S., M.D., Ph.D.
Chief of Rheumatology,
Duke University Medical Center.
[Health Updates and Resources:
Bone and Joint Disorders]

Rinehart, Rebecca D.
Director of Publications,
American College of Obstetricians
and Gynecologists.
[Health Updates and Resources:
Pregnancy and Childbirth]

Roodman, G. David, M.D., Ph.D.
Professor of Medicine,
Associate Chair for Research,
University of Texas Health Science
Center at San Antonio.
[Health Updates and Resources:
Blood]

Stephenson, Joan, B.S., Ph.D.
Associate Editor,
*Journal of the American Medical
Association.*
[A Healthy You: *A Breath-Taking
Ailment: Learning to Control
Asthma*]

Thompson, Jeffrey R., M.D.
President,
Dallas Kidney Specialists.
[Health Updates and Resources:
Kidney]

Tideiksaar, Rein, Ph.D.
Director of Geriatrics,
Sierra Health Services, Inc.
[Health Updates and Resources:
Aging]

Trubo, Richard, B.A., M.A.
Free-lance Medical Writer.
[Health Updates and Resources:
*AIDS; Child Development;
Diabetes; Ear and Hearing*]

Waddell, Christie, B.A.
Free-lance Medical Writer.
[A Healthy You: *A New Look for
Braces*]

Woods, Michael, B.S., Ph.D.
Science Editor, Washington Bureau,
*Pittsburgh Post-Gazette, Toledo
Blade.*
[A Healthy You: *Oh, My Aching
Back!*; Health Updates and Re-
sources: *Dentistry; Eye and Vision;
Infectious Diseases; Safety*]

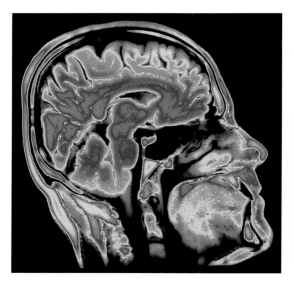

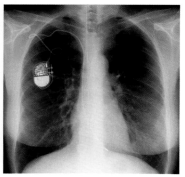

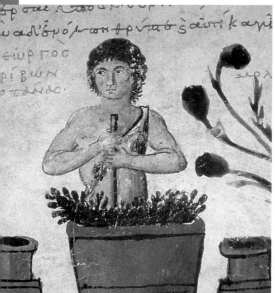

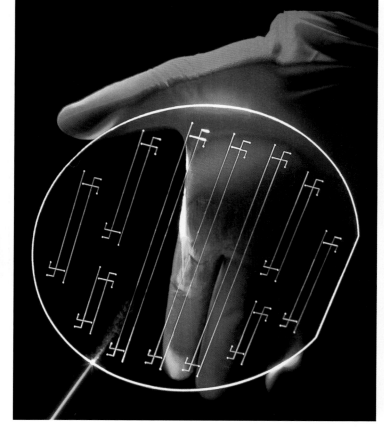

SPOTLIGHT ON THE MILLENNIUM

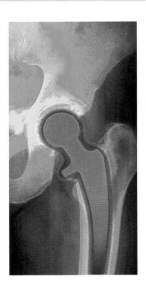

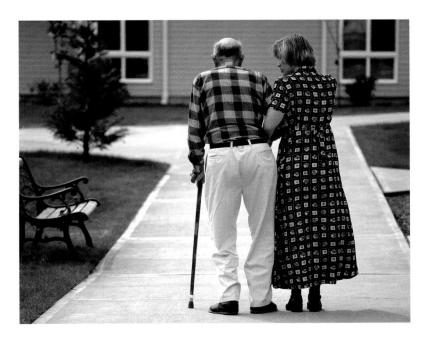

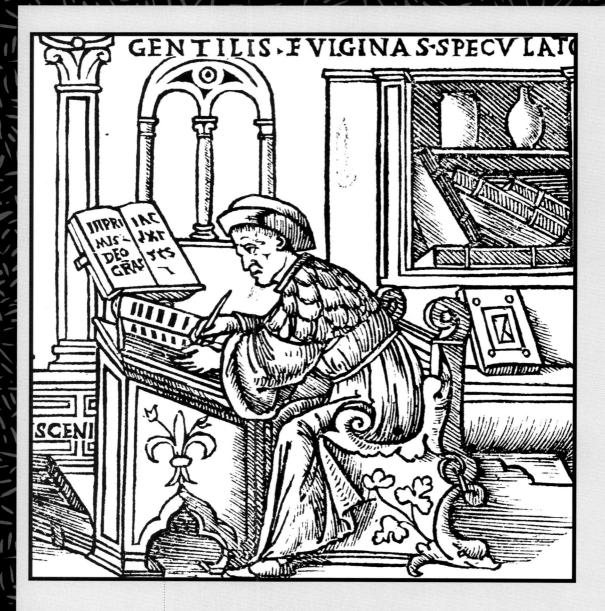

In the year 1000, medicine relied more on religious beliefs than on scientific foundation.

Medicine in the YEAR 1000

By Jeffrey Courtouise

A N ITALIAN BOY WOKE ONE MORNING WITH A TERRIBLE PAIN in his stomach. The pain was so severe that he could not dress himself. His concerned parents rushed him to a local monastery, where priests who also served as physicians mixed up an herbal tonic for the boy to drink. When the drink did not ease the pain, the monks consulted a medical text that suggested the pain might be relieved by balancing the boy's body fluids. A monk produced a knife, tested the sharpness of the blade with his thumb, and cut the boy's arm to drain blood from his body.

Although this type of treatment would be viewed as bizarre by today's standards, it was typical medical practice in the Western world of A.D. 1000. One thousand years ago, physicians had not yet learned to recognize individual illness as doctors do today. Although they treated the signs and symptoms of disease, physicians had no idea of what actually caused most diseases. They thought that disease was spread by bad odors or that illness was the result of sins of the soul.

At the dawn of the millennium in western Europe, hospitals were religious foundations and most physicians were priests, whose understanding of medicine relied more on religious beliefs than on scientific foundation. European physicians in the year 1000, however, were beginning to transcend the barriers of religion and superstition. Christian monks were translating medical and scientific literature written by Islamic scholars, which provided the Western world with ideas and practices that eventually gave rise to early modern medicine.

The Middle Ages

The year 1000 marked the mid-point of a historical period known as the Middle Ages, which lasted from the 400's to the 1500's. The Middle Ages, also known as the medieval period, bridged ancient and modern times in Western Europe. The early part of the Middle Ages—sometimes referred to as the Dark Ages—was a time characterized by widespread ignorance and lack of social progress. During this period, civilization sank low in Western Europe. Knowledge from the ancient Romans survived only in a few monastery, cathedral, and palace schools. Knowledge from ancient Greece almost disappeared. Few people received schooling. Many artistic and technical skills were lost. Population decreased, and life became more primitive.

While such darkness existed in Western Europe, life was brighter elsewhere. The Islamic empire of Southwest and Central Asia, for example, contributed greatly to medicine during the early Middle Ages. Rhazes, a Persian-born physician of the late 800's and early 900's, wrote the first accurate descriptions of measles and smallpox. Avicenna, an Arab physician of the late 900's and early 1000's, produced a vast medical encyclopedia called *Canon of Medicine*. It summed up the medical knowledge of the time and accurately de-

Translation of scientific literature

Christian monks, *left*, in the year 1000 were translating literature written by Islamic scholars, which provided the Western world with ideas from which early modern medicine eventually rose.

The author:

Jeffrey Courtouise is a medical historian.

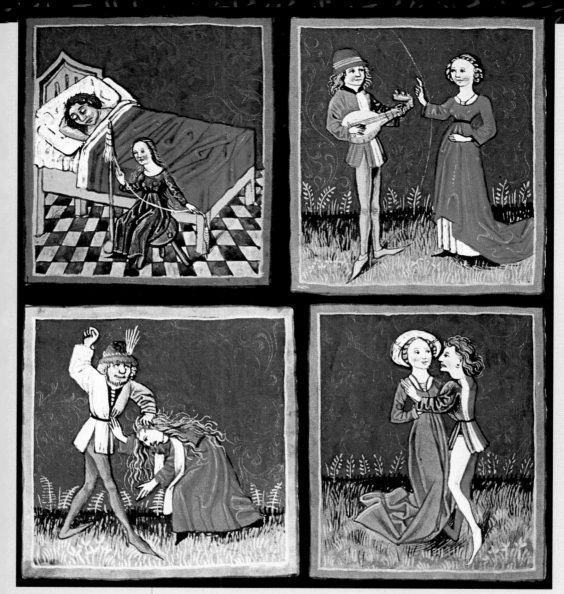

Humoralism

Humoralism viewed illness and personality as arising from a disturbance in the natural balance of four body fluids, *above*, clockwise, phlegm (slothful), black bile (sad), blood (jolly), and yellow bile (violent).

scribed meningitis, tetanus, and many other diseases. Much of the information in these writings was based on the scientific foundations established hundreds of years before by ancient Greek and Roman scholars—knowledge that had been lost to the Western world during the early Middle Ages.

By the year 1000, the opening of trade routes revived economic and political life in Western Europe. The Crusades, a series of holy wars against the Muslims, encouraged European trade with the Middle East. Merchants traveled far to trade with the peoples of the Byzantine Empire in southeastern Europe. Italians in Genoa, Pisa, Venice, and other towns built great fleets of ships to carry merchants' goods across the Mediterranean Sea to trade centers in Spain and northern Africa. Leaders in towns of northern Germany created the Hanseatic League to organize trade in northern Europe.

The opening of trade routes speeded passage of medical and scientific texts from the East to the West. These writings reintroduced what was to become one of the most enduring concepts of Western medicine: humoralism. This concept was established by the Greek physician Hippocrates (460?–380? B.C.), the first physician known to consider medicine a science and art separate from the practice of religion. Humoralism viewed illness as arising from a disturbance in the natural balance of four body *humors* (fluids)—phlegm, yellow bile, blood, and black bile.

Diseases of the Middle Ages

European physician-monks in the 1000's began learning how to make diagnoses in the manner of Hippocrates. They wrote numerous reports about illnesses. Based on these reports, medical historians know that the infant mortality rate was extremely high—around 45 percent. And life expectancy at birth was scarcely 30 years. People commonly suffered from cases of blindness, infectious dis-

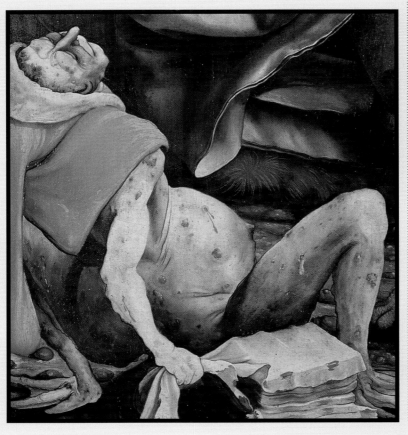

The scourge of leprosy

Leprosy was one of the most feared diseases of the 1000's. Lepers, *left*, were thought to be highly contagious. As a result, they were relegated to the margins of society.

eases, mental illness, deafness, and paralysis. Most of the paralysis, according to medical historians, can be accounted for by the dietary deficiencies of the time, especially vitamin deficiencies. And many other diseases were the result of poor sanitation.

As the population of medieval towns and cities increased after the early Middle Ages, hygienic conditions worsened, leading to a vast array of health problems. People drank water polluted by human waste, and swamps proliferated as cultivated land was abandoned. The result was an upsurge in polio, malaria, and paratyphoid fever. People also suffered from smallpox, dysentery, respiratory illness, measles, scarlet fever, tuberculosis, and syphilis, among other diseases.

Leprosy was one of the most feared diseases of the time. It was thought to be extremely contagious. Lepers were relegated to the margins of society and had to abide by many restrictions. These restrictions included not touching anything or anyone, except his or her spouse. In public, lepers announced themselves by sounding bells and rattles to warn people away. Thousands of people were sent to leper colonies scattered all over the world.

Herbal remedies

Books available in the early 1000's provided recipes for herbal medications, *below*. Health practitioners used herbal tonics to treat a variety of ills.

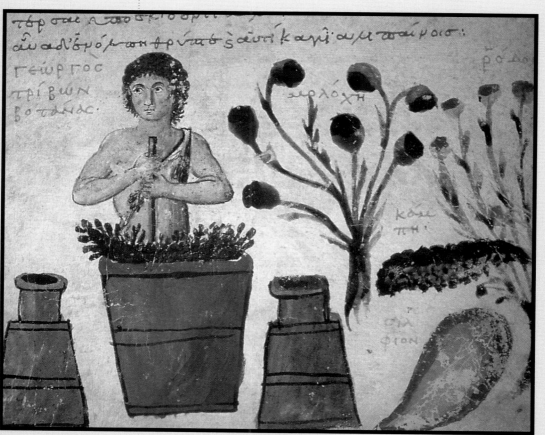

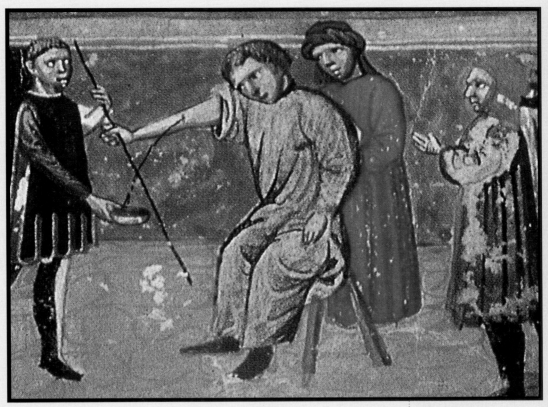

Treatment of illness

Medical practitioners in the year 1000 extolled the idea of *vis medicatrix naturae*, or the power of nature to cure itself. They believed that there was a natural tendency for things to get better on their own. Medieval physicians, like doctors today, strongly believed in the power of preventive medicine. They used diet and exercise regimes as their first line of defense against disease. And this was a wise strategy, because many of the treatments caused more discomfort than the illness itself, and few treatments actually worked.

Treatments for most diseases were a mishmash of humoral medicine, folklore, religious cures, and sorcery. For example, draping colored cloths around a person infected with smallpox was a treatment that may have been related to magic and witchcraft. Or it could have been related to the fact that smallpox patients suffered from *photophobia* (sensitivity to light) and the clothes may have protected them from light.

Remedies were often prepared from herbs, but also included ground earthworms, urine, and animal excrement. One medicine that *apothecaries* (forerunners of pharmacists) dispensed was called treacle. It consisted of more than 60 ingredients, including the roasted skin of vipers. Physicians considered treacle a cure-all. It was said

Bloodletting

A standard cure for almost any ill was bloodletting. A surgeon opened a vein to let out the excess or "bad humors." This was accepted medical theory and practice until the mid-1800's.

European hospitals in the Middle Ages

Hospitals in the Middle Ages were religious foundations and most physicians were priests. By the year 1000, Christian groups had established hundreds of charitable hospitals.

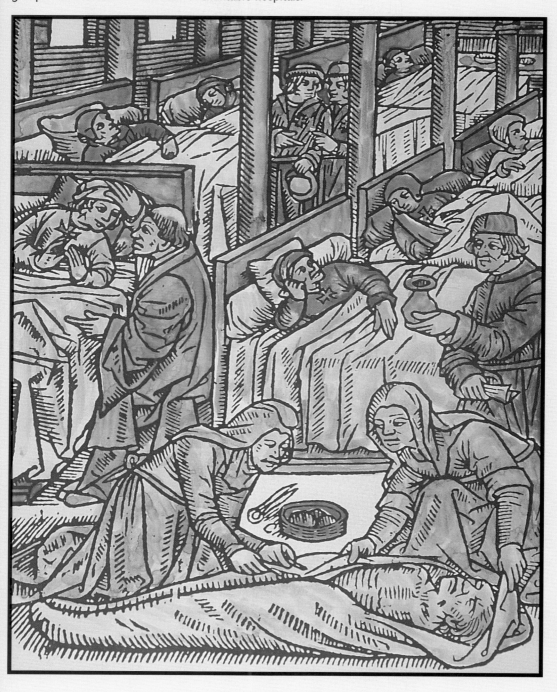

to prevent internal swellings; cure fevers; alleviate heart problems, blemishes, epilepsy, and palsy; induce sleep; improve digestion; strengthen limbs; heal wounds; remedy snake bites; and cure most other diseases.

Modern scientists analyzing the recipes used by medieval doctors have found that some of the ingredients contain chemicals that in fact do have healing properties. For example, medieval doctors often treated infected wounds with applications of moldy bread. Today, we know that bread molds contain the ingredients for the antibiotic penicillin.

Physicians believed that natural functions, such as sneezing, sweating, or excretion, were the best way of balancing body fluids and, thus, maintaining health. They would wrap patients in blankets to induce sweating or give them an herbal diuretic to increase urination. They also prescribed laxatives and medicines that would cause vomiting.

Medieval doctors believed that a buildup of blood caused fevers, apoplexy, and headache and that venesection—or bloodletting—was the obvious remedy. The normal method of bloodletting was to tie a bandage around the patient's arm to make the forearm swell up, and then open the exposed vein with a lancet. This procedure, which remained popular until the 1800's, was commonly referred to as "bleeding a vein."

Most surgery performed in the year 1000 remained small scale, if agonizing. Surgical procedures were mainly used to pull teeth and treat and dress wounds. However, medical historians have found evidence of successful surgeries in cases of breast cancer, fistula, hemorrhoids, gangrene, and cataracts.

The rise of hospitals

Most treatments were administered at the patient's home or at a local monastery. A few hospitals, however, were in existence in the year 1000. Historians, in fact, consider the founding of hospitals and the first university medical schools to be among the chief medical advances in Europe during the Middle Ages. Christian religious groups established hundreds of charitable hospitals for victims of leprosy. In the 900's, a medical school was started in Salerno, Italy. It became the chief center of medical learning in Europe during the 1000's and 1100's. Other important medical schools opened in Europe after 1000. During the 1100's and 1200's, many of these schools became part of newly developing universities, such as the University of Bologna in Italy and the University of Paris in France.

Many of the medical procedures and concepts used in the year 1000 remained in practice until the mid-1800's. It was not until then that scientific discoveries turned doctors toward the practice of a more scientific form of medicine.   •••

Medical discoveries from the 1100's to the 1800's

Medicine and science began to change after the 1000's, when a new scientific spirit developed during the Renaissance, the great cultural movement that swept across Western Europe from about 1300 to the 1600's. Before this time, most societies had strictly limited the practice of *dissecting* (cutting up) human corpses for scientific study. But laws against dissection were relaxed during the Renaissance. As a result, the first truly scientific studies of the human body began.

During the late 1400's and early 1500's, the Italian artist Leonardo da Vinci performed many dissections to learn more about human anatomy. He recorded his findings in a series of more than 750 drawings. Andreas Vesalius, a physician and professor of medicine at the University of Padua in Italy, also performed numerous dissections. Vesalius used his findings to write the first scientific textbook on human anatomy, a work called *On the Structure of the Human Body* (1543).

Other physicians also made outstanding contributions to medical science in the 1500's.

A French army doctor named Ambroise Pare improved surgical techniques to such an extent that he is considered the father of modern surgery. For example, he opposed the common practice of *cauterizing* (burning) wounds with boiling oil to prevent infection. Instead, he developed the much more effective method of applying a mild ointment and then allowing the wound to heal naturally. Philippus Paracelsus, a Swiss physician, stressed the importance of

Illustrations of dissected bodies, *above*, appeared in the first textbook on human anatomy, *On the Structure of the Human Body* (1543).

chemistry in the preparation of drugs. He pointed out that in many drugs consisting of several ingredients, one ingredient made another useless.

The English physician William Harvey performed many experiments in the early 1600's to learn how blood circulates through the body. Before Harvey, scientists had studied only parts of the process and invented theories to fill in the

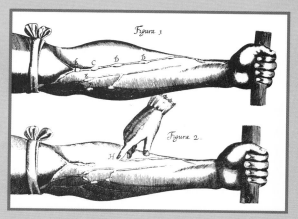

English physician William Harvey provided the first accurate description of how blood circulates, *above*, in 1628.

gaps. Harvey studied the entire problem. He performed dissections on both human beings and animals and made careful studies of the human pulsebeat and heartbeat. Harvey concluded that the heart pumps blood through the arteries to all parts of the body and that the blood returns to the heart through the veins.

Harvey described his findings in *An Anatomical Study of the Motion of the Heart and of the Blood in Animals* (1628). His discovery of how blood circulates marked a turning point in medical history. After Harvey, scientists realized that knowledge of how the body works depends on knowledge of the body's structure.

In the mid-1600's, a Dutch amateur scientist named Anton van Leeuwenhoek began using a microscope to study organisms invisible to the naked eye. Today, such organisms are called microorganisms, microbes, or germs. In the mid-1670's, van Leeuwenhoek discovered certain microbes that later became known as bacteria. Van Leeuwenhoek did not understand the role of microbes in nature. But his research paved the way for the eventual discovery that certain microbes cause disease.

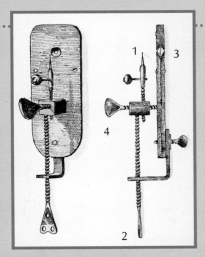

In 1673, Anton van Leeuwenhoek developed a microscope, above, to study organisms invisible to the naked eye.

Smallpox was one of the most feared and highly contagious diseases of the 1700's. It killed many people every year and scarred others for life. Doctors had known for hundreds of years that a person who recovered from smallpox developed lifelong *immunity* (resistance) to it. To provide this immunity, doctors sometimes inoculated people with matter from a smallpox sore, hoping they would develop only a mild case of the disease. But such inoculations were dangerous. Some people developed a severe case of smallpox instead of a mild one. Other inoculated persons spread the disease.

In 1796, English physician Edward Jenner discovered a safe method of making people immune to smallpox. He inoculated a young boy with matter from a cowpox sore. The boy developed cowpox, a relatively harmless disease related to smallpox. But when Jenner later injected the boy with matter from a smallpox sore, the boy did not come down with the disease. His bout with cowpox had helped his body build up an immunity to smallpox. Jenner's classic experiment

was the first officially recorded vaccination. The success of the experiment initiated the science of *immunology*—the prevention of disease by building up resistance to it.

For thousands of years, physicians tried to dull pain during surgery by administering alcoholic drinks, opium, and various other drugs. But no drug had proved really effective in reducing the pain and shock of operations. Then in the 1840's, two Americans—Crawford Long and William T. G. Morton—discovered that ether gas could safely be used to put patients to sleep during surgery. Long, a physician, and Morton, a dentist, made the discovery independently. With an effective anesthetic, doctors could perform operations never possible before.

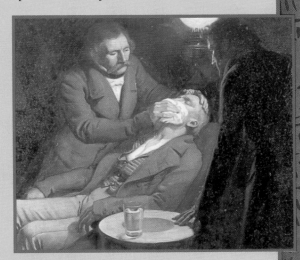

In 1846, dentist William Morton, *above*, used ether to anesthetize a patient, who was then operated on by a surgeon.

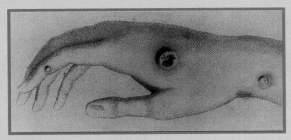

In 1796, Edward Jenner used fluid from the cowpox sores of a dairymaid, *above*, to create the first vaccine against smallpox.

The scientific study of disease, called pathology, developed during the 1800's. Rudolf Virchow, a German physician and scientist, led the development. Virchow believed that the only way to understand the nature of disease was by close examination of the affected body cells. He did important research in such diseases as leukemia and tuberculosis. The development of much improved microscopes in the early 1800's made his studies possible.

The discovery that microscopic organisms cause infection and disease led to germ theory, which paved the way for the great medical advances of the 20th century.

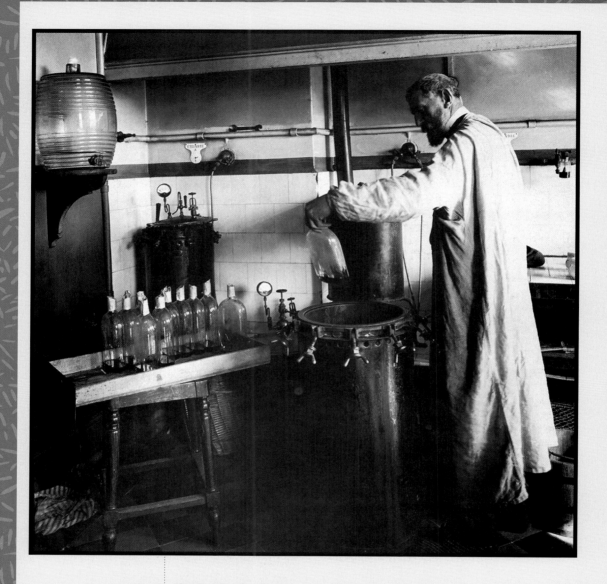

There were more medical discoveries in the 1900's than in all other centuries combined.

MEDICAL ADVANCES
of the 20th Century

By Jeffrey Courtouise

IN THE 20TH CENTURY THERE WERE MORE DISCOVERIES and advances in medical science than in all previous centuries put together. Everyone's life has been touched by at least one of three broad areas of medical achievement: the conquest of infectious disease; the almost-miraculous advances in surgery; and the birth of genetic medicine.

Before the 1900's, medicine consisted mainly of amputation saws, morphine, and crude remedies such as bloodletting. And life expectancy was short. A baby born in 1900 could expect to live only until age 47. Health hazards were especially prevalent in cities and towns. New towns throughout Europe and the United States, spawned by the Industrial Revolution, became reservoirs of water-borne, bug-borne, and air-borne diseases, such as typhus, typhoid, diphtheria, and tuberculosis. As a result, a series of pandemics orbited the world. In 1866, a cholera epidemic killed thousands of people in the United States. It was the 18th consecutive year that the country experienced such an outbreak.

But, as the result of medical progress, life expectancy increased dramatically between 1900 and 2000. An infant born in 1960 could expect to live about 70 years, and life expectancy reached 76.5 years in 1997. In 1900, an infant had only an 80 percent chance of surviving to age 15. By 1999, that probability approached 99 percent.

People live longer because of progress in the control of infectious diseases; improvements in health care programs for mothers and children; and better nutrition, sanitation, and living conditions. As a result of new drugs, medical technologies, and surgical operations, doctors can now save lives, often easily, where before they could only watch patients die.

French chemist Louis Pasteur, *left*, revolutionized medicine by firmly establishing in the late 1800's that microbes, or germs, cause infectious disease.

The author:

Jeffrey Courtouise is a medical historian.

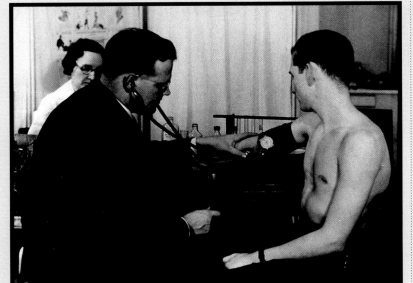

Investigating and treating disease

In the 1900's, doctors in hospitals, *left*, began to study patients, to analyze differences between them, and to distinguish the symptoms of different diseases.

The great advances of 20th century Western medicine were founded on basic sciences developed in the 1800's. Before then, scientists were usually practicing physicians or amateurs working in their homes.

The establishment of germ theory

By the end of the 1800's, however, a new breed of scientist was working in laboratories and making dramatic progress in learning about the causes of infectious disease. The research of two men in particular, French chemist Louis Pasteur and German physician Robert Koch, firmly established that microbes, or germs, cause infectious disease. Microbes include bacteria, viruses, and one-celled animals called protozoa.

In his laboratory, Koch invented a method for determining which bacteria cause particular diseases. This method enabled him in 1876 to identify the bacterium that causes anthrax, a deadly disease that affects people and animals. Koch also identified the bacterium that causes tuberculosis, a discovery for which he won the 1905 Nobel Prize for physiology or medicine.

Pasteur showed that weakening bacteria and other microbes and then inserting them into an animal's body creates immunity against the disease caused by the microbe. Using this method, he created a safe and effective vaccine against anthrax in sheep. Four years later, he used this approach to develop a vaccine against rabies. Pasteur also proved that specific microbes that spoil food or spread disease in food can be killed with heat. This method of treating food is called pasteurization.

The work of Koch and Pasteur was based not on chance observation but on the theory that germs cause infectious disease and on rigorous experimental techniques. Other research scientists followed the lead of these two pioneers. From then on, they focused on iden-

Modern milestones in medicine

The 20th century has seen thousands of discoveries and advances in medical science. This timeline illustrates some of the most important discoveries of the past 150 years.

1857—Louis Pasteur developed the germ theory of disease after proving that certain bacteria cause certain diseases.

1858—Rudolf Virchow showed that all tissues and organs are made of cells, *right*, and that many diseases are the result of changes in cells.

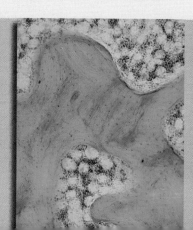

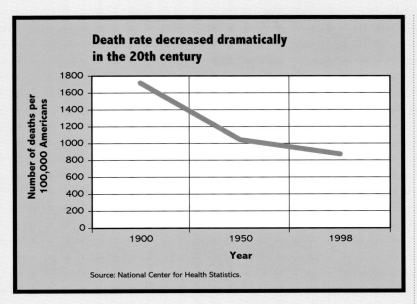

Death rate decreased dramatically in the 20th century

Number of deaths per 100,000 Americans

| | 1900 | 1950 | 1998 |

Year

Source: National Center for Health Statistics.

The death rate for people in the United States dropped dramatically in the second part of the 1900's, *left.* In 1900, approximately 1,750 per 100,000 Americans died annually. By 1998, that number fell to approximately 850.

tifying the specific germs causing distinct diseases. Interest shifted from the patient who had the disease to the disease itself. And researchers could study the disease and the microbes that caused it with the aid of inventions such as ever more powerful microscopes and special stains for examining bacteria on glass slides.

Discovery of bacteria and viruses

By the beginning of the 1900's, researchers had discovered the kinds of microbes called bacteria that are responsible for such infectious diseases as plague, cholera, diphtheria, dysentery, gonorrhea, leprosy, pneumonia, and tetanus, in addition to tuberculosis.

The study of another type of microbe, the virus, began in 1898, when Martinus Beijerinck, a Dutch botanist, realized that something smaller than bacteria could cause disease. He named the particle a *virus,* a Latin word meaning poison. In 1927, three research physicians proved for the first time that a virus caused a human disease—yellow fever. Scientists soon learned that viruses also caused smallpox, measles, poliomyelitis, rabies, and viral meningitis.

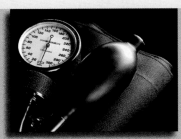

1860—Etienne Marey designed the sphygmomanograph to measure blood pressure.

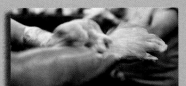

1864—George Harrington invented the first motor-driven dental drill.

1865—Joseph Lister introduced antiseptic methods to surgery.

1865—Gregor Mendel formulated the basic laws of heredity.

1866—Clifford Allbutt invented the medical thermometer.

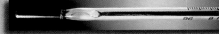

25

Development of the modern hospital

While laboratories were transforming medical science, the development of modern hospitals was also supporting the rise of scientific medicine. By the 1900's, the hospital, once an appalling place that took in poor, sick people with nowhere else to go, had evolved into an institution that investigated and treated disease. Doctors in hospitals began to study patients, to analyze differences between them, and to distinguish the symptoms of different diseases. Physicians came to recognize that certain symptoms were signs of a disease common to all who suffered from that disease rather than afflictions unique to each individual.

Hospitals also offered a chance to make statistical studies of disease. When many ill people were gathered together, the similarities of symptoms and other factors such as age or gender among sufferers became apparent. Doctors began to describe, measure, and count these similarities. Their studies were based on physical examinations by hand, eye, and ear and, increasingly, with instruments that measured such vital signs as heartbeat and blood pressure.

Drugs that revolutionized medicine

Once scientists discovered the cause of an illness, they began developing drugs to combat the disease or vaccines to prevent it. The use of drugs revolutionized medicine. Pharmacology developed into a major science in the 1900's. A major advance in pharmacology came in 1910 when the German physician and chemist Paul Ehrlich introduced a new method of attacking infectious disease. Ehrlich's method, called chemotherapy, involved searching for chemicals to destroy the microbes responsible for particular diseases. He discovered that salvarsan, a compound containing arsenic, was effective against the bacteria that cause syphilis. This was the first drug that did not merely alleviate symptoms but actually cured a serious disease. Ehrlich's work laid the foundations for the discovery of the so-called wonder drugs.

The first of these wonder drugs were sulfa drugs. In 1935, German doctor Gerhard Domagk discovered the ability of sulfa drugs to cure infections in animals. His discovery led to the development of sulfa drugs to treat diseases in human beings.

Another historic breakthrough came in 1928, when British bacte-

1867—Wilhelm Waldeyer-Hartz discovered that cancer is formed when cell division becomes uncontrolled.

1869—Jacques Reverdin performed the first human tissue graft.

1877—Max Nitze invented the cystoscope, a type of endoscope that allowed doctors to look inside the body.

1879—William Macewen pioneered successful brain surgery.

1881—Louis Pasteur developed the first successful vaccine against rabies.

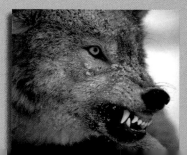

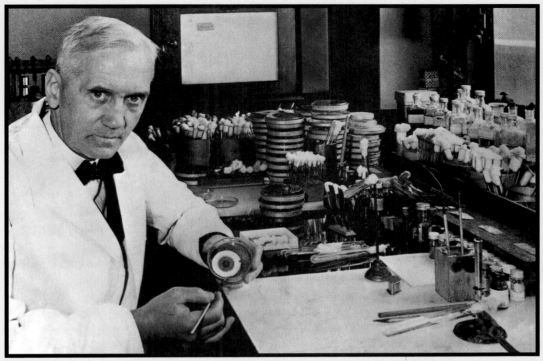

Pioneer in drug research

riologist Alexander Fleming observed that a mold of the genus *Penicillium* produced a substance that destroyed bacteria. He called the substance penicillin.

In the late 1930's, two British scientists, Ernst B. Chain and Howard W. Florey, developed a method of extracting and purifying penicillin. The first successful medical treatment with penicillin occurred in 1941, when a British policeman suffering from bacterial blood poisoning received the drug. Since the discovery of penicillin, scientists have developed dozens of antibiotics.

These powerful drugs drastically brought down the number of deaths caused by meningitis, pneumonia, and scarlet fever. Before the 1940's, about 30 percent of all pneumonia victims in the United States died of the disease. The new drugs quickly reduced the death rate from pneumonia in the United States to less than 5 percent.

In 1928, Alexander Fleming, *above*, observed that a mold of the genus *Penicillium* produced a substance that destroyed bacteria. This discovery led to the development of penicillin and other antibiotics.

1882—Robert Koch identified the bacteria that causes tuberculosis.

1892—Elie Metchnikoff discovered white blood cells, and suggested that these cells attack invading germs.

1893—Daniel Hale Williams performed the first open heart surgery.

1895—William Roentgen discovered X rays, used in diagnosing diseases and treating cancer.

1897—Scientists introduced immunology, the study of the body's specific responses to foreign substances.

1898—Pierre and Marie Curie discovered radium, used in treating cancer.

Vaccines opened another front in the war on disease. Vaccines developed during the 1900's largely eliminated many diseases that were previously prevalent and dangerous, including whooping cough, measles, diphtheria, and poliomyelitis. American physician and researcher Jonas Salk introduced the first polio vaccine in 1955. At that time, the polio virus infected about 30,000 to 50,000 people every year in the United States. By 1999, poliomyelitis had been eradicated in the United States.

Researchers in the 1900's also used basic medical research to develop drugs for replacing hormones and other substances produced by the body. A hormone was first isolated in 1898. That year American pharmacologist John J. Abel isolated epinephrine, also called adrenaline. Scientists isolated several other hormones during the next 20 years. Then in the early 1920's, a research team led by Frederick Banting, a Canadian physician, discovered the hormone insulin, important in regulating the level of sugar in the blood. Since then, insulin injected as a drug has saved the lives of millions of diabetics.

Many other important drugs have been discovered since 1900. Barbiturates, which reduce the activity of the nervous system and the muscles, were introduced in 1903. Amphetamines, which stimulate the nervous system, were first used medically in the early 1930's. Scientists developed several important tranquilizers in the 1950's, and birth control pills appeared in 1960.

Conquering nutritional diseases

Understanding about the importance of human nutrition also advanced in the early 1900's. In 1906, British biochemist Frederick G. Hopkins published a study showing that certain foods contain substances that are vital for the development of the body. Hopkins called these substances "accessory food factors," to distinguish them from already known basic food factors—carbohydrates, fats, proteins, minerals, and water. Later, these accessory substances were called vitamins. Vitamins in foods and supplements helped conquer such diseases as beriberi, rickets, and scurvy. Researchers by the 1990's had learned that other substances in food, such as fat and fiber, play a role in causing or preventing heart disease and cancer.

1899 — The drug company Bayer introduced aspirin.

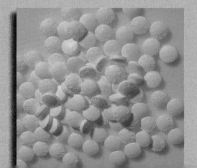

1900 — Sigmund Freud developed the psychoanalytic method of treating mental illness.

1902 — Karl Landsteiner determined that human blood has four different types: O, A, B, and AB.

1902 — Ernest Starling and William Bayliss discovered the function of hormones.

1906 — Eduard Zirm successfully transplanted a human cornea onto the eye of a patient.

How vaccines have prevented disease and death

Smallpox

A vaccine against smallpox was developed in the 1780's.

- The average annual number of smallpox cases in 1900–1904: 48,164.
- The number of smallpox cases in the United States since 1950: 0.
- The number of smallpox cases worldwide since 1977: 0.

Diphtheria

A vaccine against diphtheria was developed in the 1920's.

- The average annual number of diphtheria cases in the United States in 1920–1922: 175,885.
- The number of U.S. cases of diphtheria in 1998: 1.

Pertussis

A vaccine against pertussis was developed in the late 1920's.

- The average annual number of pertussis cases in the United States in 1922–1925: 147,271.
- The number of U.S. cases of pertussis in 1998: 6,279.

Source: National Center for Health Statistics.

A young patient, *right*, receives a vaccination against polio.

Poliomyelitis

A vaccine against poliomyelitis was developed in the 1940's and licensed for use in the 1950's.

- The average annual number of poliomyelitis cases in the United States in 1951–1954: 16,316.
- The number of U.S. cases of poliomyelitis in 1998: 0.

Tetanus

A vaccine against tetanus was developed in the 1940's.

- The average annual number of tetanus cases in the United States in 1922–1926: 1,314.
- The number of U.S. cases of tetanus in 1998: 34.

Measles

A vaccine against measles was licensed for use in the 1960's.

- The average annual number of measles cases in the United States in 1958–1962: 503,282.
- The number of U.S. cases of measles in 1998: 89

Mumps

A vaccine against mumps was licensed in the late 1960's.

- The average annual number of mumps cases in the United States in 1968: 152,209.
- The number of U.S. cases of mumps in 1998: 606.

Rubella

A vaccine against rubella was licensed in the early 1970's.

- The average annual number of rubella cases in the United States in 1966–1968: 47,745.
- The number of U.S. cases of rubella in 1998: 345.

Haemophilus influenzae type b (Hib)

A vaccine against Hib was licensed in the 1980's.

- The estimated average annual number of Hib cases in the United States before vaccine licensure: 20,000.
- The number of U.S. cases of Hib in 1998: 54.

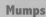

1906—Frederick Hopkins demonstrated the existence of vitamins.

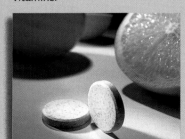

1910—The first chemotherapy treatment cured syphilis in mice.

1912—Harvey Cushing published *The Pituitary Body and its Disorders*, which marked the beginning of the science of endocrinology.

1921—Frederick Banting and Charles Best developed insulin to treat diabetes, *below*.

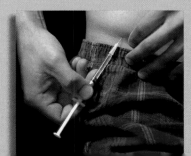

Insulin offers hope to diabetics

In the 1920's, scientists discovered the hormone insulin, important in regulating the level of sugar in blood. The drug has saved the lives of millions of diabetics. Pictured, *near right*, is a girl with diabetes before treatment with insulin, and, *far right*, four months after beginning insulin treatment.

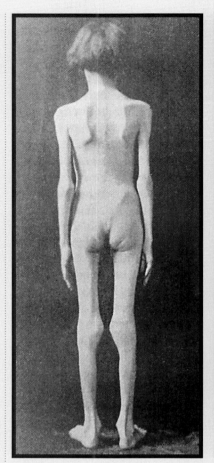
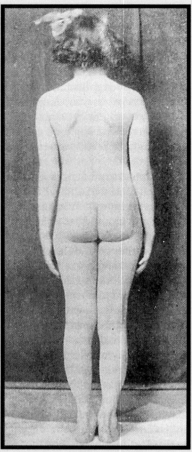

Early progress in surgery

While great progress was being made in diagnosing and treating illnesses with drugs, dramatic advances were also being made in the field of surgery. Until the late 1800's, up to half of all surgical patients died of infections. Then in the 1860's Joseph Lister, a Scottish surgeon, learned how to reduce the risk of wound infection. Because of Pasteur's work on bacteria, Lister became convinced that germs caused many of the deaths of surgical patients. In 1865, Lister began

1928 — Alexander Fleming discovered penicillin, the first antibiotic drug.

1932 — German engineers developed the electron microscope, which was capable of magnifying objects 17 times.

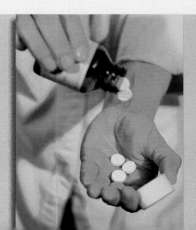

1935 — Gerhard Domagk discovered sulfa drugs, which fight bacterial infections.

1943 — Willem Kolff invented the first kidney dialysis machine for human patients.

using carbolic acid, a powerful disinfectant, to kill germs and thus sterilize surgical wounds. This method was later replaced by a more efficient technique known as aseptic surgery. In aseptic surgery, everything in the operating environment is sterilized before surgery begins. Surgeons wash thoroughly before an operation and wear surgical gowns, gloves, and masks.

A second important development was improved anesthesia. Before the use of modern anesthetics, surgeons tried to deaden the pain by giving large quantities of alcoholic beverages or by using compounds containing opium. But the relief from pain was not complete and lasted only a short time. As a result, surgeons could perform only short operations and these were usually amputations. After ether's anesthetic properties were discovered in the 1840's, surgeons were able to perform longer, more complex operations.

But during operations, the loss of blood can cause the body's circulation system to fail, inducing fatal shock. Two discoveries helped solve this problem. One was the discovery of the main blood groups A, B, AB, and O in 1902. Knowing about blood groups allowed doctors to determine whether blood from a particular donor could be given to a patient without their immune system rejecting it.

The second development occurred in 1935. English doctors developed a method to continuously drip blood into the vein of a surgical patient, replacing body fluids lost during surgery.

Surgeons explore new territories

Improved surgical techniques allowed doctors to perform ever more complex operations on every part of the body. As late as the 1870's, most surgeons would not consider operating on the abdomen, chest, or brain. But with anesthetics, reduced infection risk, and safer transfusions, such caution rapidly dissolved. In the 1900's, surgeons began to see the infinite possibilities of cutting disease out and repairing internal defects. They developed operations for diseases of the pancreas, liver, and gallbladder. They pioneered surgical treatments for peptic ulcers, cancers, bowel inflammations, and abdominal traumas due to knife and gunshot wounds.

By the mid-1950's, surgeons who once were concerned only with cutting disease out of the body, turned their attention to replacing body parts. The development of drugs that would suppress the

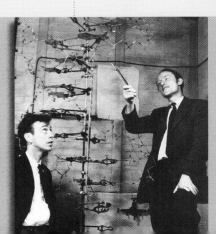

1948 — Lewis Sarett synthesized cortisone, which led to new treatments for arthritis and other diseases.

1949 — Lithium, a tranquilizing drug, was first used to treat patients suffering from mental illness.

1953 — Jonas Salk developed the first successful polio vaccine.

1953 — James Watson and Francis Crick, *right*, devised a model of the molecular structure of deoxyribonucleic acid (DNA).

Medicine before aseptic surgery

Until the late 1800's, surgeons did not realize that wearing surgical gowns, gloves, and masks helped reduce the spread of germs, *right*. As a result, up to half of all surgical patients died of infections.

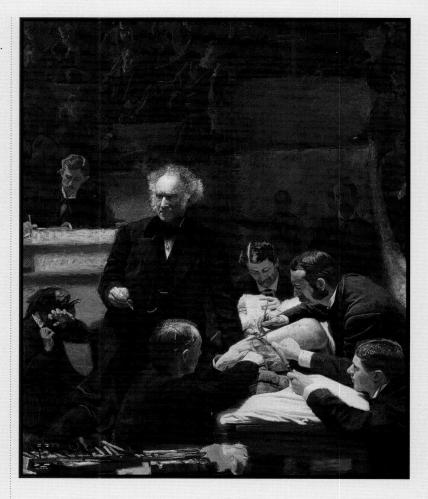

body's immune response made it possible for surgeons to transplant organs. Ordinarily a patient's immune system would attack and destroy replacement organs because they were foreign to the body.

Organ transplants began in 1950, when Richard H. Lawler performed the first kidney transplant. Lawler's pioneering efforts laid the groundwork for transplantation of other organs, including the liver and the heart.

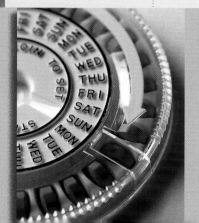

1954 — American surgeons transplanted a kidney—the first successful organ transplant.

1955 — Gregory Pincus developed the birth control pill, *left*.

1957 — Ultrasound was first used for diagnosis.

1958 — Engineers invented the artificial pacemaker, *below*.

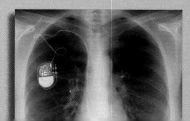

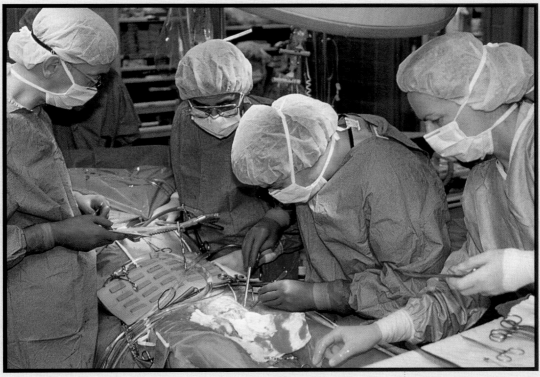

Advances in heart repair

In the 1900's there were spectacular advances in cardiovascular medicine. In 1938, Robert E. Gross, an American surgeon, performed the first successful repair of a congenital heart defect. Gross sewed up the hole in the artery of a child. In 1944, Helen Brooke Taussig and Alfred Blalock, two American physicians, developed an operation to help correct abnormal circulation of *blue babies* (newborn infants whose skin appears blue because their blood contains less than the normal amount of oxygen).

But more daring heart-repair operations could not be undertaken because surgeons faced a basic problem: how to stop the heart long enough to repair it but still keep blood circulating through the body to keep the patient alive. The first attempt to get around this prob-

Opening the heart

Spectacular advances in cardiovascular medicine made procedures such as open heart surgery, *above*, relatively safe and routine by the late 1990's.

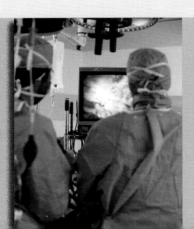

1960—Doctors perform the first successful laser surgery.

1964—James Black developed the first beta blocker drug to treat heart conditions.

1967—A British engineer developed the first computed tomography (CT) scanner.

1967—Christiaan Barnard performed the first successful human heart transplant.

1968—A Japanese research team used a surgical technique that pioneered the science of microsurgery.

Facts about transplantation in the United States

Cornea and sclera

More than 44,000 cornea and 6,200 sclera (coating around the eyeball) operations for repair and re-placement take place every year in the United States.

Cartilage

Latest technique uses cells cultivated from humans, then grafted onto joints.

Lung

Approximately 75 percent of all patients who receive lung transplants report good lung function after one year. Doctors performed 849 lung transplants in 1998.

Liver

Approximately 70 percent of adults and 85 percent of children survive for more than two years after a liver transplant. Doctors performed 4,450 liver transplants in 1998.

Pancreas

Doctors performed 253 pancreas transplants in 1998. The world's longest living recipient survived 18 years.

Kidney-pancreas

Doctors performed 965 kidney-pancreas transplants in 1998. The survival rate is more than 90 percent in the first year.

Kidney

Of the 11,990 kidney transplants performed in 1998, 4,016 kidneys were taken from living donors.

Blood

Approximately 14 million pints of blood are donated every year by 8 million volunteers.

Knees

Doctors rebuild 150,000 knees annually.

Pericardium

In 1998, there were more than 350 replacements of this membrane sac, which encloses the heart and the vessels leading into and out of it.

Heart-lung

Doctors performed 45 heart-lung transplants in 1998.

Heart valves

Doctors perform approximately 71,000 replace-ments annually.

Heart

In 1998, doctors performed 2,340 heart trans-plants. The one-year survival rate is 82 percent; the two-year survival rate is 78 percent.

Hip replacements

On average, new hips last 10 to 15 years after surgery.

Bone marrow

Approximately 1,100 people receive bone marrow transplants annually.

Skin

Scientist are using tissue engineering to grow hu-man skin in laboratories to help repair burns and ulcers. Approximately 7,000 square feet of artificial skin is grafted annually.

Muscles and tendons

Total muscle transfers move whole muscles (includ-ing tendons and vessels) to other parts of the body, where they are reconnected.

Sources: American Heart Association; American Lung Association; American Liver Foundation; American Association of Tissue Banks; Eye Bank Association of America; National Marrow Donor Program; United Network for Organ Sharing.

1968 — Bone marrow trans-plant was first performed to cure immunodeficiency disease.

1969 — Denton Cooley per-formed the first successful im-plant of a temporary artificial heart.

1977 — American researchers tested the first magnetic reso-nance imaging (MRI) scanner.

1978 — The first successful in vitro fertilization produced Louise Brown, the world's first "test tube" baby.

1980 — The World Health Organization announced that smallpox had been eliminated.

1981 — Doctors use artificial skin for the first time on human patients.

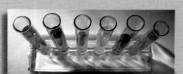

lem was carried out by Floyd Lewis at the University of Minnesota in 1952. He was able to slow down the heart rate by lowering the patient's body temperature to reduce the need for oxygen. Slowing the heartbeat gave Lewis the opportunity to sew up a hole in the patient's heart. Then in 1953, John Gibbon of Philadelphia succeeded in stopping the heart altogether. He routed blood through a special heart-lung machine that did the job of the heart and lungs by sending oxygen-rich blood through the arteries and removing waste gases from blood returning through the veins.

Eventually, a combination of the two techniques—a heart-lung machine that also cooled the blood—helped pave the way for such spectacular operations as the first transplantation of a human heart in 1967 by Christiaan Barnard of South Africa.

Technology's role in medical triumphs

Other technological advances also aided surgeons. High-energy light beams called lasers were developed into scalpels of light that surgeons began using in the 1970's to make delicate cuts in body tissues. Lasers cut tissue by burning fine lines in organs.

Another technological advance of the late 1990's was the development of microsurgery. Miniature instruments and light guided on fiber-optic strands allowed surgeons to operate through tiny incisions. Eliminating the need for large incisions enabled many patients to have a shorter hospital stay or avoid hospitalization altogether.

Meanwhile, imaging techniques that produce amazingly detailed views of internal body structures allowed doctors to "see" inside the body. The X-ray machine, first invented in the late 1890's, allowed doctors to diagnose a range of ills from broken bones to tumors. By the late 1990's, biomedical engineers had developed very sophisticated imaging techniques such as *computerized axial tomography* (an X-ray system used to produce three-dimensional images), *magnetic resonance imaging* (a technique used to produce images of tissue using a magnetic field instead of radiation), and *ultrasound* (a device that uses high-pitched sound waves to distinguish different types of tissue in the body) for diagnosis and treatment.

Biomedical engineers also made great progress in creating artificial replacements for worn or damaged body parts. These replacements include artificial limbs, joints, and heart valves.

1983 — A team of French and U.S. researchers discovered HIV, the virus that causes AIDS.

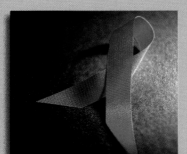

1990 — The Human Genome Project, an international effort to analyze all human genes, began.

1990 — Researchers successfully used gene therapy to treat a disorder of the immune system.

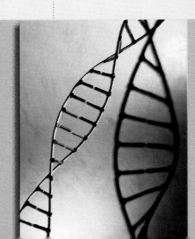

A better view inside the body

Improved imaging techniques, such as computerized axial tomography, *right*, allowed doctors in the late 1900's to view internal body structures in incredible detail.

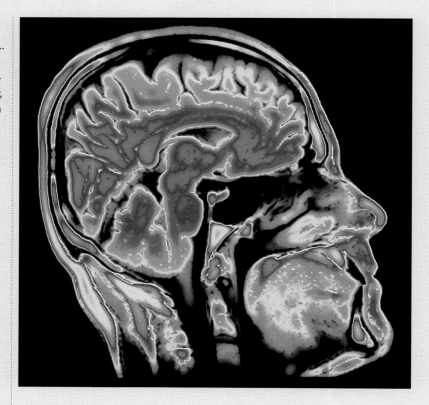

Genetic medicine—the next revolution

By the end of the 1900's, medicine was on the verge of another revolution—genetic medicine. Genetic medicine is based on the manipulation of genes, which contain the blueprint of the cell. Genes carry hereditary traits and also guide the manufacture of proteins by which cells regulate all their functions. In 1953, American biologist James D. Watson and British physicist Francis H. C. Crick proposed a model of the molecular structure of deoxyribonucleic acid (DNA), the material of which genes are made. Knowing the structure of DNA enabled biologists to probe the mysteries of the gene and eventually to alter genes, a process called genetic engineering. This opened new avenues for the diagnosis and treatment of disease.

In 1982, human insulin "manufactured" by the gene that codes

1997—Ian Wilmut successfully cloned a sheep.

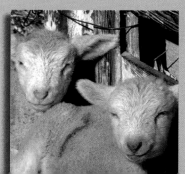

1997—Doctored announced a technique to grow new organs for transplantation from a patient's own cells.

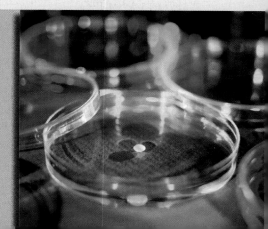

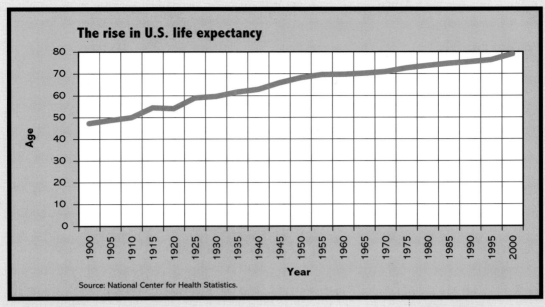

The rise in U.S. life expectancy

Age

Year

Source: National Center for Health Statistics.

for this hormone became the first genetically engineered drug approved by the U. S. Food and Drug Administration for use on people. Other genetically engineered drugs followed, including human growth hormone, which is used to treat children whose growth is seriously below average; and tissue plasminogen activator, used to treat heart attacks by breaking up blood clots.

Preparing for the 21st century

As a result of the medical advances of the 1900's, people in the United States and other developed nations were living longer by the year 2000. With people living longer, older people began to make up a larger percentage of the population. Physicians grew concerned about quality of life issues in senior citizens. As a result, doctors began to put a greater emphasis on preventive medicine, which they hoped would help people stay healthy well into their old age.

People alive during the 1900's witnessed a dazzling array of medical advances, including reproductive technologies that allowed previously infertile couples to have children; drugs that attack, conquer, and control infectious and malignant diseases; repair of heart defects, transplantation of organs; the reconstruction or replacement of diseased blood vessels; the development of artificial joints; and the alleviation of crippling diseases of the nervous system. As the new century—and the new millennium dawned—the remarkable advances of medicine in the 20th century gave great promise that even more marvelous advances, perhaps unimaginable now, are yet to come. ●●●

Life expectancy on the rise

As a result of advances in science and medicine, life expectancy in the United States nearly doubled in the 20th century. In 1900, people lived an average of 47 years. Population experts predicted that by 2000, the average person would live approximately 80 years.

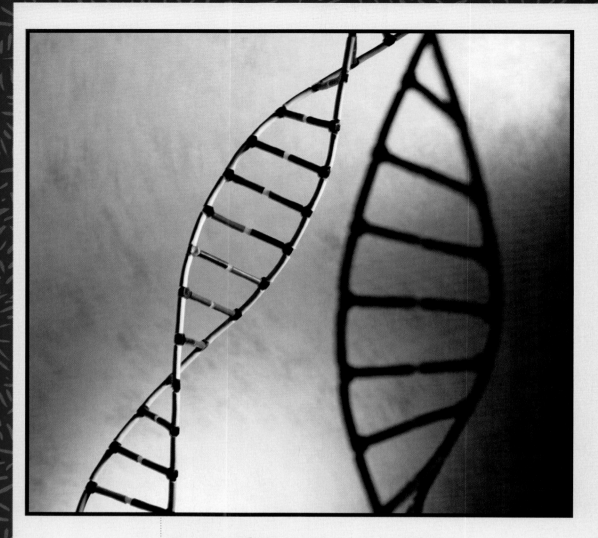

Medicine in the 21st Century:
THE PROMISE OF GENETICS

Science's rapidly growing power to read our genes is having a momentous impact on medicine.

By Laura Bushie

A N INFANT GIRL LIES ON AN EXAMINING TABLE awaiting her first checkup. The doctor collects a sample of mucus from the inside of the girl's cheek and then inserts it into a machine. The machine extracts genetic material from the mucus cells, analyzes it, and then provides a printout of every gene in the infant's body. The doctor explains the results to the baby's mother. He tells her that all but a few of the genes are labeled "normal." The genetic information shows, however, that the baby may be susceptible to cardiovascular disease later in life. To lessen her risk, the doctor advises a lifelong low-fat, high-fiber diet.

Incredible as it seems, this scenario may soon be commonplace. Science's rapidly growing power to read our genes is having a momentous impact on medicine. Medicine is in the midst of a revolution that in the 2000's promises to change not only the ways in which physicians heal, but the very concept of health itself. Scientists are identifying specific disease-causing genes, creating tests for those genes, and developing treatments for previously incurable ills. And the maps they are making of genes may one day give healthy people advance warning of potential genetic trouble ahead.

How genes work

An understanding of this new era requires some basic information about genes and how they work. Genes are the units that carry hereditary information from generation to generation. They are located on the *chromosomes*, threadlike structures found in the nucleus of the cell. Human cells contain 23 pair of chromosomes, one member of each pair comes from the mother, the other comes from the father.

The information carried by the genes is written in a code that controls the body's production of proteins. Some proteins serve as structural material for the body's tissues and determine the color of eyes or hair. Other proteins enable the body to carry out the thousands of minute-by-minute chemical reactions that sustain life.

How do genes encode the instructions for making proteins? The answer lies in molecular structure. Genes are made up of a compound called deoxyribonucleic acid (DNA). The DNA molecule resembles a ladder twisted into a spiral, a shape called a double helix. Each "rung" of the ladder consists of a pair of simple molecules called bases, and it is the order of base pairs in a gene that carries the code for each protein. Each gene is a segment of DNA, ranging from a few hundred to several thousand base pairs.

One of the miracles of life is that the genes in the human body dictate the production of thousands of proteins without making a mistake. But if a single gene is defective, the effects can be devastating. For example, because hemophiliacs are born with one defective gene, they are unable to produce a protein crucial for blood clotting. As a result, they suffer prolonged bleeding when they are injured, because their blood clots very slowly.

The author:

Laura Bushie is a physician and a free-lance writer specializing in science issues.

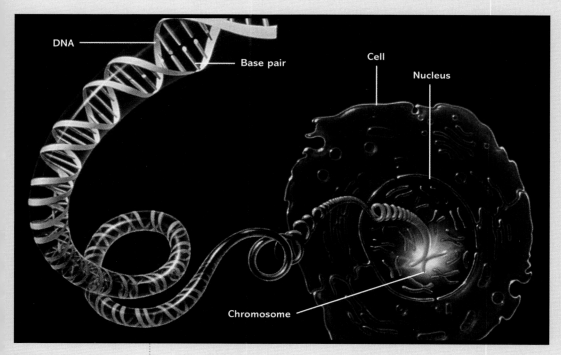

DNA

Base pair

Cell

Nucleus

Chromosome

What genes are

Genes, which carry instructions for all our physical characteristics, are carried on structures called chromosomes, located in the nucleus of every cell. Each chromosome contains a long strand of DNA, with rungs made up of two interlocking substances called bases. A gene is a particular sequence of these base pairs.

Mapping the human genome

By 1999, scientists had cataloged more than 4,000 hereditary diseases and identified the defective proteins in several hundred of them. And researchers were engaged in one of the most important medical research projects of all time—deciphering the human genome, the 50,000 to 100,000 genes made up of some 3 billion base pairs. Coiled in the nucleus of the human cell, the genome is in effect a blueprint of the human body.

Aided largely by grants from the federally funded Human Genome Project, researchers raced to map the genome by 2005. When the human genome is fully mapped, it will provide for medicine the kind of dramatic insights that the periodic table contributed to chemistry. The periodic table categorized chemical elements so that scientists could predict how they would react. By the time the human genome is complete, science will at last have access to the "book of life"—the precise biochemical code for every gene, which largely determines every physical characteristic in the human body. Once researchers know that, they will be able to figure out how each gene normally functions and exactly how changes in a particular gene trigger deadly illnesses from heart disease to cancer.

Testing for genetic disorders

Once a gene is located and its sequence of chemical code letters discerned, scientists can devise a test for the presence of that gene in any patient. To conduct a gene test, doctors take a blood sample and then extract DNA from some of the cells. The DNA sample is mixed with a chemical that causes the two strands of the DNA molecule to "unzip." A *gene probe* (segments of a disease-causing gene that have been tagged with a radioactive compound or a special dye) is added to the mixture. If the DNA sample contains the defective gene, the probe will attach to the DNA strand. Scientists can then use tests to detect whether the probes have attached to strands of DNA.

Researchers hope to develop a technology that will analyze millions of genetic sequences simultaneously. Using *DNA chips* (a tiny array of DNA) with hundreds of different DNA probes scientists might be able to identify genetic errors almost as quickly as a supermarket scanner prices a load of groceries. By 1999, genetic researchers were trying to use DNA chips to look for any number of genetic characteristics, including the complex web of genes that may lurk behind familial patterns of heart disease and stroke, cancer, diabetes, Alzheimer's disease, various kinds of mental disorders, and even gingivitis.

There were a number of genetic tests available by the late 1990's. One form of genetic testing, called carrier identification, helps couples learn whether they carry certain disease-related genes they could pass on to their children. Cystic fibrosis, the most common hereditary disease among people of northern European background, and Tay-Sachs disease, a fatal hereditary central nervous system disorder that affects primarily children of eastern European ancestry, are conditions for which carrier testing is used. Other carrier identification procedures include tests for an inherited form of amyotrophic lateral sclerosis (Lou Gehrig's disease), fragile X syndrome, Gaucher's disease, Huntington's disease, two types of muscular dystrophy, and polycystic kidney disease.

A procedure known as predictive gene testing seeks to determine whether a person may develop a particular disease in the future. For example, there are predictive tests for many genes linked with various types of cancer that run in families, including breast, colorectal, ovarian, and thyroid cancers, melanoma, and retinoblastoma.

The most common use of genetic testing in the late 1990's was to screen newborns for certain disorders. The effects of several fairly common dis-

How genetic defects lead to disease

Genes contain the instructions that a cell uses in the production of proteins, molecules that are essential to the cell's structure and functioning. A gene with damaged DNA may result in an abnormal protein or no protein at all. Malfunctioning proteins are the underlying cause of genetic diseases.

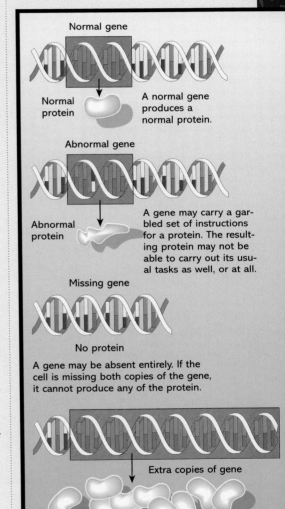

Normal gene

Normal protein

A normal gene produces a normal protein.

Abnormal gene

Abnormal protein

A gene may carry a garbled set of instructions for a protein. The resulting protein may not be able to carry out its usual tasks as well, or at all.

Missing gene

No protein

A gene may be absent entirely. If the cell is missing both copies of the gene, it cannot produce any of the protein.

Extra copies of gene

Too much protein

Extra copies of a gene may cause the cell to produce too much of the protein. The excess protein can overwhelm the cell.

eases can sometimes be prevented if the conditions are discovered at birth and treatment is begun immediately. For example, all 50 states require a test for phenylketonuria, a disorder that causes mental retardation unless treated in infancy.

Prenatal screening has helped to reduce by more than 95 percent the number of Tay-Sachs births. As a result of early identification, some congenital conditions, such as *spina bifida* (a disabling hole in the spinal cord), are being surgically treated in the womb. And sex selection techniques based on in-vitro fertilization can reduce the risk of giving birth to a baby with sex-linked disorders, such as Duchenne muscular dystrophy and hemophilia, which affect only males.

If a couple know they carry genes for a life-threatening illness that they don't want to pass on to the next generation, they can opt for a remarkable procedure called preimplantation genetic diagnosis. In this process, sperm from the father are mixed with eggs collected from the mother in a Petri dish. The fertilized eggs are subjected to intense DNA analysis. Only those that pass the test are implanted.

Genetically engineered drugs

Researchers have made good use of gene discoveries and new technology to develop an array of genetically engineered drugs. By 1999, researchers had identified 500 biological targets for drugs. They expected to identify another 500 targets by 2005.

Researchers use genetic information to develop drugs that target very specific conditions. For example, researchers know that there are at least three or four forms of Alzheimer's disease, each of which may be caused by a different defective gene. If scientists develop a drug for gene A, it may not have any influence on a patient who has a defect on gene B. So genetics research is critical to the development of very precise and effective drugs. Focusing on receptors in brain cells for *serotonin* (a chemical that carries nerve impulses between brain cells), for example, led to the development of Prozac and other drugs for the treatment of depression. Targeting receptors in the stomach for *histamine* (a chemical that stimulates gastric secretion) produced Tagamet and Zantac to relieve severe acid indigestion.

Along with drugs, scientists have been working on the development of genetically engineered vaccines. A vaccine works by stimulating the immune system to recognize a particular bacterium, virus, or other foreign invader. A conventional vaccine consists of killed or weakened microbes responsible for a particular disease, such as measles. The killed or weakened organism cannot cause the disease, but when it is injected into a person, the immune system recognizes identifying proteins on the surface of the microbe and produces molecules called antibodies to immobilize and help kill it. Then, if the natural microbe invades, the immune system is primed to respond quickly before the germ can multiply and cause disease.

Selected conditions for which genetic tests are available

Disease	What genetic testing may reveal	Possible action
Breast cancer	A woman's risk for this form of cancer, especially hereditary breast cancer.	Frequent mammograms and breast self-examinations to check for lumps.
Colorectal cancer	A person's risk for some forms of the cancer.	Colonoscopy once a year to check for growths, especially after age 30.
Cystic fibrosis	Whether a prospective parent is carrying a copy of the flawed gene.	Avoiding pregnancy if both members of a couple are found to be carriers of the defective gene and may thus produce a child with cystic fibrosis.
Fragile X syndrome	The presence of the defective gene that can result in this form of mental retardation.	Avoiding pregnancy if either member of a couple is found to be carrying the defect.
Gaucher's disease	Whether a prospective parent is carrying a copy of the flawed gene associated with this severe enzyme deficiency.	Enzyme replacement therapy for children who have inherited two copies of the gene and thus have developed the disease.
Huntington's disease	Whether a person has inherited the defective gene and will develop the disorder, which causes mental and physical deterioration.	No known cure, though drug therapy can lessen some symptoms.
Phenylketonuria (PKU)	Whether a child has inherited two defective copies of a gene, causing loss of a crucial enzyme, which—if left untreated—will lead to mental retardation.	A carefully restricted diet followed from birth to head off the disease.
Polycystic kidney disease	Whether a person has a copy of the flawed gene, which will eventually lead to the development of cysts in both kidneys.	No known cure, but condition can be treated with dialysis or kidney transplant.
Sickle-cell anemia	Whether prospective parents are carriers of the gene causing this serious blood disorder, which afflicts primarily African Americans.	Avoiding pregnancy if both members of a couple carry the flawed gene.
Tay-Sachs disease	The presence of the gene responsible for the disease, a fatal hereditary brain disorder affecting the nervous system.	Avoiding pregnancy if both members of a couple are found to be carriers of the gene.

Source: National Institutes of Health.

The vaccines of tomorrow are likely to be far more sophisticated concoctions, made up of snippets of DNA from the genome of a virus, bacterium, or parasite. Using DNA, as opposed to proteins made from a microbe, elicits a more vigorous, aggressive response from the immune system.

While most of the conventional vaccines do a good job of marshaling antibodies against invading cells, they often do not reliably coax the body into producing killer T cells, the attack agents of the immune system that strike at the offending microbes with great specificity. But, in early tests, DNA-based vaccines initiated the production of T-cells. For example, immunologists reported in 1998 that patients injected with an experimental DNA-based malaria vaccine showed not just malaria antibodies but also significant levels of killer T cells.

Moreover, genetic engineering techniques might solve the problem of creating vaccines against organisms that mutate rapidly, such as the influenza virus or the virus that causes AIDS. Because gene-based vaccines can easily be manipulated by adding or deleting DNA, researchers were attempting to apply the technique to treat various forms of cancer. The work in 1999 was still limited to animals, but researchers were able to develop inoculations made up of tumor cells that acted as a red flag to rally an animal's immune system against the tumor.

Progress in gene therapy

Another major advance being brought about by genetic medicine is the treatment of disease through gene therapy. Gene therapy, simply defined, is the placement of beneficial genes into the cells of patients. Introducing the gene and, consequently, the protein it codes for will either eliminate the defect, slow the progression of the disease, or in some way interfere with the disease.

In 1990, physicians at the National Institutes of Health (NIH) in Bethesda, Maryland, performed the first federally approved gene therapy. The experiment involved a 4-year-old girl who suffered from an inherited disorder called adenosine deaminase (ADA) deficiency, in which a defective ADA protein leaves the immune system defenseless against infections. NIH researchers decided to treat the girl with normal copies of the ADA gene.

From a sample of her blood, the researchers filtered out *white blood cells* (the cells of the immune system that normally fight infection). In the laboratory, they spliced a copy of the normal human ADA into the DNA of a harmless mouse virus, then infected the girl's white blood cells with the virus.

They hoped that the virus would carry the ADA gene into the DNA of some of the white blood cells, which they then returned to the girl's blood. One year later, they reported that the girl's immune system was producing ADA and fending off infection better. The therapy was a success.

Correcting genetic abnormalities

Scientists are searching for safe, effective ways of giving patients copies of new genes that produce normal proteins. One method uses viruses to carry new genes into cells. Researchers used the method to replace a faulty gene in white blood cells of two girls, *right*, with an immune system disorder called adenosine deaminase.

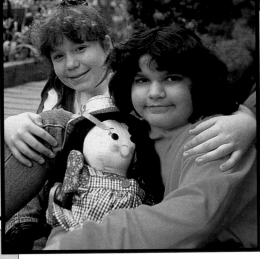

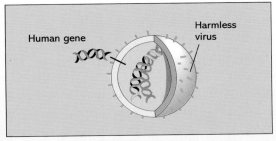
Human cells

Blood is taken from the patient. The white blood cells are extracted and grown in a dish in the laboratory.

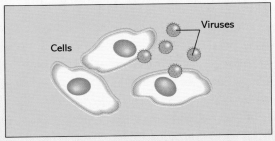
Human gene
Harmless virus

A normal copy of the faulty gene is spliced into the DNA of a harmless virus.

Viruses
Cells

The genetically engineered viruses are mixed with the patient's white blood cells in the laboratory, and the viruses enter the cells.

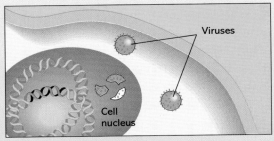
Viruses
Cell nucleus

The viruses transfer copies of the human gene into the DNA of the patient's white blood cells. These cells are then injected back into the patient, where they produce the missing immune system protein.

The field of genetic medicine exploded after the ADA trial. The widely heralded success of that treatment raised public expectations that permanent cures achieved by gene therapy would soon be commonplace. But researchers struggled with a host of technological problems in subsequent human trials. By 1999, gene therapy had yet to live up to its promise, despite more than 250 experiments involving several thousand people.

The main roadblock to gene therapy was the inability to devise an effective means of delivering genes to the nucleus of cells so that the genes can reproduce themselves. Viruses were a favorite delivery vehicle. Viruses can be stripped of harmful genes while preserving the virus's ability to enter cells. Scientists then insert human genes into the viral DNA and use the virus to infect the patient's cells. The altered virus inserts its own now harmless genes, as well as the beneficial one, into the cellular DNA. If all goes well, the beneficial gene directs the cell to produce the needed protein.

The problem is that the altered viruses infect only certain types of cells, and even then, they infect at a low rate. Second, they insert their genes at random in a human cell's chromosomes. However, the location of a gene is important to its proper expression, so inserted genes do not tend to work as well as naturally inherited copies.

Finally, because the viruses are not selective about where they insert their DNA, they may inadvertently damage properly working cells.

Scientists can do incredible things with a cell in a laboratory dish. They can get genes into the cell, change the cell's properties, and do other spectacular things that ought to enable doctors to treat disease successfully. But they have not had the same success in treating cells within the human body. One problem is that the body's immune system regards the viral carrier as foreign invaders. The immune system attacks the carrier and causes inflammation and swelling at the injection site.

In an early gene therapy trial for cystic fibrosis, inflammation caused by the viral carrier was so severe that the Food and Drug Administration (FDA) ordered a halt to the effort. Other trials failed, as well. Many of these gene therapy trials failed during what the FDA calls Phase I, in which the safety of

DNA drugs

Vitravene, *below*, a drug that fights eye infection in AIDS patients, is one of the first of a new breed of genetically engineered drugs.

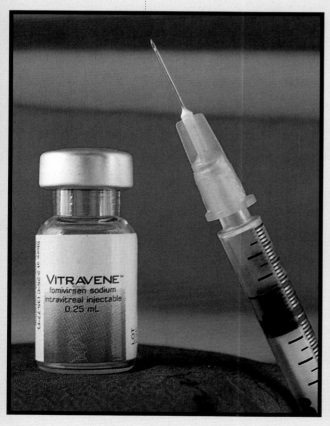

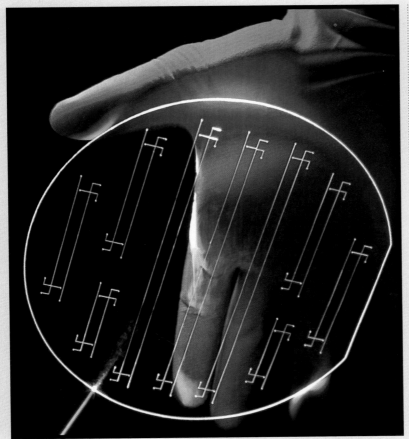

Faster diagnosis

Scientists are designing microchips, *left*, to swiftly analyze fragments of DNA. Doctors hope to use microchips to screen their patients for thousands of genetic disorders.

the procedure is evaluated on a handful of patients. Others proved ineffective and faltered during Phase II trials, which test a larger group to determine the effectiveness of the therapy.

A mixed blessing?

Some people view the genetics revolution as a mixed blessing because of the social and ethical issues it provokes. The ability to detect genes that predispose people to health problems may open a Pandora's box of social controversy. On the one hand, detecting such genes will permit people to adopt lifestyles that reduce their risk of developing the diseases to which they are susceptible. On the other hand, insurance companies and employers might demand to know what diseases a person is genetically prone to develop.

But despite these concerns, few people would suggest turning our backs on the revolution of medical genetics. With its promise of new ways to diagnose, treat, and cure devastating diseases, genetic medicine seems destined in the 21st century to write a new chapter in the history of medicine. ● ● ●

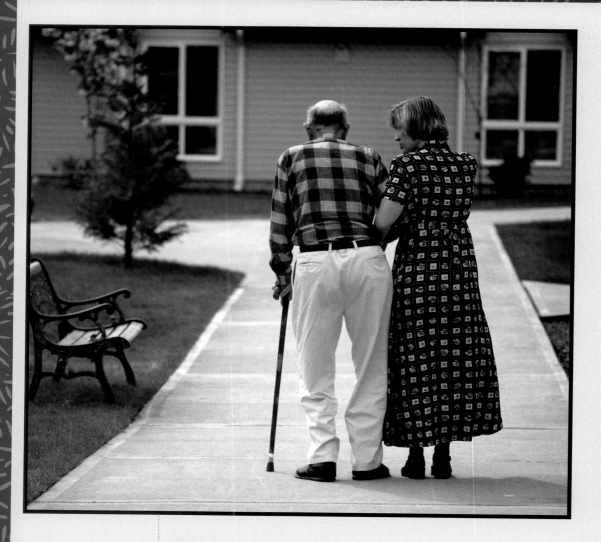

THE AGING POPULATION:

A Medical Challenge for the Next Century

By Laura Bushie

T HE AGE OF AGING IS UPON US. By 2000, average life expectancy in the United States was almost 80 years, up from 47 years in 1900. This longer life expectancy has result-ed in a growing elderly population. In the 1990's alone, the 65-and-older crowd increased 7 percent to reach 34 million, or 13 percent of the U.S. population, according to the National Center for Health Statistics. The growth rate of this group was almost twice the growth rate of those under age 65. Demographers project that after the first *baby boomers* (individuals born between 1945 and 1964) hit retire-ment in 2011, the numbers will explode, with people age 65 and older numbering 1 in 5 by the middle of the 2000's.

That is only part of the story. The 3.8 million seniors who cele-brated their 85th birthday before the year 2000 constituted the fastest-growing segment of the population. The U.S. Census Bureau projects that by 2030, this group will number 9 million, and then will swell to 19 million by 2050.

These statistics frame one of the greatest challenges the medical community faces in the 2000's—how to improve the quality of peo-ple's later years and perhaps even extend them. Scientists now be-lieve that much of the physical deterioration brought on by age is far from inevitable. Fast-paced advances in physiological and biomedi-cal research give hope that old age may finally cast off its pall and become a healthier and more active time for millions of people.

To ensure that those added years continue to be a blessing rather than a painful and expensive curse, physicians and scientists are pursuing two different strategies to retard the aging process. One is a preventive approach that assumes that people have a maximum natural lifespan of approximately 120 years but believes attendant disease, disability, and decline can be delayed or staved off through exercise, diet, and medical advances. The other, more radical strate-gy focuses on greatly increasing the human lifespan by aiming to halt or reverse degeneration in the body's cells.

Improving mobility

As the population ages, doctors and scientists have increasingly turned their attention to treating and preventing *chronic conditions*, conditions that persist over time and affect the ability to live inde-pendently. Arthritis, osteoporosis, Alzheimer's disease, cardiovascu-lar disease, cancer, general memory loss, vision and hearing loss, and loss of muscle mass that results in frailty and weakness are con-ditions that frequently make life more difficult for older people. In 1998, people age 65 or older represented nearly half of the almost 50 million Americans disabled by chronic conditions, according to the National Center for Health Statistics.

The medical breakthroughs in this area that have already had the deepest impact are those that enhance sight and mobility. In the United States, more than 1 million cataract procedures are per-formed each year to correct clouding in the lens of the eye, accord-

The author:
....
Laura Bushie is a physi-cian and a free-lance writer specializing in science issues.

49

Rise in aging and age-related health care costs

The U.S. Census Bureau predicts that by 2030 there will be 9 million people age 85 and over in the United States. The cost of caring for the elderly population will nearly double by 2030.

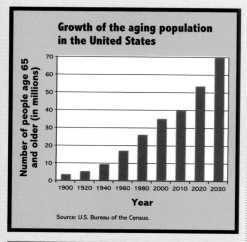

Growth of the aging population in the United States

Source: U.S. Bureau of the Census.

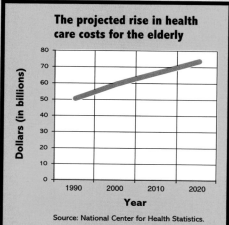

The projected rise in health care costs for the elderly

Source: National Center for Health Statistics.

ing to the American Society of Cataract and Refractive Surgery. Until the late 1970's, the main treatment was the removal of the patient's lens and its replacement with a thick pair of cataract glasses to correct vision. Since then, ophthalmologists have learned how to implant an artificial lens behind the iris, a procedure that by 1999 had become so routine that it was usually done on an outpatient basis.

Surgery to replace the body's injured or worn-out joints has also risen dramatically. Between 1983 and 1996, the total number of hip replacements swelled from 49,000 to 83,000 and knee replacements almost quadrupled, to 131,000, according to the National Center for Health Statistics. Hip replacement surgery following fractures typically restored patients to the level of mobility they enjoyed before the bone was fractured. The surgery liberated them from a walker or wheelchair—and from housebound existence.

Such surgery carries the risk of precipitating a stroke or heart attack, however. In addition, rehabilitation can be long and painful. And though artificial joints are generally durable for 10 years or more, they sometimes fail far earlier—resulting in more surgery, rehabilitation, and pain.

Physicians see the real battle as preventing such fractures in the first place. Many hip fractures, especially among women, involve *osteoporosis*, a disease that makes the bones brittle. Among menopausal women, estrogen-replacement therapy, which can help prevent bone loss, came into wide usage by 1999. However, the therapy carries risks of depression and endometrial cancer.

In December 1997, women gained a new option in preventing osteoporosis when the Food and Drug Administration approved raloxifene, a drug that mimics estrogen's bone-saving effects without increasing the risk of breast cancer.

Advances in ways to halt bone loss could substantially pare the medical bills of the elderly, which totaled $50 billion annually by 1999 and accounted for 30 percent of the nation's health-care tab, according to the National Center for Health Statistics. Fully one-fifth of those dollars were applied to the costs that accumulate after a senior takes a fall, because brittle bones break easily. The average bill for emergency treatment resulting from a fall was $11,000.

New focus on preventive medicine

By 2000, researchers were attempting to identify ways to forestall bone loss and other types of degeneration though preventive measures, such as nutrition. Physicians had come to believe that the type of foods a person eats plays an important role in protecting against disease and other physical effects of aging. For example, studies have shown that calcium taken throughout life reduces bone loss as women grow older. And numerous studies have indicated that a diet low in fat and high in fiber can decrease the risk of the two leading causes of death among senior citizens in the United States: cancer and cardiovascular disease.

Many *biogerontologists* (researchers who study the biological processes associated with aging) and nutritionists believe that certain nutrients act as antioxidants, chemicals that may intercept and react with potentially damaging molecules called free radicals, and render them harmless. Among

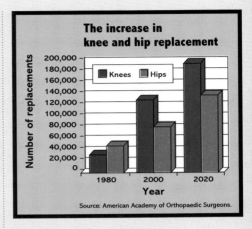

The increase in knee and hip replacement

Number of replacements / Year

■ Knees ■ Hips

Source: American Academy of Orthopaedic Surgeons.

New hope for old joints

Surgery to replace worn-out joints, *below*, has risen dramatically in the late 1900's. Physicians predict that by 2020 more than 300,000 people will have either an artificial hip or knee.

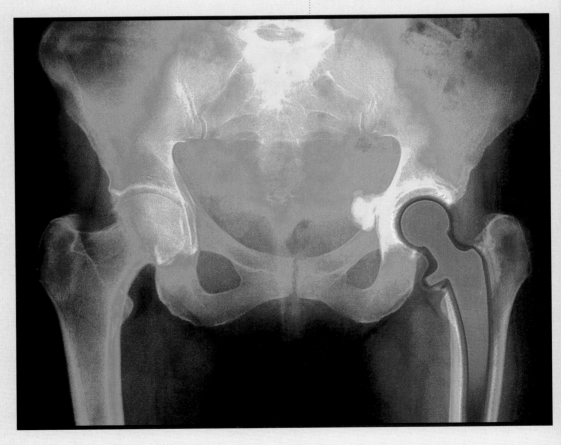

such antioxidants are *beta-carotene* (a substance the body turns into vitamin A) and vitamins C and E, all found in many fruits and vegetables.

Other studies have focused on how exercise slows or reverses some effects of aging. Since 1993, physiologist Ethan Nadel and epidemiologist Loretta DiPietro, both of Yale University in New Haven, Connecticut, have studied the effects of exercise on people over age 65. Their research focused on whether exercise can slow the effects of aging, and if so, which effects. One of the focuses of the study was to determine why people who exercise feel better than other people. To find answers, the researchers were looking, for instance, at the effects of stretching exercises on the taste buds. If, as they suspected, such exercise enhances the sense of taste, that could be a great boon for the elderly. A common problem of aging is a lessening sense of taste, which makes eating less appealing and can lead to unwanted weight loss, even malnutrition.

Researchers also found evidence that exercise may help prevent Type II diabetes—the most common form of diabetes mellitus. In this disorder, the body is unable to use insulin efficiently. Insulin is a hormone that is important in using and storing sugar. The risk of developing Type II diabetes increases with age, and complications from it can irreversibly damage the heart, blood vessels, kidneys, eyes, and nerves.

Researchers at the University of California at Berkeley in 1997 reported that among 6,000 healthy men, those who exercised most vigorously were less than half as likely as those who were the least active to develop Type II diabetes. A study of 87,000 middle-aged women reported in June 1998 by researchers at Harvard Medical School came to similar conclusions.

Improving mental function

Studies have also found that lifestyle factors may improve mental fitness. This has punctured some long-standing myths about aging's effects on the brain. Neurologists acknowledge that the brain loses some of its cells and shrinks somewhat with age, possibly causing some impairment of memory. But substantial mental decline is no longer considered an inevitable consequence of growing older. In fact, studies have shown that most elderly people who show marked signs of mental deterioration actually have some underlying disorder, such as depression or Alzheimer's disease.

In addition, scientists have revised their belief that the brain's nerve cells cannot rejuvenate themselves. Researchers at the University of California at Irvine reported in the early 1990's that the brains of old rats were just as adept at repairing damaged nerve cells and growing new connections between them as were the brains of young rats. This finding was confirmed by a number of similar studies in the 1990s. In October 1998, a team of American and Swedish researchers reported that they had discovered for the first time that

Osteoporosis fact box

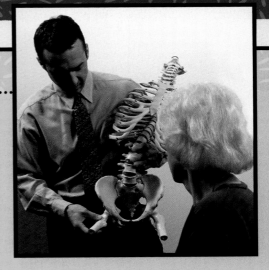

- Osteoporosis, or porous bone, is a major public health threat for more than 28 million Americans, 80 percent of whom are women. In the United States in 1999, 10 million individuals have the disease and 18 million more have low bone mass, placing them at increased risk for osteoporosis.

- Osteoporosis is often called the "silent disease" because bone loss occurs without symptoms. People may not know that they have osteoporosis until their bones become so weak that a sudden strain, bump, or fall causes a fracture or a vertebra to collapse.

- Collapsed vertebrae may initially be felt or seen in the form of severe back pain, loss of height, or spinal deformities such as kyphosis or stooped posture.

- Women can lose up to 20% of their bone mass in the five to seven years following menopause, making them more susceptible to osteoporosis.

- One in two women and one in eight men over age 50 will have an osteoporosis-related fracture in their lifetime.

- White women 65 or older have twice the incidence of fractures as African American women.

- Osteoporosis is responsible for more than 1.5 million fractures annually, including approximately 300,000 hip fractures, 700,000 vertebral fractures, 250,000 wrist fractures, and 300,000 fractures at other sites.

- The rate of hip fractures is two to three times higher in women than men; however, the one-year mortality following a hip fracture is nearly twice as high for men as for women.

- A woman's risk of hip fracture is equal to her combined risk of breast, uterine, and ovarian cancer.

- In 1991, about 300,000 Americans age 45 and over were admitted to hospitals with hip fractures. Osteoporosis was the underlying cause of most of these injuries.

- An average of 24% of hip-fracture patients age 50 and over die in the year following their fracture. One-fourth of those who were ambulatory before their hip fracture require long-term care afterward.

- The health-care costs for osteoporotic and associated fractures was approximately $14 billion in 1997.

- Specialized tests called bone density tests can measure bone density in various sites of the body. A bone density test can detect osteoporosis before a fracture occurs; predict your chances of fracturing in the future; and determine your rate of bone loss and/or monitor the effects of treatment if the test is conducted at intervals of a year or more

- Although there is no cure for osteoporosis, there are four medications approved by the FDA for postmenopausal women to either prevent and/or treat osteoporosis: Estrogens are approved for both the prevention and treatment of osteoporosis; Alendronate, a bisphosphonate, is approved for prevention and treatment; Calcitonin is approved for treatment; Raloxifene, a selective estrogen receptor modulator (SERM), is approved for prevention.

Source: National Osteoporosis Foundation.

brain cells in adults are continually dividing and producing mature new cells. This finding may lead to methods for mending brains damaged by disease or treating diseases caused by a damaged brain, according to researchers at the Salk Institute for Biological Studies in San Diego, California.

Neurobiologists also have found that when rats are kept in isolation and are sedentary, with nothing to interest them, the number of connections between the brain's nerve cells declines. But when the animals are required to perform a complex task, such as finding their way through a maze, new connections sprout between their brain and nerve cells. Researchers suspect that mental stimulation might have a similar effect on human beings.

Why do people age?

While some researchers sought ways to cope with aging, others tried to understand the aging process itself, and they proposed several hypotheses to explain this phenomenon. *Genetic makeup* (traits passed in genes from parents to their offspring) lies at the heart of a number of theories on aging.

Genes in the human body orchestrate growth and maturation and the maintenance and repair of cells. Studies have shown that these processes proceed simultaneously until about age 30. At that point, growth has stopped, and the body does not work as efficiently to repair and replace cells.

A cell's genes tell the cell how and when to divide, and one theory of aging proposes that each of our many types of cells has a built-in limit to the number of times the cell can divide. Experiments to support this theory were first done in the 1960's by geneticists Leonard Hayflick and Paul Moorhead, then at the Wistar Institute in Philadelphia. They reported that normal human embryo cells placed in laboratory cultures divided about 50 times before dying. Normal adult cells, however, divided only about 20 times. Hayflick's experiment suggests that messages contained in genes control how long cells live, which may dictate how long human bodies survive.

Aging might reflect the accumulation of errors in genes, according to some biogerontologists. Researchers suggest that external factors, such as pollutants or radiation and even the oxygen we breathe, can cause these errors by damaging the components of genes. Most genes contain the recipe to create proteins. The recipe is DNA (deoxyribonucleic acid), the molecule of which genes are made. If external factors damage a cell's DNA, the recipe can become garbled, and the proteins the cell makes may be abnormal. A cell with abnormal proteins may not be able to perform its particular task adequately, whether it is to fight infection, refurbish body parts, digest food, or communicate with other cells.

Other researchers suggest that we age because the body's ability to handle proteins deteriorates. Studies indicate that as the body gets older, it produces certain proteins more slowly than it did in the

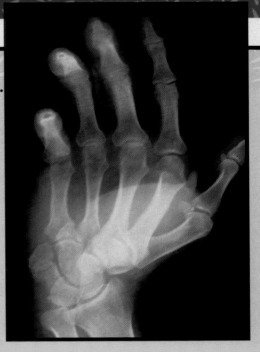

Arthritis fact box

- Arthritis refers to more than 100 different diseases that cause pain, swelling, and limited movement in joints and connective tissue throughout the body.

- The three most prevalent forms are osteoarthritis (OA), fibromyalgia, and rheumatoid arthritis (RA).

- Arthritis is one of the most prevalent chronic health problems and the number one cause of limitation in movement in the United States.

- Arthritis is second only to heart disease as a cause of work disability.

- More than 43 million Americans have arthritis; 27.5 million of these Americans are over age 45.

- For nearly 7 million Americans, arthritis limits such everyday activities as walking, dressing, or bathing.

- The condition takes an especially heavy toll among women; nearly two-thirds of people with arthritis are women.

- The incidence of arthritis is growing. In 1985, 35 million Americans had arthritis; in 1990, 37.9 million people had the disease. By 1995, the figure rose to 40 million. The U.S. Centers for Disease Control project that 59.4 million Americans—or almost 20 percent of the population—will have arthritis in 2020.

- Arthritis costs the U.S. economy $65 billion per year in medical care and lost wages.

- Arthritis results in 39 million physician visits and more than half a million hospitalizations.

- Many treatment approaches can be used to help manage arthritis. Most treatment programs include a combination of exercise, drugs, and diet therapies.

Source: The Arthritis Foundation.

past. Furthermore, the aging body becomes less efficient at clearing out old protein molecules. And the longer a protein stays in a cell, the more likely it is to react with a blood sugar called glucose or with other proteins. This theory, first proposed in 1981 by scientists at Rockefeller University in New York City, suggests that this phenomenon, called cross-linking, gums up the cell and interferes with its normal functions. But scientists do not yet understand why the body becomes less efficient at making and removing proteins in the first place.

Another theory of cell aging holds that cells "rust" as a result of interactions with oxygen. Just as oxygen takes its toll on iron, interacting with and chewing up the surface to create rust, the oxygen that is continuously fed through the body may take its toll on tis-

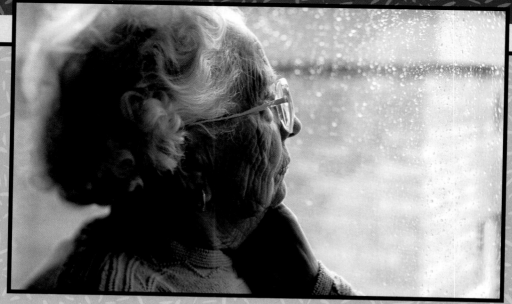

Alzheimer's disease fact box

- Alzheimer's disease is a progressive, degenerative disease of the brain, and the most common form of dementia.

- Approximately 4 million Americans have Alzheimer's disease. A survey conducted in 1993 indicates that approximately 19 million Americans say they have a family member with Alzheimer's, and 37 million know someone with the disease.

- 14 million Americans will have Alzheimer's by the middle of the next century unless a cure or prevention is found.

- One in 10 persons over 65 and nearly half of those over 85 have Alzheimer's disease. A small percentage of people in their 30s and 40s develop the disease.

- A person with Alzheimer's lives an average of 8 years and as many as 20 years or more from the onset of symptoms.

- U.S. society spends at least $100 billion a year on Alzheimer's disease. Neither Medicare nor private health insurance covers the type of long-term care most patients need.

- Alzheimer's disease costs American businesses more than $33 billion annually— $26 billion is attributed to lost productivity of caregivers plus $7 billion related to costs for health and long-term care.

- More than 7 out of 10 people with Alzheimer's disease live at home. Almost 75 percent of the home care is provided by family and friends. The remainder is "paid" care costing an average of $12,500 per year, most of which is covered by families.

- Half of all nursing-home patients suffer from Alzheimer's or a related disorder. The average per patient for nursing home care is $42,000 per year, but can exceed $70,000 per year in some areas of the country.

- The average lifetime cost per patient is estimated to be $174,000.

- The federal government estimates spending approximately $400 million for Alzheimer's disease research in 1999. This represents $1 for every $250 the disease now costs society.

- There is no medical treatment currently available to cure or stop the progression of Alzheimer's disease. Two drugs—donepezil and tacrine—may temporarily relieve some symptoms of the disease and have been approved by the FDA.

Source: The Alzheimer's Association.

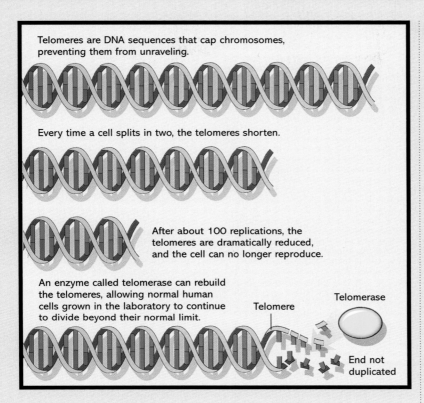

Telomeres are DNA sequences that cap chromosomes, preventing them from unraveling.

Every time a cell splits in two, the telomeres shorten.

After about 100 replications, the telomeres are dramatically reduced, and the cell can no longer reproduce.

An enzyme called telomerase can rebuild the telomeres, allowing normal human cells grown in the laboratory to continue to divide beyond their normal limit.

Telomere

Telomerase

End not duplicated

Fountain of youth?

Scientists theorize that a cell's biological clock lies in its telomeres, *left*. Researchers are using an enzyme called telomerase to repair damaged telomeres in hopes of extending the life of human cells.

sues. Highly reactive free-radical molecules routinely form when the cell uses oxygen to produce energy. Free radicals can also form in other ways, such as through exposure to radiation. Some scientists think that free-radical damage to the cells of the immune system may explain the elderly's increased susceptibility to disease.

Attempts to slow the aging process

Researchers have long sought ways to extend the life span of humans. Throughout the 1990's, for example, biologists experimented on rats and rhesus monkeys to see if restricting the intake of calories would slow the metabolic rate, producing a lower body temperature that in turn would decrease oxygen consumption. The studies showed that animals on restricted diets lived nearly 30 percent longer than other animals. However, the animals on restricted diets also had lower bone mass, a dangerous condition that leads to osteoporosis for older people. Moreover, because lab animals do not have the same life span as humans, these experiments remain highly speculative.

Researchers also have sought substances that can slow or even reverse the aging process. In the 1990's, the National Institutes of Health in Bethesda, Maryland, supported research into the risks and benefits of boosting the levels of three hormones that decrease as

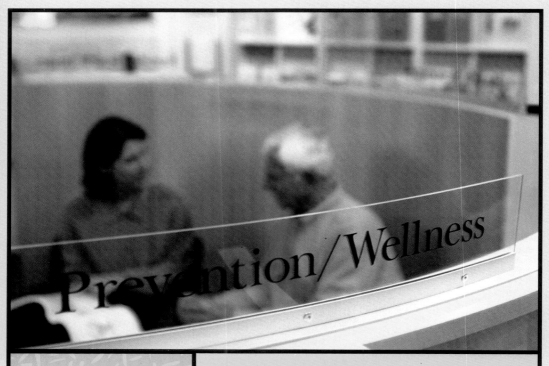

Tips for healthy aging

No known substance can extend life, but the odds of staying healthy and living longer may be improved by following these suggestions:

- Eat a balanced diet, including five helpings of fruits and vegetables a day.

- Exercise regularly. Check with a doctor before starting an exercise program.

- Get regular health check-ups.

- Don't smoke. It's never too late to stop.

- Practice safety habits at home to prevent falls and fractures. Always wear your seat-belt in a car.

- Stay in contact with family and friends. Stay active through work, play, and community.

- Avoid overexposure to the sun and the cold.

- If you drink alcohol, drink only in moderation.

- Keep a positive attitude toward life.

Source: The National Institute on Aging.

people age: melatonin, which affects sleep cycles; dehydroepiandros-terone, a product of the adrenal glands that converts to estrogen and testosterone; and human-growth hormone, which affects bone and organ development, as well as metabolic rate.

Limited lab tests on animals suggested to some investigators that melatonin may serve as an antioxidant, wiping out free radicals that can harm the body's cells. But scientists were cautious because as of 1999, results had not been repeated in other animal studies. Also, because the metabolism of animals is different from that of humans, scientists may never be able to replicate such results in humans.

Studies in the 1990's reported that human growth hormone increased muscle mass in older people. However, the treatments caused side effects, including joint pain and water-weight gain.

The promise of telomeres

A major breakthrough in extending lifespan at the cellular level came in 1997, when researchers announced they had unlocked the secrets of a powerful enzyme with the potential to rejuvenate the human body's aging tissues. Scientists had long theorized that a cell's biological clock lies in its *telomeres*, tiny strips of DNA that coat the tips of the chromosomes (which carry the DNA) and, much like the plastic cuffs of shoelaces, prevent the strands from unraveling. Every time a cell splits in two, the telomeres shorten, until finally, after about 40 to 90 divisions, they are reduced to stubs. Because any further divisions would fray the chromosomes, the cells settle into a twilight stage and eventually die. Only an enzyme called telomerase, first discovered in 1984, can repair the damaged telomeres. However, most human cells, with the exception of reproductive cells, stop making the compound during the fetal stage.

In 1997, however, three different groups of researchers cloned a gene that makes it possible to reactivate telomerase in human-tissue samples. Researchers from the Geron Corporation, a biotech company in Menlo Park, California, and the University of Texas Southwestern Medical Center in Dallas infected normal cells with a virus that had been genetically engineered to switch telomerase on. In every case the cells' telomeres lengthened instead of shortening, while the cells stayed healthy and continued to divide.

Researchers are already familiar with cells that live indefinitely: they are called cancer cells. Apparently one reason why malignant tumors expand aggressively is that their cells are full of telomerase. So, unless scientists carefully control cell division, activating human telomerase may not prolong life but just create cancers.

It may be years before researchers in biomedical science will be able to reverse the aging process at the cellular level. Biomedical researchers all agree that until then, the best offense against the ravages of time is level-headed defense: watch your weight, drink alcohol only in moderation, don't smoke, get plenty of sleep and exercise, and maintain a proper diet. ●●●

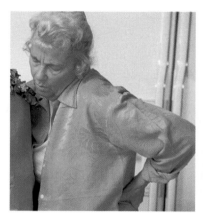

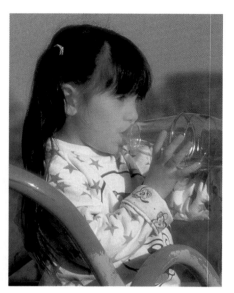

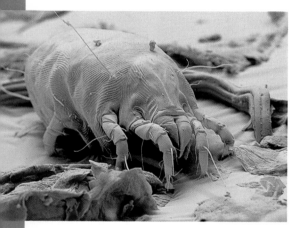

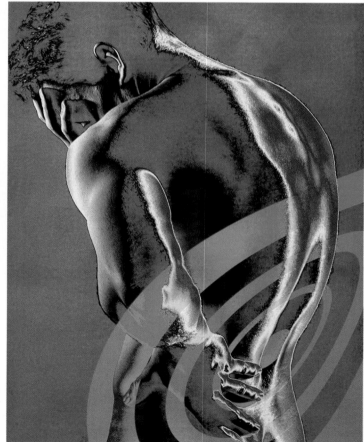

A HEALTHY YOU

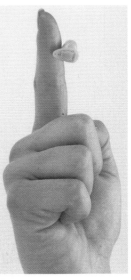

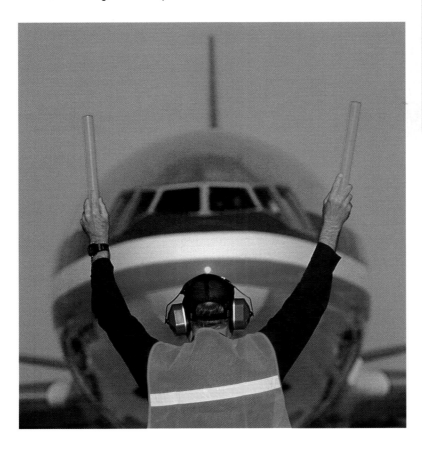

Low back pain is one of the most
common health problems, but
simple treatments and precautions
can make it go away for good.

Oh, My Aching Back!

By Michael Woods

AFTER SITTING AT THE COMPUTER IN HER OFFICE FOR HOURS, Jen leaned across the desk to pick up a book. She cried out in agony as pain pierced her back like a white-hot knife. On the loading dock, Stanley lifted a heavy crate. In mid-lift, he twisted to answer a coworker's question and heard the pop in his back just before he froze stiff with pain.

Jen and Stanley have a lot of company. More Americans visit doctors for back pain each year than for any other problem except respiratory infections, according to the Agency for Health Care Policy and Research (AHCPR), an arm of the United States Department of Health and Human Services. AHCPR reports that low back pain is the leading cause of disability in people under the age of 45. This problem is a pain in the pocketbook as well. Low back pain costs U.S. society as much as $50 billion each year in health care bills and time lost from work.

In the late 1990's, changes were underway in the treatment of back pain. More patients were taking over-the-counter medications and exercising instead of undergoing surgery and being confined to bed. Furthermore, physicians were placing a greater emphasis on preventing back problems from developing in the first place.

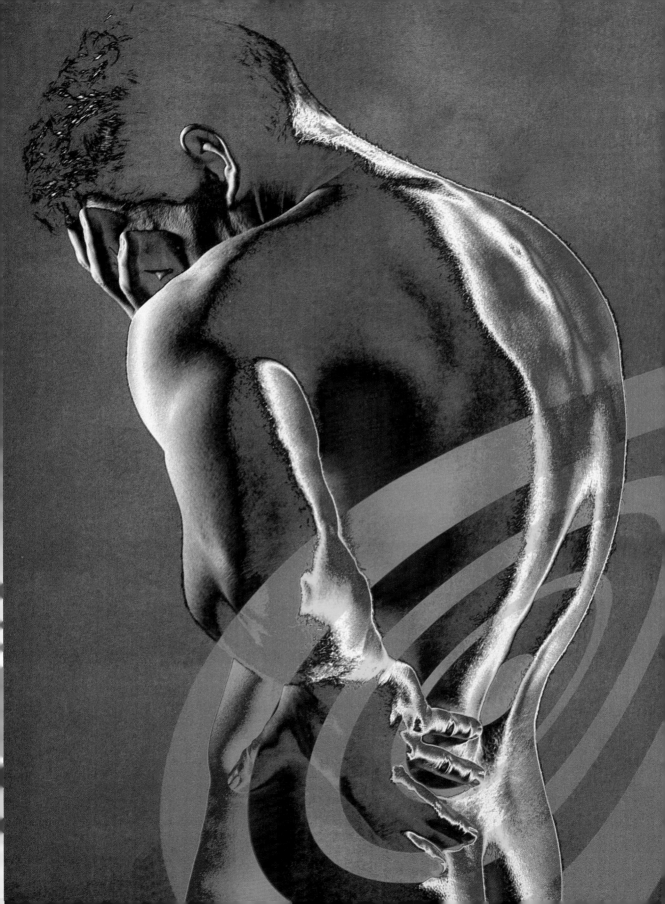

The human spine

To understand the causes of back pain, it is necessary to know something about the spine. The human spine consists of 33 bones, called vertebrae, stacked on top of one another to form the spinal, or vertebral, column. Seven cervical vertebrae in the neck support the head. Twelve thoracic vertebrae in the upper part of the back serve as attachment points for the ribs. The five lumbar vertebrae in the lower back bear the load of the entire upper body. Most back pain occurs in the lumbar region. When a person lifts an object, the weight presses down on the lumbar vertebrae. If a person leans forward while lifting, the strain is magnified in the lumbar vertebra.

The lumbar vertebrae connect to the sacrum, which forms the back of the *pelvis* (hipbone). The sacrum consists of five vertebrae that in most adults are fused into one flat bone. Finally, the *coccyx* (tailbone), consisting of four small vertebrae, ends the spine.

Each vertebra consists of an oval block of bone with winglike projections. The projections form a large tunnel, called the spinal canal, along the entire length of the column. Inside the spinal canal is the *spinal cord* (the large bundle of nerves that carries electrical signals between the brain and the nerves serving the rest of the body).

We can twist, stretch, and flex the back because tough, elastic pads of tissue called intervertebral disks separate one vertebra from another, providing cushions for the bones. Each disk consists of an outer covering of tough, fibrous tissue surrounding a soft inner core. The outer covering, or *annulus fibrosus,* holds the disk together, while the core, or *nucleus pulposus,* has a shock-absorbing effect that cushions the stress of walking, lifting, and other activities. The vertebrae are bound together with *ligaments* (elastic, connective tissue) and muscles, which keep the spine in proper alignment.

What causes back pain?

Most back pain is caused by mechanical problems, which involve damage to the bones, ligaments, muscles, or other structures in the *spine* (backbone). A small amount of back-pain cases are *pathological* (caused by disease).

The major mechanical problems responsible for back pain are strains or sprains in ligaments or muscles. Such damage may result in severe inflammation or cramplike spasms.

Another mechanical problem behind back pain is a herniated, or slipped, intervertebral disk. A herniated disk occurs when a weak spot develops in the annulus fibrosus. If the annulus fibrosus ruptures, or tears, the nucleus pulposus oozes out like toothpaste from a tube. If this disk material touches a spinal nerve, it will cause irritation and pain.

Painful pressure is also placed on spinal nerves by a condition called *segmental instability,* in which two adjacent vertebrae become unstable and shift in position. This movement can inflame vertebral joints and irritate spinal nerves.

The author:

Michael Woods is the Science Editor of the *Pittsburgh Post-Gazette* and *Toledo Blade,* Washington Bureau.

A common back condition in people over age 65 is spinal stenosis. In this disorder, the spinal canal narrows, usually as a result of disk degeneration and joint swelling, and this leads to compression of spinal nerves.

A condition that is most common in women over age 50 is *osteoporosis* (a bone-thinning disease that drains bones of the minerals that give them strength). The disease also sometimes occurs in older men. Although osteoporosis is painless, it weakens the vertebrae and might lead to vertebral fractures that put pressure on spinal nerves.

But age is only one of several factors that determine the risk for back problems. Pregnant women, for example, are at increased risk for back problems because the extra weight of the unborn baby adds strain to the lower back. In addition, ligaments and muscles in the pelvic area stretch to make room for the birth of the baby. Stretching may leave the structures weakened, increasing the risk of back pain in the months after birth.

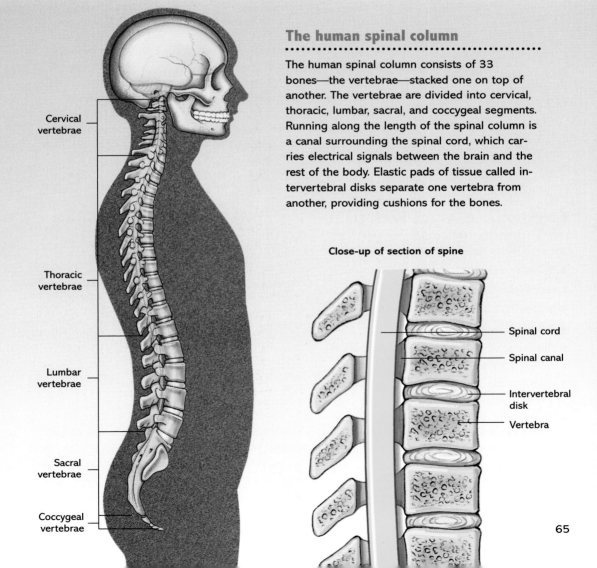

The human spinal column
···

The human spinal column consists of 33 bones—the vertebrae—stacked one on top of another. The vertebrae are divided into cervical, thoracic, lumbar, sacral, and coccygeal segments. Running along the length of the spinal column is a canal surrounding the spinal cord, which carries electrical signals between the brain and the rest of the body. Elastic pads of tissue called intervertebral disks separate one vertebra from another, providing cushions for the bones.

Cervical vertebrae

Thoracic vertebrae

Lumbar vertebrae

Sacral vertebrae

Coccygeal vertebrae

Close-up of section of spine

Spinal cord

Spinal canal

Intervertebral disk

Vertebra

65

Women may engage in activities at home that increase the risk of low back pain. They lean to pick up children, carry children and heavy bags of groceries, and twist into awkward positions while lifting, cooking, and cleaning. Wearing high-heeled shoes puts strain on disks and muscles by causing changes in posture. Frequent carrying of heavy purses, briefcases, backpacks, or tote bags can also strain the lower back.

Although various kinds of home and office activities may lead to back pain, jobs that require heavy physical labor present the greatest risk of back pain. The National Institute for Occupational Safety and Health (NIOSH), an agency of the U.S. Centers for Disease Control and Prevention, identifies five workplace risk factors for low back pain. Besides doing heavy physical work, these factors include making frequent lifts, pushes, pulls, or other forceful movements; bending, twisting, or working in an awkward posture; working in the same position for long periods of time; and experiencing frequent whole-body vibration (as from riding in trucks or other vehicles).

Other factors that increase the risk of low back pain include being more than 20 pounds (9 kilograms) overweight—which puts excessive strain on the lower back—and smoking. Nicotine *constricts* (narrows) blood vessels, and health authorities warn that this can reduce the supply of oxygen and nutrients going to intervertebral disks, thus weakening the disks.

Finally, psychological stress and anxiety are hidden factors in some cases of low back pain. People under emotional stress may unconsciously tense their muscles, triggering muscle spasm and pain. Sudden, forceful movement of a stiff, tense muscle or ligament may cause a strain.

Common causes of back pain

Some common causes of back pain include:

- Strain or sprain of back muscles or ligaments
- Herniated (ruptured) intervertebral disk
- Segmental instability
- Spinal stenosis
- Degenerative disk disease, in which the intervertebral disks deteriorate
- Osteoporosis, a disease in which vertebrae and other bones lose their strength
- Pathological conditions, such as cancer and infections affecting the spine or body organs, including the kidneys and pancreas

Source: American Medical Association.

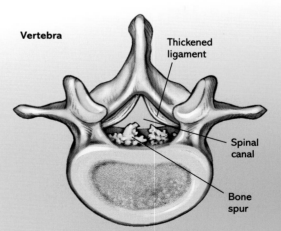

Spinal stenosis. The *spinal canal* (the canal through which the spinal cord passes) narrows. This is usually caused by disk degeneration that results in *bone spurs* (bony outgrowths) and ligament thickening. Narrowing of the canal may lead to compression of spinal nerves.

Most back pain lasts for only a short period. Doctors define back pain as acute if it lasts less than three months. Acute back pain sometimes results from a specific event, such as lifting a heavy object, twisting the body, or falling down. In other cases, it appears for no apparent reason. Back pain that lasts longer than three months is classified as chronic. It may occur steadily over a long period, or it may disappear briefly and then return. Chronic back pain often results from weak back muscles, injuries that never healed, or some underlying disease.

Diagnosis and treatment

Low back pain that has lasted for only a few days or weeks can sometimes be diagnosed in the doctor's office without expensive tests. To diagnose such cases of back pain, a physician will take the patient's medical history and perform a physical exam. However, back pain that has persisted for several weeks almost always must be diagnosed with sophisticated medical imaging techniques. X rays, *computerized tomography* (an X-ray system used to produce three-dimensional images), and *magnetic resonance imaging* (a technique used to produce images of tissue using a magnetic field instead of radiation) are some of the ways in which long-lasting cases of back pain are diagnosed.

In diagnosing back pain, physicians must determine if a serious pathological condition may be producing the pain as a symptom. Such pain can be caused by cancer, infection, or other diseases of body organs, including the kidneys and pancreas. Very few cases of low back pain are caused by pathological conditions, however.

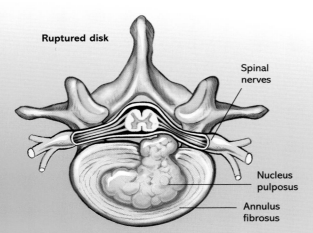

Ruptured disk

Spinal nerves

Nucleus pulposus

Annulus fibrosus

Herniated disk. A tear develops in the *annulus fibrosus* (the outer covering of the cushiony disk that separates two verte-brae), and the *nucleus pulposus* (the inner core) oozes out. Pain results when the nucleus pulposus touches a spinal nerve.

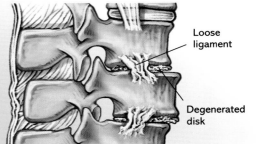

Misaligned vertebrae

Loose ligament

Degenerated disk

Segmental instability. Two adjacent vertebrae become unstable and shift in position. This often results from disk degeneration and ligament slackening. An unstable vertebra may irritate spinal nerves, causing pain.

Most people who have low back pain need no treatment beyond over-the-counter pain relievers to recover fully within two to six weeks. AHCPR officials state that acetaminophen, aspirin, and ibuprofen are all effective in relieving back pain, but the agency warns that some people may get stomach irritation or allergic reactions from aspirin or ibuprofen.

If nonprescription medicines don't work or if symptoms are severe, a physician may recommend stronger drugs, such as prescription nonsteroidal anti-inflammatory drugs or corticosteroid injections. Although some physicians prescribe muscle relaxants, most studies have concluded that these drugs are no more effective than over-the-counter medicines in relieving back pain.

Several other treatments, to be used either alone or in combination with drugs, are available for back pain. These include the application of cold or heat, exercise, spinal manipulation, and surgery.

Cold or heat can provide temporary relief of symptoms for some patients, according to AHCPR. A cold pack or ice bag should be applied to the painful area of the back for 5 to 10 minutes at a time during the first 48 hours of symptoms. Cold acts as first aid for a back injury by reducing swelling in damaged muscles and minimizing the extent of the injury. If symptoms continue after 48 hours, a hot shower or heating pad may help, notes AHCPR. Heat increases blood flow to the injured area, speeding healing.

Extended bed rest once was a common part of back treatment, but physicians now recognize that lying down for long periods may actually slow recovery by weakening muscles, ligaments, and bones. AHCPR reports that most patients do not require bed rest. However, the agency states that patients with unusually severe back pain may benefit from two to four days of bed rest.

Exercise is the best treatment

Physicians now believe that exercise is the best thing you can do for a bad back. AHCPR recommends *aerobics* (exercises designed to promote the use of oxygen by the body), such as walking, riding a stationary bicycle, and swimming. According to the agency, these exercises should be started gradually within the first few weeks following recovery. After that, the patient can gradually increase the amount of time spent doing aerobics to as much as 20 to 30 minutes every day. AHCPR also notes that various stretching exercises may help relieve back pain, but the agency warns that these exercises should not be performed during the first few weeks of symptoms because they may be too stressful to the back. A patient should always get a doctor's permission before doing exercises.

Physicians sometimes prescribe physical therapy to patients suffering from low back pain. Although some patients report temporary relief of symptoms from physical therapy, AHCPR maintains that the benefits of this type of treatment for cases of acute back pain remained unproven as of 1999.

Risk factors for back pain

Several factors increase a person's risk of developing back pain, including:

- Age—in older people, muscles and ligaments are more likely to become weakened or strained, and bones are more likely to fracture.
- Pregnancy—carrying the extra weight of pregnancy adds strain to the lower back.
- Homemaking—picking up children, carrying groceries, and twisting while cooking and cleaning all add strain to the lower back.
- Body weight—being more than 20 pounds (9 kilograms) overweight increases strain on the back.
- Heavy physical work, including frequent lifting, pushing, pulling, or other forceful movements.
- Bending, twisting, or working in an awkward posture.
- Standing or sitting in the same position for long periods.
- Frequent whole-body vibration, such as that caused by riding in trucks or other vehicles.
- Smoking—nicotine *constricts* (narrows) blood vessels, reducing the supply of oxygen and nutrients going to intervertebral disks.
- Psychological stress—stress and anxiety may tense back muscles, increasing the chance that they might become damaged.

Source: United States Department of Health and Human Services.

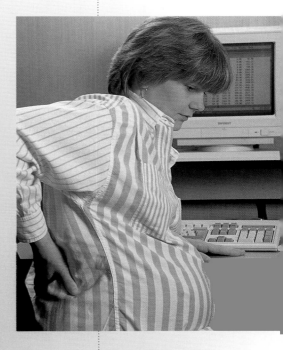

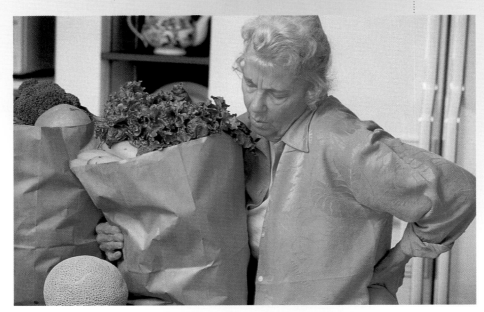

In a method of back treatment called spinal manipulation, practitioners, such as osteopathic physicians and chiropractors, use their hands to apply force in ways that adjust the vertebrae into proper alignment. AHCPR has concluded that spinal manipulation is both safe and effective in the first month of acute back problems. However, for symptoms lasting longer than a month, the agency states that spinal manipulation had not yet proven its effectiveness as of 1999.

Government health authorities say the effectiveness of a number of other forms of back treatment are also in question. These treatments include massage, traction, *acupuncture* (the use of thin needles to relieve pain), *transcutaneous electrical nerve stimulation* (the passing of a mild electric current through the skin to block pain), *biofeedback* (a method of monitoring and controlling one's own brain waves or other body functions), and *ultrasound* (the use of high-frequency sound waves to reduce pain). According to AHCPR, these treatments may bring relief from back pain for only short periods of time, and none has proven effective in speeding recovery or keeping acute back problems from returning.

Surgery is the last resort for patients with severe long-lasting back pain. AHCPR states that surgery is useful in only 1 percent of back-pain cases.

The most common reason for back surgery is to remove pressure on nerves from a herniated lumbar disk. To relieve the pressure, a

Although some patients find that physical therapy temporarily eases their low back pain, government health authorities said the benefits of physical therapy for cases of acute back pain remained unproven as of 1999.

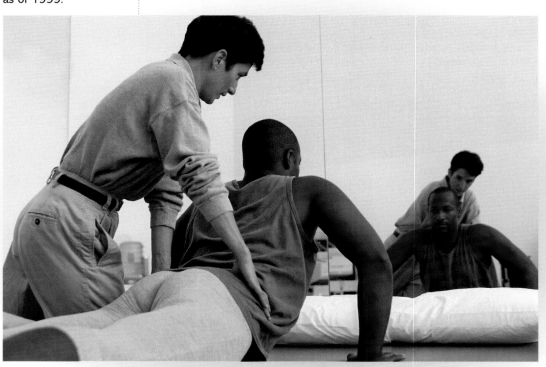

Exercises for people with back pain

Physicians recommend various exercises for spinal care and back pain relief. People who have hurt their backs in the past or have been diagnosed with specific back problems should get medical advice before exercising.

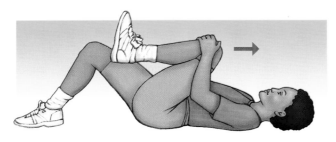

Knee to shoulder stretch. Lie on your back on a firm surface with your knees bent and feet flat. Pull one knee toward your chest with both hands. Hold for 15 to 30 seconds. Return to starting position. Repeat with other leg. Do three to four times with each leg.

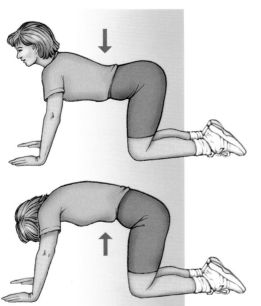

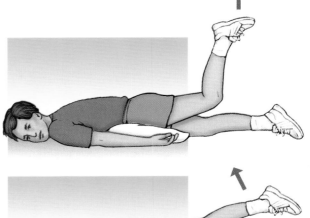

Cat stretch. Get down on your hands and knees. Slowly let your back and abdomen sag toward the floor, *top*. Then slowly arch your back away from the floor, *bottom*. Repeat several times.

Leg lifts. Lie face down on a firm surface with a large pillow under your hips and lower abdomen. Keeping your knee bent, raise one leg slightly off the surface and hold for five seconds, *top*. Repeat several times. Then, keeping your legs straight, repeat the exercise, *bottom*.

Source: Mayo Foundation for Medical Education and Research.

surgeon may perform a minimally invasive operation called endo-scopic diskectomy. In this procedure, which involves only local anesthesia, the surgeon operates through a small incision using an *endoscope* (a thin, hollow tube with a viewing lens on one end and a bright light on the other). The hollow center of the endoscope serves as an opening for the passage of miniature surgical instruments needed to remove any torn or bulging disk material that is applying pressure on nerves. Patients usually return home after a few hours and go back to work in a few days.

Some operations on patients with low back pain, however, require general anesthesia and larger incisions. In one such operation, called *laminectomy*, surgeons remove the bone arches, or laminae, of one or more vertebrae in order to gain access to and remove herniated disks, thereby relieving pressure on spinal nerves. In another type of surgery, called *fusion*, surgeons join two or more vertebrae to eliminate movement of parts of the spine that irritate spinal nerves. The vertebrae are joined with screws, plates, rods, and bone grafts.

Avoiding back problems

Avoiding a health problem is always better than treating one. Physicians advise that the best way to prevent future bouts of back pain is to exercise. Combine walking, biking, or other aerobic exercises with stretching exercises to condition the back muscles. But,

Tips to prevent back pain

- When sitting, keep your back straight with your lumbar spine supported by the chair back. Prop your feet on a stool.

- Don't sit for long periods. Stand or walk at every opportunity.

- While standing, prop one foot and then the other on a stool.

- Stand straight, with your spine centered over your pelvis.

- Wear comfortable, low-heeled shoes.

- Don't lift by bending over an object. Lift objects by bending knees to a squatting position while keeping the back straight.

- Don't twist your body while holding a heavy load. Turn your entire body in the direction you want to move.

- Don't push a heavy object in front of you. To move a heavy object, place your back against it and push.

- Maintain proper body weight, and exercise regularly.

- Don't smoke.

- Learn to cope with stress.

Source: United States Department of Health and Human Services.

The wrong way and the right way to prevent back injury

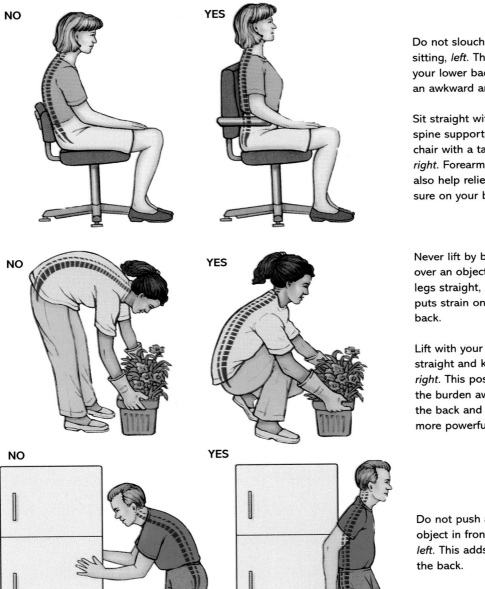

NO   **YES**

Do not slouch while sitting, *left*. This pushes your lower back out at an awkward angle.

Sit straight with your spine supported by a chair with a tall back, *right*. Forearm rests will also help relieve pressure on your back.

NO   **YES**

Never lift by bending over an object with your legs straight, *left*. This puts strain on the lower back.

Lift with your back straight and knees bent, *right*. This position shifts the burden away from the back and to the more powerful legs.

NO   **YES**

Do not push a heavy object in front of you, *left*. This adds strain to the back.

Always push a heavy object backward, *right*. This allows the legs to do the work.

Source: American Medical Association.

as always, a physician's advice should be obtained before starting an exercise program.

Back-injury prevention is very important for workers who do heavy lifting. However, not all prevention techniques are effective. Many employers, for example, encourage such workers to wear an industrial back belt, a corsetlike elastic band fastened around the lower back and abdomen, to decrease stress on the spine during lifting. But NIOSH studies have found no evidence that back belts prevent injury in people with healthy backs. Furthermore, says NIOSH, back belts may give workers a false sense of security, leading them to lift heavier loads and take greater risks.

Rather than relying on back belts, NIOSH recommends that employers place more emphasis on identifying lifting hazards and encouraging safer lifting techniques. NIOSH also recommends that companies implement *ergonomics* (the study of the relationship between individuals and their work environment) programs and redesign jobs that require much lifting, bending, twisting, pushing, or pulling.

Many people do not lift objects safely. They keep their legs stiff, bend over the object, and lift by straightening the back. Lifting with the back strains the lumbar muscles, ligaments, and disks. Twisting while lifting increases the strain. To lift an object safely, according to NIOSH, you should bend your knees to a squatting position while keeping your back straight. Do not twist your body while holding the heavy load. Instead of twisting, point your toes in the direction you want to move, and turn your entire body in that direction.

Other precautions

NIOSH, AHCPR, and other health authorities recommend a number of other precautions to prevent back problems. One of these precautions is avoiding long periods of sitting. Sitting puts more stress on the lumbar disks than standing. A person should get out of the chair and stand or walk at every opportunity to reduce this stress. For example, office workers can stand at their desks while talking on the telephone.

While sitting, your spine should be supported by the chair back or a pillow. Health officials recommend using a chair with a high back and armrests, which help take strain off the lower back. If possible, sit with your feet on a stool to increase the bend in your knees. This position eases the spinal curvature in the lower back, taking pressure off the disks.

Prolonged standing in one position can also lead to back problems. Back experts advise bending the knees by alternately propping one foot and then the other on a stool. This helps reduce strain on the lumbar vertebrae.

Maintaining good posture is very important, according to health officials. Many people tend to stand with the pelvis and buttocks arched slightly backward. That position increases curvature in the lower back and strain on the lumbar disks. Stand straight with your spine centered over your pelvis. Officials also warn that maintaining proper body weight is important to avoid straining the lower back.

Finally, health authorities advise people not to smoke and to learn how to better manage the stresses of everyday life. Following both of these tips can help prevent physical problems that lead to back pain.

Low back pain is one of the most common medical conditions, causing misery for millions of people each year. Fortunately, most cases of back pain are not serious. With simple treatments, regular exercise, and proper precautions, low back pain should go away and stay away. ● ● ●

For additional information:

Books and periodicals

Deyo, Richard A. "Low-Back Pain." *Scientific American,* August 1998, pp. 48-53.

Fishman, Loren and Ardman, Carol. *Back Talk: How to Diagnose and Cure Low Back Pain and Sciatica.* W. W. Norton & Company, 1997.

Hochschuler, Stephen and Reznik, Bob. *Treat Your Back Without Surgery: The Best Non-Surgical Alternatives to Eliminating Back and Neck Pain.* Hunter House, Incorporated, 1998.

Johns Hopkins University. *Back Pain: What You Need to Know.* Time-Life Books, 1999.

Miller, Robert H. and Opie, Christine A. *Back Pain Relief—The Ultimate Guide: A Comprehensive Pain Management Program.* Capra Press, 1997.

Sobel, Dava and Klein, Arthur C. *Backache: What Exercises Work.* St. Martin's Press, 1996.

Web sites

http://www.vh.org/Patients/IHB/Ortho/BackPatient/Contents.html (Acute Low Back Problems in Adults—AHCPR)

http://www.cdc.gov/niosh/ergtxt6.html (Musculoskeletal Disorders and Workplace Factors—NIOSH)

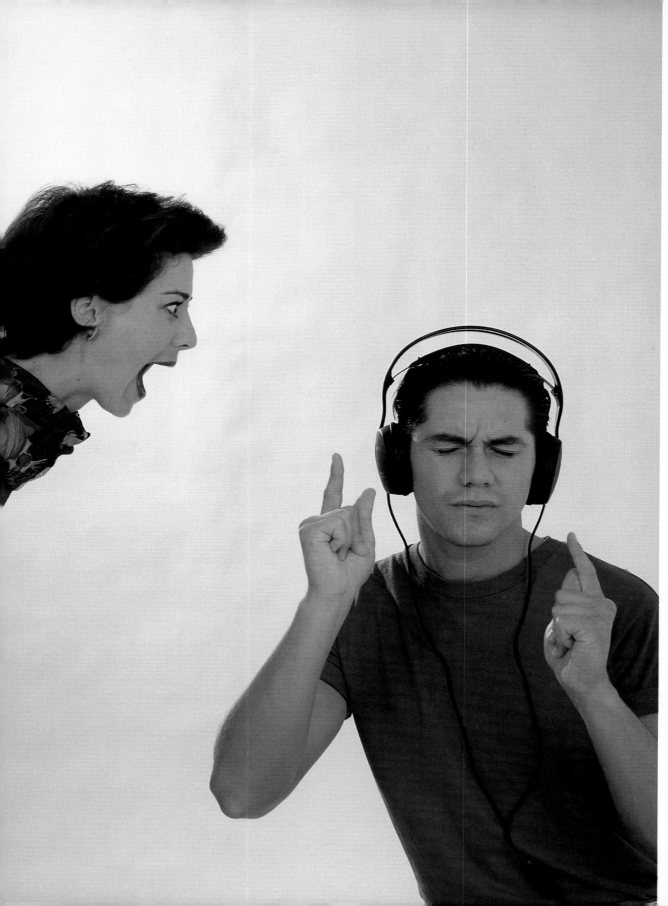

While hearing loss can be a normal part of the aging process, exposure to excess noise can threaten hearing in the young.

Can You Hear What I'm Saying?

By Dennis Connaughton

PRESIDENT RONALD REAGAN EXPERIENCED A SIGNIFICANT LOSS of hearing while in the White House. Before leaving the presidency in 1989, Reagan began wearing a hearing aid to improve his perception of sound. His physicians did not consider the hearing loss unusual, considering the president's age. (Ronald Reagan became president at the age of 69 and left office at age 77.) The hearing loss experienced by Mark Herndon, drummer for the popular country band Alabama, however, was unexpected. Herndon was only 27 when he discovered that he had lost hearing in higher frequencies. Physicians diagnosed the loss as the result of years of performing in front of stacks of blasting speakers. Herndon now wears earphones or earmuffs on stage to protect his hearing.

More than 28 million people in the United States—nearly 10 percent of the population in 1999—have experienced hearing loss to some degree, according to the Better Hearing Institute, a nonprofit, educational organization based in Washington, D.C. Traditionally, the elderly make up the largest percentage of those 28 million people. In 1998, age-related hearing loss affected 30 to 35 percent of the population between the ages of 65 to 75 years and 40 percent over age 75. However, in the 1990's, researchers discovered a sharp increase in hearing loss among younger people. The Better Hearing Institute reported in 1998 that as much as 10 percent of the U.S. population aged 40 to 65 had experienced some degree of hearing loss. Loud music blasting from stereos and radio boomboxes, sound effects blaring from video games, booming sound systems in movie theaters, and the high-intensity sounds of everyday life can cause almost anyone to lose some of his or her hearing over time.

Types of hearing loss

Physicians categorize most hearing losses as either sensorineural, conductive, or "mixed." Approximately 95 percent of all hearing loss in the United States is classified as sensorineural, according to the Better Hearing Institute. This type of hearing loss is produced by damage to the structures of the inner ear. The structures include the *cochlea* (the organ in the inner ear that transforms sound to electric nerve impulses) and the sensory hair cells and nerve fibers that transmit nerve impulses to the brain. Inner ear damage is most commonly the result of aging or prolonged exposure to loud noises. Age-related hearing loss is called *presbycusis*, a condition in which the sensory hair cells in the inner ear die.

Traumatic head injuries and sharp blows to the ear can also result in sensorineural hearing loss. Damage to the inner ear can be triggered by certain diseases and medical conditions, including viral infections, such as mumps or measles; Meniere's disease, which increases fluid pressure in the inner ear; bacterial meningitis, a brain infection that can damage the acoustic nerve; and acoustic neuroma, a benign brain tumor. Certain antibiotics, such as streptomycin, gentamicin, and neomycin, can result in sensorineural hearing loss. Aspirin, if taken in large quantities, also can cause hearing loss. The condition is also associated with certain birth defects and inherited inner ear abnormalities.

Conductive hearing loss is produced by sound blockage between the outer and inner ear. Sound travels in waves from the outer ear through the ear canal to the eardrum, a thin membrane of tissue that vibrates when hit by sound. Vibrations travel from the eardrum through the middle ear. The middle ear contains tiny bones that pass the vibrations to the inner-ear membrane. In the inner ear, the vibrations are converted to electric impulses that are transmitted to the brain through the acoustic nerve.

A number of medical conditions produce conductive hearing loss. The most common, especially among children, is otitis media. This inflammation of the middle ear is most often caused by colds or other upper respiratory tract infections. Sticky fluids build up behind the eardrum, which can become infected.

Otosclerosis is another disorder that causes progressive conductive hearing loss. The condition, which is usually inherited and occurs for unknown reasons, produces an overgrowth of bone in the middle ear that eventually immobilizes the stapes (the innermost bone of the middle ear). Sound cannot pass to the inner ear if the stapes is unable to vibrate. A perforated eardrum, tumors, changes in air pressure, and a foreign body in the middle ear, such as a wax blockage, are also common causes of conductive hearing loss.

Mixed hearing loss is a combination of the sensorineural and conductive types of hearing loss. It can result from infections, tumors, genetic disorders, and head and ear injuries. A middle ear infection can damage the eardrum and the tiny bones that conduct sound waves and then move into the inner ear. Certain tumors can block the flow of sound waves in the ear canal or middle ear and then spread to the inner ear.

How the ear works

The ear is made up of three sections—the outer, middle, and inner ear. The outer ear, which includes the pinna and ear canal, captures sound waves. The middle ear includes the eardrum and an air-filled chamber containing tiny bones, the stapes, incus, and malleus. The three bones amplify sound waves and carry them to the cochlea. The inner ear, which consists of the cochlea and the semicircular canals, converts the sound waves from the middle ear into nerve impulses that travel to the brain through the auditory nerve.

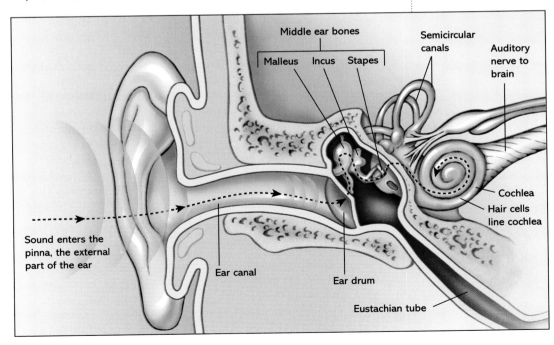

Middle ear bones
Malleus   Incus   Stapes

Semicircular canals

Auditory nerve to brain

Cochlea
Hair cells line cochlea

Sound enters the pinna, the external part of the ear

Ear canal

Ear drum

Eustachian tube

Preventing hearing loss

Some forms of hearing loss cannot be prevented, and noise, the most common cause of hearing loss after aging, is also the most easily preventable. Most experts agree that hearing loss among people 40 to 65 years old is generally the result of exposure to excessive levels of noise. The National Institute on Deafness and Commun-ication Disorders (NIDCD), a privately-funded, research foundation located in Washington, D.C., reported in 1998 that as many as 20 million Americans were exposed annually to hazardous levels of noise or worked in dangerously noisy environments.

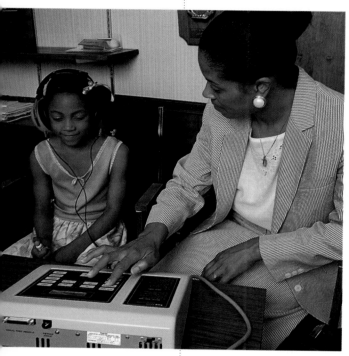

A child's hearing is tested during a routine checkup at the office of a family physician with the use of an audiometer, a machine that measures the intensity of sounds, *above.*

Research in the late 1990's also re-vealed that noise-induced hearing loss was affecting the nation's school-age population. The Centers for Disease Control and Prevention (CDC), locat-ed in Atlanta, Georgia, reported in 1998 that hearing loss among school-age children has become widespread in the United States. In 1998, 15 percent of all children between the ages of 6 and 19 had experienced hearing loss to some degree. A significant propor-tion of incidences resulted from avoid-able noise, such as prolonged loud music and video games.

Noise is measured in decibels. The higher the decibel level, the greater the effect on hearing. A whisper regis-ters at 30 decibels (db). Normal con-versation ranges from 50 to 65 db. A hairdryer or vacuum cleaner produces 70 db. None of these sounds damage hearing.

Damage occurs after prolonged ex-posure to sounds at 80 db or higher. City traffic can hit 80 db. Noise from lawnmowers ranges from 85 to 90 db. Subway and motorcycle sounds reach 90 db. Stereo volume set at the half-way mark registers 100 db. Rock concerts often hit 110 db. A jet taking off produces 120 db, a radio "boombox" can reach 120 db, a jackhammer 130 db, and a shotgun 140 db. The higher the decibel level, the less expo-sure time it takes to damage human hearing.

Physical effects of excessive noise levels

Prolonged exposure to noise at hazardous levels eventually injures the sensory hair cells in the inner ear. This injury causes swelling of the nerve endings in the cochlea, particularly at the base, where the nerve endings are extremely sensitive to high-intensity sound.

Excessive noise levels initially produce a short-term hearing loss,

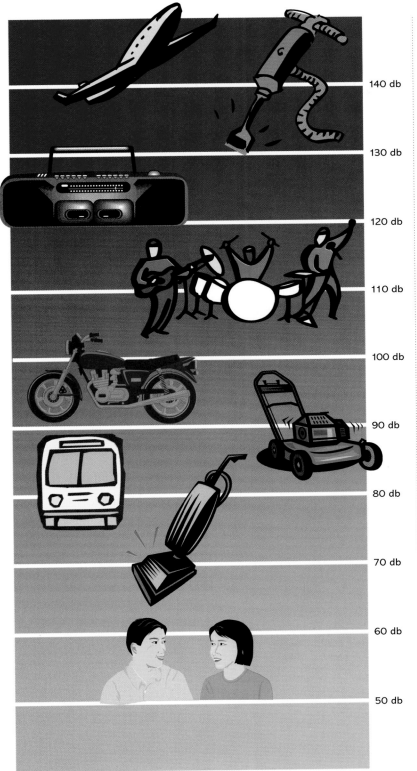

140 db

130 db

120 db

110 db

100 db

90 db

80 db

70 db

60 db

50 db

Measuring noise

Noise is measured in decibels. Normal conversation ranges from 50 to 65 decibels (db). A vacuum cleaner produces 70 db. Damage occurs after prolonged exposure to sounds at 80 db or higher. Motorcycles can hit 85 to 90 db. A jet taking off produces 120 db. A radio "boombox" can also reach 120 db. A jackhammer normally registers at 130 db. The higher the decibel level, the less exposure time it takes to damage human hearing.

known as a temporary threshold shift. Sounds are muffled, usually for a few hours or a day. People who attend a rock concert, for example, often experience temporary threshold shift. They hear ringing or buzzing sounds and feel a sense of fullness in their ears. Normal hearing returns after damaged hair cells repair themselves, which usually begins the first day after exposure to the noise.

Hair-cell repair, however, can take as long as a month, depending on the damage done and an individual's sensitivity to noise. If exposure to loud noises is constant or frequent, inner ear hair cells may lose the ability to bounce back. They die, producing irreversible hearing loss.

A second type of noise-induced hearing loss is acoustic trauma, which is produced by a single exposure to a noise of very high intensity, such as an explosion. Such a sound can rupture the ear-

Reasons for hearing loss	Type	Causes
acoustic trauma	sensorineural	one-time exposure to explosion or loud noise
barotrauma	conductive	unequal air pressure on two sides of eardrum in air or under water
drugs	sensorineural	use of certain antibiotics, diuretics, aspirin, quinine
eardrum, perforated	conductive	otitis media; sharp object; blow to ear; explosion; skull fracture; air pressure change; tumor
earwax	conductive	overproduction of cerumen (earwax)
foreign body in ear canal	conductive	children insert small objects in ears; flying or crawling insects
injury	sensorineural	blunt blow to external ear
mastoiditis, acute	conductive	spread of untreated otitis media to surrounding bone
Meniere's disease	sensorineural	unknown
myringitis, infectious	conductive	inflammation of eardrum from a viral or bacterial infection
noise	sensorineural	prolonged exposure to noise
otitis media	conductive	complication of a cold
otosclerosis	conductive	hereditary disease
presbycusis	sensorineural	aging
tumors	conductive	sebaceous cysts; bone tumors; and growths of excess scar tissue

drum and blow apart the structures of the inner ear. A person who is experiencing acoustic trauma may become dizzy, feel pain, and hear ringing in the ear. The ear closest to the explosion usually suffers more damage than the opposite ear. A person suffering hearing loss due to acoustic trauma may regain some or all of his or her hearing over time.

Recognizing hearing loss

How do people know they are losing their hearing? There are a number of warning signs. The first sign may be asking other people to repeat what they are saying or missing parts of conversations, especially when there is a lot of background noise, such as at a restaurant or party.

Physical characteristics	Treatments
damage or death of sensory hair cells	hearing aid; cochlear implant
rupture of blood vessels in middle ear or sinuses	antibiotic for possible infection; other treatments usually necessary
damage to cochlea and/or labyrinth	discontinue use of drugs
hole in eardrum	antibiotic drugs for possible infection; eardrum usually heals by itself
blockage of outer ear canal	removal by physician
	removal of foreign object by physician; mineral oil kills insects
bruising between cartilage and connective tissue	painkilling drugs; rest
bacterial infection of prominent bone behind the ear	antibiotics; surgical drain of bone abscess
increase in fluid in the canals in the inner ear; damage to cochlea and/or labyrinth	bed rest; drugs to relieve nausea and ringing; surgery
fluid-filled blisters on eardrum	antibiotics; painkilling drugs
damage to or death of sensory hair cells in inner ear	hearing aid; cochlear implant
infection in middle ear	antibiotic drugs and pain killers; removal of infected debris by physician
bone overgrowth immobilizes stapes in middle ear	hearing aid; stapedectomy operation to replace stapes
degeneration of hair cells/nerve fibers in inner ear	hearing aid; cochlear implant
growth blocks ear canal, causing earwax build-up	surgical removal of tumor

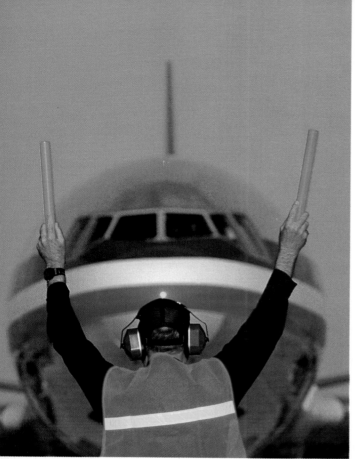

An airport employee wears earphones to protect his hearing while a jet is readied for take-off, *above*. Jets routinely produce 120 decibels on take-off, a noise level that can produce hearing loss.

Other warning signs of possible hearing loss include being unable to hear over the telephone; finding oneself unable to follow a conversation involving two or more people; turning the TV or radio volume higher in order to hear it; being unable to determine where sounds are coming from; deciding that other people are not speaking clearly; responding incorrectly to a misunderstood question; or not hearing ringing of doorbells or telephones.

Babies born with impaired hearing may fail to turn their head or move their eyes in response to voices or other sounds. An infant with impaired hearing may not form sounds or words at the right time and may have difficulty learning to speak. A child with hearing loss may have trouble carrying on a conversation or may constantly turn one ear to hear a voice or other sounds.

Individuals who experience hearing loss may withdraw socially and experience confusion, depression, and feelings of inadequacy. They often deny or attempt to cover their loss. They may also exhibit embarrassment, frustration, impatience, and guilt.

Diagnosing a loss of hearing

While sensorineural and conductive hearing loss can be permanent, proper treatment helps many people with hearing loss improve their hearing. The first step is to see a physician. A family physician, in turn, may refer a patient with hearing problems to an *audiologist* (a specialist trained to evaluate hearing problems) or to an *otolaryngologist* (ear, nose, and throat doctor) or *otologist* (another ear specialist) to determine the kind of hearing loss.

During a hearing test, the audiologist seats a patient in a sound-proof booth and places a set of headphones over his or her ears. The audiologist broadcasts various tones and various noise levels through the headphones. An *audiometer*, a machine that measures the intensity of sounds, plots test results on an *audiogram*, a sheet on which hearing impairment is classified on a scale from mild to profound.

A person with normal hearing can pick up sounds that range between 0 to 20 db. A person who is unable to hear sounds below 20 to 45 db is classified as having suffered a minor hearing loss. Moderate loss involves sounds between 45 and 60 db and moderately severe, between 60 and 75 db. Individuals with severe hearing loss are unable to hear sounds ranging from 75 to 90 db, and people with profound hearing loss do not hear sounds as loud as 90 db and above. With the audiogram results and other tests, the audiologist determines the degree of hearing loss and recommends appropriate treatment.

Treating hearing loss

Treatment for hearing loss can range from the removal of earwax to corrective surgery. Physicians use a syringe and warm water to remove a build-up of earwax, which can cause temporary conductive hearing loss. When otitis media causes conductive hearing loss, resulting in a collection of sticky fluid in the middle ear, the individual may need an operation to drain the fluid through a hole created in the eardrum. If there is no build-up of fluid, antibiotics may be given to clear the infection.

Surgical procedures for hearing loss include tympanoplasty, to repair perforated eardrums, and stapedectomy, to remove a bone damaged by otosclerosis and replace it with an artificial bone. Physicians also recommend hearing aids in some cases of otosclerosis.

Hearing aids

Hearing aids are battery-operated electronic instruments that collect sound waves, amplify them electronically, and aim the sound into the ear. They are most often used to treat sensorineural hearing loss. They do not cure the loss but increase the volume of the sound that reaches the inner ear. The components of most hearing aids include an amplifier, receiver, microphone, earpiece, and batteries.

There are essentially three types of hearing aids available—the behind-the-ear type; in the ear; and in the canal. The behind-the-ear type has an amplification device with a microphone that fits in back of the ear. Amplified sound travels through a flexible plastic tube to a small plastic earmold in the ear itself. Behind-the-

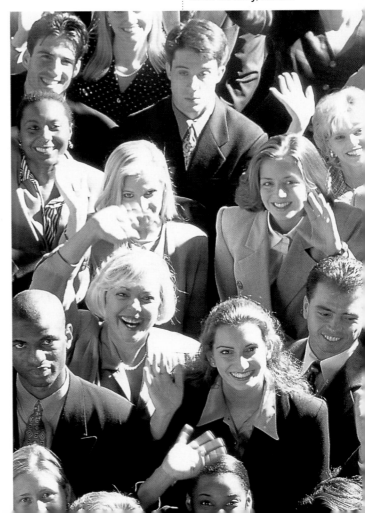

Individuals who undergo hearing loss often experience confusion, depression, and feelings of inadequacy and withdraw socially, *below*.

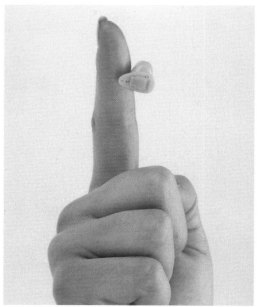

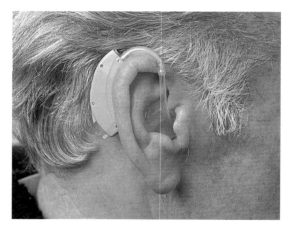

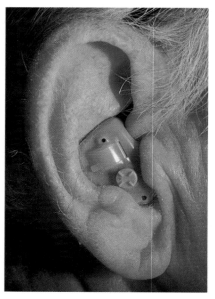

Types of hearing aids

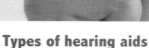

There are essentially three types of hearing aids—the completely-in-the-canal type, *above*, which fits in the lower portion of the ear canal and is the least visible of external hearing aids; the behind-the-ear type, *above right,* which has an amplification device with a microphone that fits in back of the ear; and the in-the-ear type, *right,* which has an amplifier, microphone, and speaker in a shell-shaped container on the opening to the ear canal.

ear hearing aids can also be mounted on eyeglasses.

The in-the-ear type of hearing aid is the most commonly used type. This hearing aid has an amplifier, microphone, and speaker contained in a shell-shaped container that is custom fitted to the shape of an individual's ear. It sits on the opening to the ear canal.

The in-the-canal style of hearing aid, which fits down in the lower portion of the ear canal, is considerably smaller and less powerful than the in-the-ear style. One type of in-the-canal device can be placed deeply in the ear canal. Only a tiny portion of it shows at the opening to the ear canal. The in-the-canal styles are popular because they are the least visible of all external hearing aids.

Hearing aids are equipped with a variety of electric circuitry. The majority of hearing aids are made with analog circuits, which is the same technology used to transmit television signals. When sound waves enter analog hearing aids, they are amplified across the entire spectrum of sound.

Hearing aids are also made with digital circuits, which convert incoming sound to binary numbers that are processed by a computer chip. Digital devices separate background noise from speech, eliminating some of the noise distortion that may accompany analog units.

A third type of hearing-aid circuit is a programmable or combined digital/analog circuit. They are programmed with digital circuits to adapt to a wide range of hearing loss but amplify the sound using analog circuitry. The duel technology allows the user to change settings in order to adjust to various environments.

Cochlear implants

A cochlear implant, which can be helpful to people with profound sensorineural hearing loss, is an electronic device that is surgically implanted into the inner ear. Cochlear implants compensate for the missing function of dead sensory hair cells in the inner ear. The implant consists of a small external microphone, worn behind the ear, that picks up sound. The sound travels through a wire to a speech or signal processor that converts speech into digital signals.

The best way for an individual to improve his or her hearing, however, is to avoid situations that may inflict damage. Not all types of hearing loss can be prevented, but with a little caution, the individual can help preserve his or her hearing for a long time.　•••

For further information:

Books and articles

Carmen, Richard. *The Consumer Handbook on Hearing Loss and Hearing Aids.* Auricle Ink Publishers, 1998.

Connaughton, Dennis, and Kotulak, Donna. *American Medical Association Complete Guide to Your Children's Health.* Random House, 1999.

Haaf, Wendy. "Too much noise?" *Parenting,* Nov. 1998.

Pope, Anne. *Hear: Solutions, Skills, and Sources for People with Hearing Loss.* Dorling Kindersley, 1997.

Suss, Elaine. *When the Hearing Gets Hard: Winning the Battle Against Hearing Impairment.* Insight Books, 1993.

Vernick, David M., and Grzelka, Constance. *The Hearing Loss Handbook.* Consumer Reports Books, 1993.

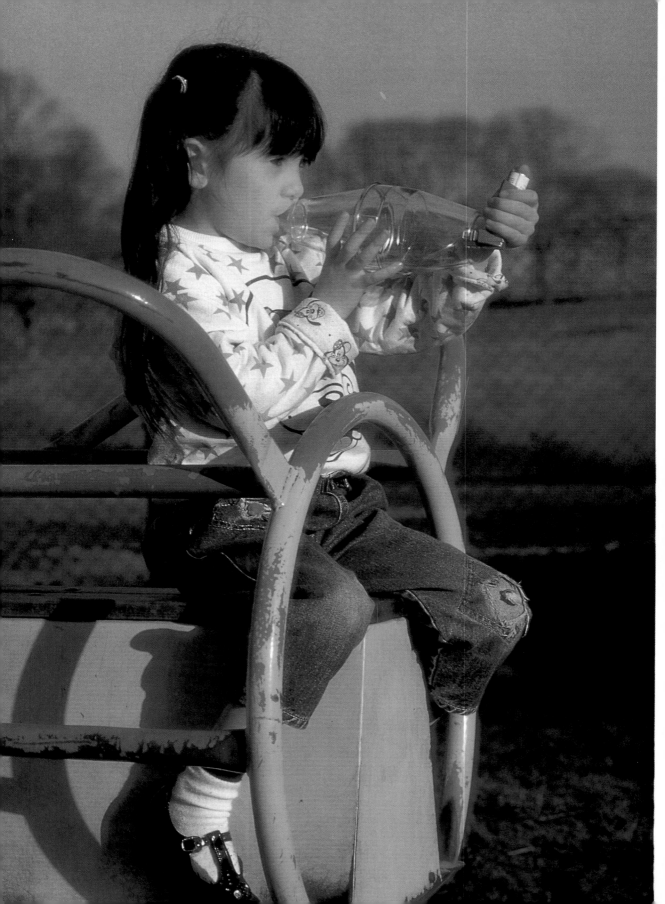

Asthma can be a life-threatening disease, but physicians and patients can work together to keep it under control.

A Breath-Taking Ailment:
Learning to Control Asthma

By Joan Stephenson

FOURTEEN-YEAR-OLD ALICIA can't imagine a life without sports. Whether it's baseball, football, or soccer, it's hard to keep the athletic teen-ager off the playing field. And so, many people would be surprised to learn that not only does Alicia have asthma, an illness that can make it difficult to breathe at times, but also that exercise is one of the factors that can trigger her symptoms.

What Alicia knows, however, is that by following the asthma action plan she has worked out with her doctor, she can decrease the likelihood of an asthma attack and lead the active life she enjoys. She has a daily routine that involves taking a combination of two long-acting asthma drugs that she inhales in a spray form. And when it's time for sports, Alicia comes prepared.

"Before I play, I 'pretreat' by taking two puffs of medication," she says. The medication is a rapid-acting prescription drug that helps open up Alicia's airways. "I wait a few minutes for it to kick in, and then go play." Even after taking these precautions, she knows that a breathless feeling or tightness in the chest is a warning sign to sit down and take another dose. If this does not help, Alicia follows her asthma action plan and asks to see the school nurse immediately to determine whether she needs additional medical attention.

Opposite page:
A girl inhales a proper dose of asthma medication from a device called a metered-dose inhaler.

Doctors have learned a great deal about how to help the 15 million to 17 million people in the United States who, like Alicia, have to live with asthma, but the disease still has a substantial impact. It causes an estimated 100 million days of restricted activity each year in the United States. With about one-third of people with asthma under the age of 18, it is the most common *chronic* (long-lasting) childhood disease and the leading cause of missed school days due to a chronic condition.

Asthma experts are also alarmed by a disturbing trend—an increase in the number of people with asthma and an increase in the number of asthma-related deaths. According to a 1998 report by the Centers for Disease Control and Prevention (CDC) in Atlanta, Georgia, the number of people with asthma more than doubled between 1980 and 1994. In that same period, the number of deaths nearly doubled as well, with more than 5,400 deaths in 1994.

Despite these sobering trends, advances in the 1990's have led to a better understanding of the disease and better ways to prevent and treat it. While there is no known cure, patients can do much with proper treatment to control their asthma and minimize symptoms.

What is asthma?

The visible face of asthma is its symptoms: *wheezing* (a whistling or hissing noise during exhalation), breathlessness, persistent coughing, and a tight feeling in the chest. These symptoms reflect the fundamental problem that underlies all asthma: chronic inflammation inside the branching network of tubes called bronchi and bronchioles that carry air from the windpipe to the tiny air sacs of the lungs. The inflamed tissues are reddened, irritated, and swollen. If the inflammation is severe, frequent, and untreated, it can irreversibly damage the airway walls. When this occurs, airway narrowing may persist and become dangerously unresponsive to medication.

Although researchers do not know what initially causes the chronic inflammation, they do know that the inflammation sets the stage for additional complications in a person's respiratory system. Chronic inflammation causes airways to become overly sensitive to specific stimuli such as *allergens* (substances to which a person is allergic, such as pollen), irritants (such as tobacco smoke), viral respiratory infections (such as the flu), and even cold air. Exposure to such a "trigger" can cause an asthma attack, or episode, by causing a variety of cells to release chemicals that contribute to and perpetuate inflammation. Some of these chemicals also cause bronchoconstriction or bronchospasm, the tightening of the bands of muscles around the airways, narrowing the passages even more. Other cells in the airways produce a thick, sticky mucus that can plug the smaller passageways, leaving even less room for air to flow into and out of the lungs.

Asthma attacks range from mild breathing difficulties to life-threatening episodes. The more severe the airway narrowing, the

The author
....

Joan Stephenson is an associate editor with the *Journal of the American Medical Association.*

more difficult it becomes to move air into and out of the lungs. Overcoming the lack of air flow requires more effort from muscles involved in breathing, which are located in the chest, neck, back, shoulders, and below the lungs. When an attack is mild, the breathing becomes somewhat more labored and slightly faster than usual. The individual may experience some mild wheezing, coughing, spitting up of mucus, shortness of breath, or tightness in the chest. In a moderate attack, these symptoms become more pronounced, the skin may become pale, and the muscles of the chest may become drawn in as the body strains to move air through the airways.

During a severe asthma attack, breathing is either very fast or slow and labored. Skin color is poor, and lips and fingernails may turn gray or blue. Neck, abdominal, and chest muscles may tighten and draw in. If the airways become completely blocked from mucus, detached airway cells, swelling, and constriction, the person is in danger of suffocation and death if he or she does not receive emergency treatment.

In some cases, an asthma attack may seem to subside with the use of medications, but potentially dangerous and subtle changes may continue to obstruct airways. For days or weeks after an initial episode, the airways can remain inflamed and continue to swell, becoming even more susceptible to asthma triggers and additional attacks.

The allergy connection

Identifying factors that trigger asthma attacks is as important as recognizing the symptoms. One of the most common triggers of asthma episodes is an allergic reaction, a kind of overreaction of the body's immune system. Although everyone with allergies does not have asthma and everyone with asthma does not have allergies, there is a significant link between the two conditions. About 75 to 80 percent of children who get asthma, for example, have allergic reactions to common environmental allergens when they are exposed to these allergens in a simple skin test.

When the immune system encounters a harmful bacteria or virus, the system usually produces antibodies, proteins that attack infectious agents. In an allergic reaction, the body deploys antibod-

Asthma statistics

Asthma is a growing health concern

Between 1980 and 1994, the number of people diagnosed with asthma in the United States more than doubled.

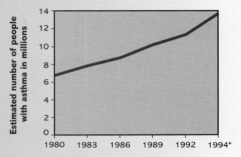

Source: U.S. Centers for Disease Control and Prevention, *Morbidity and Mortality Weekly Report*, April 24, 1998.

*Most recent data available.

Estimated number of people diagnosed with asthma in the United States by age group

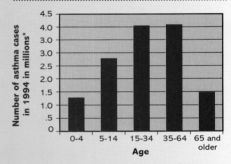

Source: U.S. Centers for Disease Control and Prevention, *Morbidity and Mortality Weekly Report*, April 24, 1998.

*Most recent data available.

Asthma-related deaths are on the rise

From 1975 to 1995, the total number of asthma-related deaths in the United States almost tripled.

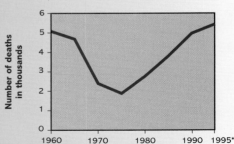

Source: U.S. Centers for Disease Control and Prevention, *Morbidity and Mortality Weekly Report*, April 24, 1998.

*Most recent data available.

Why is it difficult to breathe?

Asthma is a condition that makes it difficult for an individual to breathe because the lungs are not functioning as well as they should. The fundamental problem is inflammation of the lining of air passages in the lungs that makes it more difficult for air to move into and out of the lungs. Long-term inflammation sets the stage for other reactions that make air passages even smaller.

In a healthy lung, air can move freely through air passages called bronchi and bronchioles.

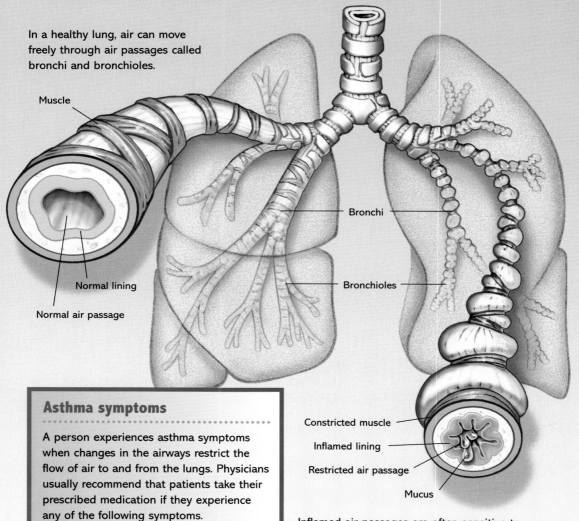

Muscle

Normal lining

Normal air passage

Bronchi

Bronchioles

Constricted muscle

Inflamed lining

Restricted air passage

Mucus

Asthma symptoms

A person experiences asthma symptoms when changes in the airways restrict the flow of air to and from the lungs. Physicians usually recommend that patients take their prescribed medication if they experience any of the following symptoms.

- Wheezing (whistling or hissing noise during exhalation)
- Breathlessness
- Coughing
- Tightness in the chest

Inflamed air passages are often sensitive to irritants or allergy-causing agents that can prompt muscles to constrict, certain cells to produce an excess of mucus, and inflammation to increase. The restricted air passages make it difficult for the person to inhale and exhale adequate amounts of air. The appearance of such events is referred to as an asthma attack or episode.

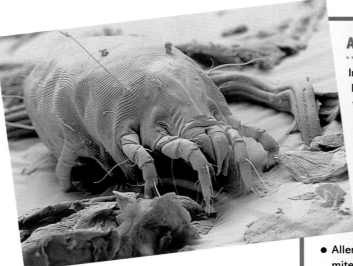

ies against harmless substances in the environment, such as dust mite feces, molds, pollen, and animal *dander* (shed skin particles). When the antibodies encounter the allergens, other specialized cells are prompted to release chemicals called mediators. One such mediator is called histamine, which causes the typical allergic reactions such as nasal congestion and sneezing. Histamine can also cause swelling of airway tissues and excessive amounts of mucus. Another group of mediators called leukotrienes can cause bronchoconstriction and swelling of the airway lining.

People who spend time outdoors and have allergy symptoms that worsen at certain times of the year are most likely allergic to pollen from trees (in early spring), grasses (particularly in late spring), and weeds (in late summer and autumn). Spores from both outdoor and indoor molds can also be allergenic.

The home can be a virtual minefield of asthma-triggering allergens. These include the dander, urine, feces, and saliva of cats, dogs, birds, small rodents, and other pets; feathers in pillows, comforters, sleeping bags, and outdoor clothing; and the feces from microscopic mites found in house dust and dust in bed mattresses, pillows, bed covers, upholstered furniture, carpets, and stuffed toys.

In America's inner cities, cockroaches are an especially important source of allergens. In 1997, researchers led by allergist David L. Rosenstreich of Albert Einstein College of Medicine in New York City published results of their study of children in eight inner-city neighborhoods. The researchers found that children with asthma who were allergic to cockroaches and lived in roach-infested homes

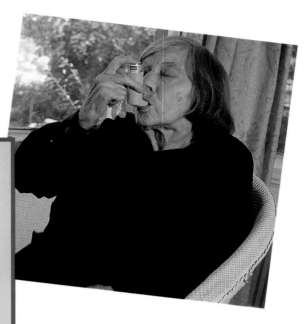

A woman, *right,* uses a metered-dose inhaler, a device that delivers certain kinds of asthma medication directly to the lungs. Doctors must educate patients on the proper technique for using inhalers.

Asthma medications

There are two general classes of asthma medications, those that provide long-term control of asthma and those that provide short-term relief from symptoms during an asthma attack.

Long-term medications

- Anti-inflammatory agents, which include corticosteroids, prevent or reduce inflammation in air passages and make them less sensitive to asthma triggers.

- Long-acting beta-agonists or bronchodilators relax the muscles around air passages to prevent or reverse the narrowing of the passages.

- Antileukotrienes interfere with an immune-system response to prevent inflammation and muscle constriction.

Short-term relief medications

- Short-acting beta-agonists act quickly to relax muscles around air passages.

- Anticholinergics interfere with a nervous-system response to relax the muscles around air passages.

- Corticosteroids may be used with other short-acting medications to reduce inflammation and mucus production.

were hospitalized three times more often and missed more days of school than the other children with the disease. Rosenstreich's team concluded that the combination of cockroach allergy and the children's exposure to high levels of roach allergen may be a key factor in explaining why so many inner-city children have asthma-related health problems and higher than average asthma-related death rates.

Other asthma triggers

Not all asthma episodes, however, are triggered by allergens. Any substance that can irritate oversensitive airways is a potential asthma trigger. The most common indoor irritant is tobacco smoke, which can irritate the airways of both smokers and nonsmokers who breathe secondhand smoke. Other common airborne irritants include pollutants such as *ozone,* a form of oxygen that can be created by the interaction of auto exhaust with sunlight; smoke from wood-burning stoves and fireplaces; household cleaners; hair spray and other aerosols; and strong odors, including perfumes. In the workplace, industrial vapors and airborne particles can irritate the lungs and trigger an asthma episode in some people.

Foods that contain sulfites—compounds sometimes used as preservatives in shrimp, dried fruit, processed potatoes, beer, and wine—can trigger asthmatic symptoms. And people who handle foodstuffs such as flour, coffee, and soybeans in the workplace often inhale food particles, which may provoke an adverse reaction. "Baker's asthma," for example, is an occupational hazard among people who are constantly exposed to flour on the job.

Viral infections of the respiratory system—the common cold, influenza, or sinus infections—are known to inflame and irritate the airways, leaving the person with asthma more vulnerable. A condition known as gastroesophageal reflux (commonly called heartburn) can also trigger symptoms. In this condition, the muscle that acts as a valve between the stomach and the *esophagus* (the passage connecting the mouth and stomach) does not work properly, allowing the acidic contents of the stomach to flow back into the esophagus. Studies suggest that over time, stomach acids can irritate and erode the esophagus, increasing the sensitivity of nerve endings. Eventually, refluxed acids can trigger a chain reaction in the esophagus that irritates the airways, which are in close proximity to the esophagus.

People can also have adverse reactions to aspirin and other pain relievers, such as ibuprofen. Such reactions can trigger an asthma attack or make one more severe—even deadly. Some beta-blocker drugs, which are used to treat such conditions as heart disorders and glaucoma, can also worsen asthma symptoms.

Even physical exercise can induce asthma symptoms. The rapid exchange of air during exercise tends to cool and dry the air passages, which can release mediators that trigger asthma symptoms. Similarly, emotional stress can trigger or aggravate asthma. If a person is crying, shouting, or feeling anxious, the irregular breathing can irritate sensitive passages much as exercise would. It is important to note, however, that while emotional stress can make asthma worse, asthma is a medical condition, not a psychological problem.

Some women with asthma are more likely to have a worsening of symptoms just before and during their monthly periods, which suggests that hormones may play a role in aggravating asthma. Additional evidence that hormones can be a factor in asthma was provided in June 1998 by medical statistician Andrea Venn and her colleagues at the City Hospital in Nottingham, England. They found that

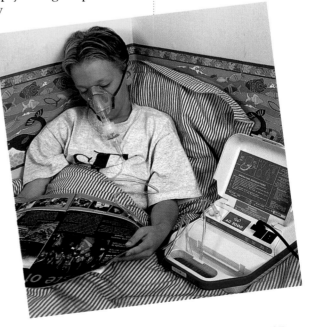

A boy, *right,* inhales asthma medication using a nebulizer, a device that delivers medicine in the form of a mist. A doctor may prescribe a nebulizer for a patient who has difficulty using other inhaling devices.

while boys were more likely than girls to experience asthma symptoms until about age 12, after that age, when most girls begin to get menstrual periods, the prevalence of asthma among girls increases.

Who is at risk for developing asthma?

There are several factors that put an individual at greater risk of developing asthma. Although the disease can develop at any age, new cases of asthma, according to the CDC, occur most frequently among children under the age of five. About one in four children with asthma becomes free of symptoms from adolescence onward, when their airways reach adult size.

Asthma tends to run in families, particularly in those with allergy-related conditions such as hay fever. People whose parents have asthma are much more likely to develop the condition themselves. Asthma specialists believe, therefore, that the condition has a genetic component, and scientists are avidly seeking to identify genes that play a role in asthma. In the 1990's, for example, researchers were studying the inhabitants of the remote island of Tristan da Cunha in the South Atlantic; at least one-third of them have asthma. Scientists hoped this study and others like it would narrow the search for genes that may increase the likelihood that a person will become an asthma sufferer.

Researchers have also noted that asthma prevalence varies considerably by race. In the United States, researchers have found asthma rates are higher in African Americans and Hispanics than in whites. Among other groups, such as certain Native American tribes, asthma is comparatively rare. Several studies have also indicated that asthma is more severe in minority populations living in America's inner cities. These findings have been attributed to several factors, including genetic susceptibility, high exposure to allergens in substandard housing, and inadequate access to regular, high-quality health care.

Being overweight may also increase a person's risk of developing asthma. In April 1998, a research team led by asthma specialist Carlos Camargo, Jr., of Harvard Medical School in Boston reported their analysis of data from a study of 89,061 nurses between the ages of 27 and 44. Between 1991 and 1995, the number of nurses who developed asthma was 1,652. After controlling for factors such as age, race, smoking, diet, and physical activity, the investigators found that women who were obese were three times more likely to develop asthma. The study did not demonstrate how obesity led to asthma, but Camargo suggested that extra weight might compress airways, making them more likely to react to asthma triggers.

Treating asthma

In 1997, an expert panel convened by the National Asthma Education and Prevention Program (NAEPP) unveiled new guidelines to help physicians and their patients formulate a treatment plan for managing asthma. (The NAEPP is a division of the National Heart, Lung, and Blood Institute in Bethesda, Maryland.) The guidelines stressed the importance of having both patients and physicians understand the role of inflammation in asthma and the need to actively treat inflammation as well as relieve symptoms during an asthma episode.

The NAEPP guidelines describe a diagnostic process for physicians to confirm whether a patient's breathing problems are due to asthma. Typically, the doctor will ask about whether the patient has asthmalike symptoms that occur in episodes, when and where such episodes occur, whether symptoms are worse under certain circumstances (such as during exercise or when a dog or cat is around), and whether other relatives have asthma or allergies. The physician will listen with a stethoscope for sounds of wheezing and look for other clues consistent with asthma, such as *eczema*, skin inflammation caused by allergies. Finally, physicians can learn about the presence and severity of airway obstruction by using a device called a spirometer, which measures the volume and rate at which air is exhaled.

Once the asthma diagnosis is established, the physician will talk with the patient about such factors as asthma triggers and the patient's lifestyle, and then formulate a treatment plan. Because asthma symptoms can improve or worsen, the NAEPP guidelines note that follow-up visits every one to six months are essential for monitoring a patient's condition and, if necessary, modifying treatment.

A man, *below,* uses a device called a peak flow meter, which measures how much air he can quickly blow out after filling his lungs with air. The reading of this test indicates how well the lungs are functioning. A physician will often recommend that a patient take a daily measurement of his or her peak flow rate and keep a record of results. This information can help the physician determine if the individual needs to make any changes in medication. Also, doctors and patients may devise an action plan, *below left,* that lets the patient know what medications to take or when to seek help.

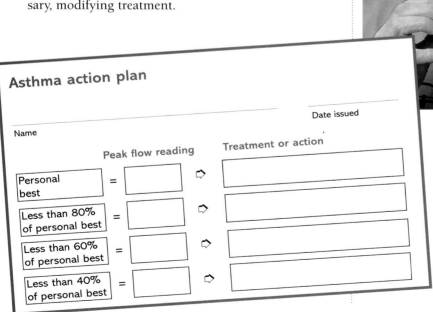

Asthma action plan

		Date issued
Name		

	Peak flow reading		Treatment or action
Personal best	=	⇨	
Less than 80% of personal best	=	⇨	
Less than 60% of personal best	=	⇨	
Less than 40% of personal best	=	⇨	

Source: *Asthma Management and Prevention: A Practical Guide for Public Health Officials and Health Care Professionals,* National Institutes of Health.

Patients are also advised to monitor their symptoms with the use of a hand-held device called a peak flow meter, which measures how quickly an individual can force air out of fully inflated lungs. Working with his or her physician, the patient determines a "personal best" peak flow rate. Then, by taking daily readings, the patient can monitor how well the lungs are working and detect early warnings of airway obstruction even before symptoms appear. In most treatment plans, the physician indicates to the patient what medications to take when a peak flow rate drops to a certain percentage of the personal best. The peak flow meter can also help the patient determine if certain medications are adequately treating the symptoms during an episode.

Asthma medications

There are two main types of asthma medications that doctors may prescribe: those aimed at providing long-term control of persistent asthma and those that provide rapid relief during a flare-up of symptoms. In general, asthma drugs are either inhaled using a device which delivers the medicine directly to the lungs or taken orally in pill or liquid form. In an emergency, however, some medications are administered by injection.

The three basic groups of long-term controller medications are anti-inflammatory agents, long-acting bronchodilators, and antileukotrienes or leukotriene modifiers. Doctors usually prescribe these drugs in various combinations and doses, depending on such factors as the patient's age, asthma severity, and side effects. The goal is to use the least medication necessary to maintain control of asthma symptoms and to reduce the patient's dependence on the medications that only provide rapid relief.

Inhaled anti-inflammatory agents—such as cromolyn sodium, nedocromil sodium, and corticosteroids—are usually taken on a daily basis to prevent or reduce airway inflammation and make the airways less sensitive to triggers. (Corticosteroids, often called steroids, are different from anabolic steroids, the muscle-building drugs that have been abused by some body builders and athletes.)

Long-acting bronchodilators relax the muscles around the airways to reverse or prevent airway narrowing. Physicians usually prescribe this medication in addition to inhaled anti-inflammatory drugs. These drugs include some members of a family of drugs called beta-agonists as well as a drug called theophylline.

In the late 1990's, the third class of long-lasting controller asthma medications, the antileukotrienes, became available. These drugs, which are taken in tablet form, prevent and reduce airway swelling and the constriction of airway muscles.

While these drugs are useful in long-term asthma control, they are not appropriate for providing rapid relief for symptoms during an asthma episode. Quick-relief medications, including inhaled short-acting beta-agonists and corticosteroids (in pill or liquid

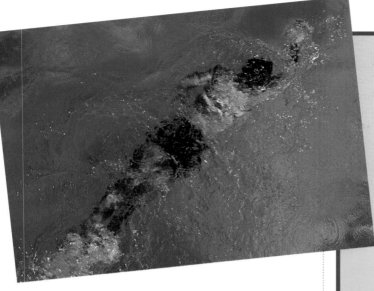

form), are taken if symptoms begin to increase or the patient's peak flow readings begin to fall. Sometimes a physician will also prescribe these medications to be taken just before exercise to prevent exercise-related asthma symptoms.

Inhaled short-acting beta-agonists, like their long-acting counterparts, relax the muscles around the airways to widen constricted airways, easing breathing difficulties. Unlike long-acting beta-agonists, however, these medications start to work within 5 to 15 minutes and last for 4 to 6 hours. Asthma experts warn, however, that patients should not use beta-agonists more often than prescribed without checking with the doctor. Such overuse indicates poor asthma control. It can also be dangerous because the temporary relief these medications offer may delay a patient from seeking help for a severe, life-threatening asthma attack.

When an asthma attack is underway and inhaled short-acting beta-agonists fail to provide enough relief, an inhaled anticholinergic drug, such as ipratroprium bromide, may be added to help reverse symptoms. Anticholinergic drugs may also be used as an alternative for short-acting beta-agonists in patients with asthma who have a lung disease such as emphysema, people who smoke, or individuals who have a lingering cough after a respiratory infection.

Other asthma management strategies

Developing a strategy for managing stress and anxiety, which can worsen or even trigger an asthma episode, is another useful component of an asthma treatment plan. Coping with the disease itself can make people feel anxious. Counseling can help people with asthma learn how to deal with stress and anxiety—asthma-related and not. Research suggests that muscle relaxation exercises—such as tensing and relaxing all of the body's major muscle groups—may blunt the intensity of an asthma attack. Ongoing research at the Center for Complementary and Alternative Medicine Research in Asthma at the University of California at Davis and other institu-

Creating a healthy bedroom

A bedroom can be a haven for *allergens* (allergy-causing agents) and irritants that can trigger asthma attacks for many people. The problem bedroom, *left,* has many features that make it difficult to reduce the levels of triggers, such as dust and dust mites. The healthier bedroom, *right,* is designed to control asthma triggers and allow an individual to breathe more easily.

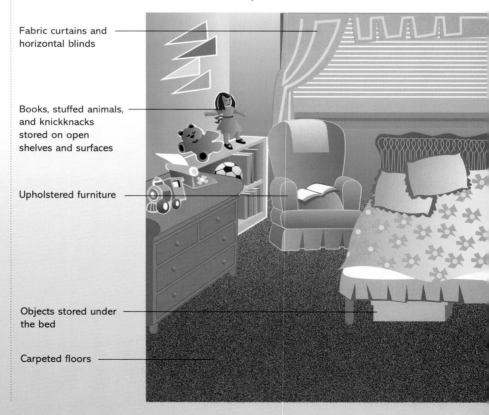

Fabric curtains and horizontal blinds

Books, stuffed animals, and knickknacks stored on open shelves and surfaces

Upholstered furniture

Objects stored under the bed

Carpeted floors

tions has suggested that biofeedback, a technique that teaches an individual how to control physical responses such as heart rate and muscle tension, may be helpful in controlling the emotional responses that can aggravate asthma.

Educational and support groups for people with asthma (as well as for the parents of children with asthma) also play a useful role in helping people cope with the stress, anxiety, and frustration of living with the condition. In addition, such groups can provide a network for learning about the disorder and advances in asthma treatment.

Another key component of asthma treatment is targeting triggers in order to prevent the fuse for an asthma attack from being ignited. Preventive measures include reducing exposure to allergens, getting an annual flu shot, and learning how to prevent exercise-induced flare-ups. If it is not clear what factors are triggering symptoms, a doctor may perform a simple skin test to identify offending allergens. Once the culprits have been identified, patients and their families can take steps to reduce or eliminate exposure to them.

If an asthma sufferer is sensitive to allergens he or she encounters at home, experts recommend minimizing these triggers to help keep symptoms at bay. If pets are a cause of asthma flare-ups, removing the animal from the home is the best strategy. If this is not accept-

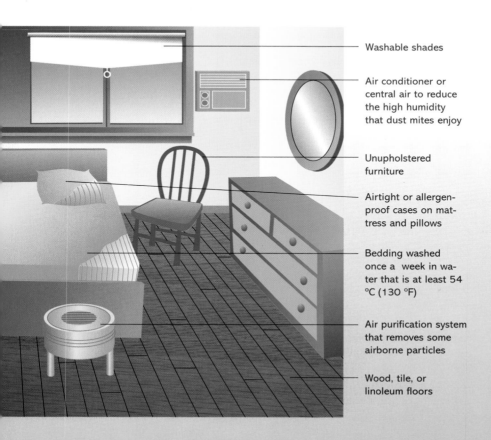

Washable shades

Air conditioner or central air to reduce the high humidity that dust mites enjoy

Unupholstered furniture

Airtight or allergen-proof cases on mattress and pillows

Bedding washed once a week in water that is at least 54 °C (130 °F)

Air purification system that removes some airborne particles

Wood, tile, or linoleum floors

Managing asthma at school

Successful asthma management depends a great deal on the individual with asthma knowing when and how to take medication and what asthma triggers to avoid. Parents can help their children who have asthma by working with school personnel to develop an asthma management plan. Most physicians recommend that parents address the following issues:

- Notify teachers, school health care professionals, and administrators of the child's asthma and need to take medication.
- Create a list of possible asthma triggers for the child, such as exercise, animal dander, or fumes from laboratory chemicals.
- Provide a list of the child's asthma medications.
- Write a description of the child's treatment program and recommendations for how school personnel can assist with the program.
- Provide a list of asthma symptoms.
- Create an emergency action plan that includes the physician's phone number.
- Ask physician to approve the entire management plan.

Source: *Asthma & Physical Activity in the School: Making a Difference*, National Asthma Education and Prevention Program.

able, the animal should be kept away from rooms the person with asthma uses most often, such as the bedroom. For people who are sensitive to cockroaches or dust mites, efforts should be made to eliminate or reduce their numbers. Dust-mite allergen control includes removing carpets; laundering bedding in hot water once a week; replacing curtains with shades; encasing mattresses, pillows, and upholstery in mite-proof coverings; giving away stuffed toys; and frequently dusting and vacuuming (preferably by someone other than the asthma sufferer). Reducing humidity with air conditioning units and dehumidifiers also can reduce the level of dust mites, mold, and fungi.

Some physicians may recommend immunotherapy—allergy shots—to try to reduce a patient's response to allergens. This treatment involves a series of injections of tiny doses of an allergen extract, typically given over a period of three to five years, with the aim of "educating" the immune system to tolerate the allergen. The NAEPP guidelines advise that immunotherapy, administered by an allergist, may be considered when there is a clear link between asthma symptoms and exposure to an allergen that the patient cannot avoid.

Other indoor triggers to be avoided include irritants such as tobacco smoke, improperly vented furnaces and stoves, and household sprays and polishes. Doctors strongly advise people with asthma not to smoke and warn parents of children with asthma to keep their children away from tobacco smoke. Similarly, people with sensitivities to outdoor allergens and irritants should avoid these triggers as much as possible, keeping windows closed and avoiding such activities as jogging or camping during pollen season or when air pollution levels are high.

Studies suggest that regular exercise also may help reduce the frequency and severity of asthma episodes. However, since exercise itself can be an asthma trigger, doctors advise patients to take precautions, such as wearing a scarf or mask over the nose and mouth on cold days. Proper warm-up for 10 to 15 minutes before vigorous exercise can reduce symptom flare-ups, and doctors can prescribe some preventive medication to be taken before working out.

Asthma experts stress that patients and their doctors should work together as partners to develop a personalized asthma action plan—a set of guidelines to help the individual avoid triggers, recognize warning signs of an attack, and use asthma medications properly. Following such a plan takes commitment, but for the majority of asthma sufferers, the reward can be an essentially normal life. That's the way Alicia, the teen-age athlete, views living with asthma. Following her own asthma action plan makes it possible for her to envision a life with few limitations.

"I can do anything a normal kid can do," she says.   •••

For further information:
Books and periodicals

Adams, Francis V. *The Asthma Sourcebook: Everything You Need to Know.* Lowell House, 1998.

The American Lung Association Family Guide to Asthma and Allergies. Little, Brown, and Co., 1997.

Perry, Angela R., Ed. *Essential Guide to Asthma.* American Medical Association/Pocket Books, 1998.

Asthma Magazine. This magazine is published for people with asthma. For subscription information, call 800-527-3284.

Web sites and phone numbers

Allergy and Asthma Network/Mothers of Asthmatics, Inc.: http://www.aanma.org; 800-878-4403 or 703-641-9595.

American College of Allergy, Asthma & Immunology: http://allergy.mcg.edu; 800-822-2762.

American Lung Association: http://www.lungusa.org; 800-LUNG-USA.

National Asthma Education and Prevention Program: http://www.nhlbi.nih.gov/nhlbi/othcomp/opec/naepp/naeppage.htm; 301-251-1222.

National Jewish Medical and Research Center: http://www.njc.org; 800-222-LUNG (The toll-free "Lung Line" is staffed by registered nurses who can answer questions about asthma and send literature to callers.)

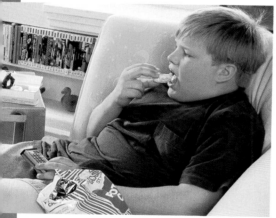

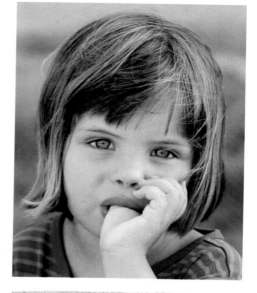

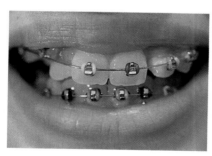

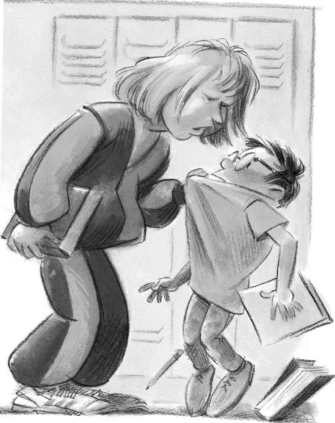

A Healthy Family

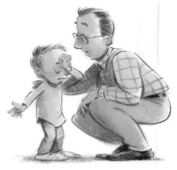

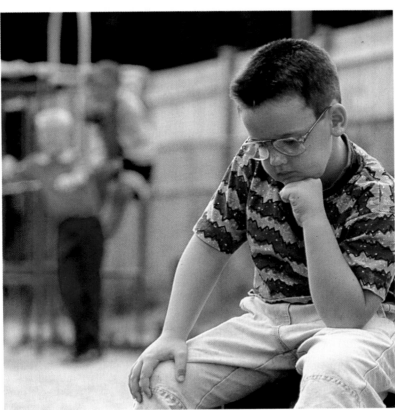

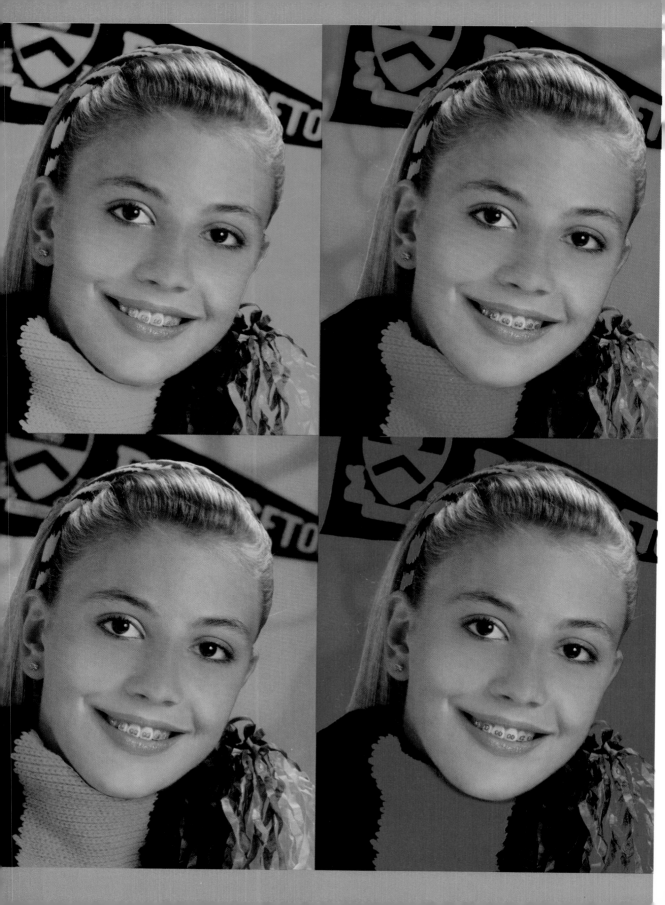

Today's high-tech braces are more comfortable, efficient, and attractive— and not just for teen-agers.

A New Look for
Braces

By Christie Waddell

THE WORD "BRACES" USED TO CONJURE UP IMAGES of teen-aged teeth encased in bulky, heavy-metal hardware; painful sessions at the orthodontist's office; and taunting with nick-names such as "metal mouth," "tin grin," and "tinsel teeth." Moreover, few adults whose teeth made them self-conscious about their smile could imagine themselves sporting braces, no matter how much an improved appearance might boost their self-esteem.

By 1999, however, advances in *orthodontics* (the branch of dentistry dealing with straightening and repositioning the teeth and reshaping and expanding the jaws using pressure) had resulted in a new image for braces and the people who wear them. New materials and new treatment strategies made braces and other orthodontic appliances more comfortable, more attractive, and—most important of all—more efficient.

One of the most significant changes involved the age at which patients were undergoing orthodontic treatment. What was once considered a rite of passage for adolescents was by 1999 a popular option for children as young as 7 or 8. Many orthodontists argued that early treatment could spare children and their parents the need for more complicated, painful, and expensive dental treatment later on.

In addition, increasing numbers of people in middle age and even their senior years were gaining a new appreciation for orthodontics. According to the American Association of Orthodontists (AAO), about 1 million of the 4.4 million Americans wearing braces in 1999 were adults, double the number in the late 1980's.

An improved appearance is probably the most common reason for having teeth straightened. But orthodontic treatment also offers health benefits. For example, straight teeth are easier to clean than crooked teeth. In addition, correcting misaligned teeth and jaws can correct chewing difficulties, unnatural wear on the teeth, and painful strain on the joint that acts as a hinge between the upper and lower jaws.

Orthodontic treatment also may offer psychological benefits, according to the AAO. An even smile can make people feel more confident about their appearance. As a result, people who have their teeth straightened often feel more comfortable in social situations and may even perform better at school and on the job.

The flexible jawbone

Although jawbones appear to be rock solid, they are actually spongy and relatively flexible, especially when children are growing. Like the rest of the skeleton, jawbones grow throughout childhood. Children also experience several bursts of jawbone growth. These occur at age 4; at age 6, when the *deciduous* (baby) teeth begin to fall out and are replaced by the permanent teeth; and in early adolescence. The growth and eruption of the permanent teeth, especially the molars, also work to expand the jawbones.

Once the jawbones quit growing at about age 13, they become more dense and teeth can be moved less easily. That is why orthodontic treatment for young children may be easier than for adolescents and why adults usually must wear braces for relatively longer periods than do children.

The pressure applied by orthodontic appliances actually stimulates a process of jawbone destruction and growth. The force of the appliances pushes the roots of a tooth being moved against nearby bone. This causes special bone cells responsible for *resorbing* (dissolving) bone to hollow out a space for the incoming roots. As this space grows larger, the roots can move along. At the same time, bone cells responsible for creating new bone fill in the space left behind by the moving roots.

Why teeth don't meet

In general, human teeth do not fit comfortably in the human mouth. One reason is human evolution. Over the past several million years, both human jawbones and teeth have grown smaller. However, jawbones have shrunk faster than teeth. The result is a general tendency to dental overcrowding. As permanent teeth come in, the roots of

The author:

Christie Waddell is a free-lance medical writer.

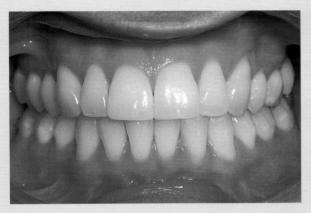

The good, the crowded, and the misaligned
··

In a normal bite, the upper front teeth slightly overlap the lower front teeth, and the molars line up and meet on both sides of the mouth. The teeth are straight, properly aligned in the mouth, and spaced slightly apart. Teeth that are *maloccluded* (fail to meet properly during a bite) fall into three main categories: crowding, overbite, and underbite.

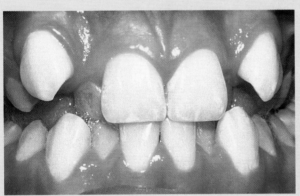

In crowding, the most common form of malocclusion, the upper and lower jaws come together properly but the teeth do not, usually because they are jammed together in the jawbones.

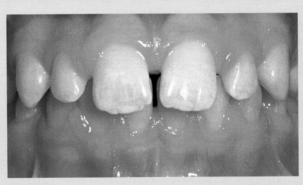

In overbite, the top teeth extend farther forward than normal in relation to the lower teeth. Serious cases of overbite are sometimes called buck teeth.

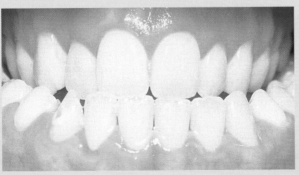

In underbite, a larger lower jaw closes in front of a smaller upper jaw, often creating a jutting jaw and chin. Underbite, among the most difficult of all dental problems to treat, may cause discomfort, chewing problems, and difficulty in talking.

teeth that have already erupted frequently take up more than their fair share of space, forcing the teeth that follow out of their proper position.

Heredity is also to blame for misaligned teeth and jaws. We are all at the mercy of our ancestors' genes when it comes to the size and shape of our jaws and teeth. Parents pass along genes for larger-than-normal teeth that further cramp an already overcrowded mouth, smaller-than-normal teeth that drift because of a lack of support from neighboring teeth, and jaws that do not grow large enough to accommodate the wisdom teeth. Inheriting a combination of these conditions from one's parents complicates the misalignment problem even more.

Behavior also may play a role in creating an uneven smile. For example, sucking on the fingers, especially the thumb, can push the upper teeth outward and the lower teeth inward, if children continue this behavior past the age of 5 or 6. The pressure from finger sucking also may push the jaws out of alignment.

Causes of malocclusion

Malocclusion is the medical term for the failure of the teeth of the upper and lower jaws to meet properly when a person takes a bite. Possible causes for this condition include:

- lack of adequate space in the mouth so that teeth are crowded;
- too much space in the mouth so that teeth shift from their correct position;
- a genetic tendency to crooked teeth or misaligned jaws;
- thumb-sucking;
- tongue-thrusting (pushing the tongue against the front teeth when swallowing);
- poor care of primary teeth;
- larger-than-normal teeth; and
- smaller-than-normal teeth.

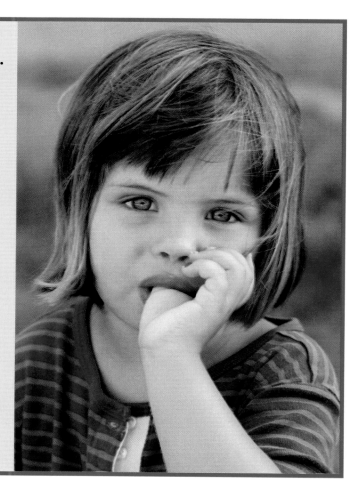

A behavior called *tongue-thrusting,* which often occurs in children who breathe through their mouth, also can affect a child's bite. Tongue-thrusting involves pushing the tongue against the front teeth while swallowing. This problem can be difficult to correct because it usually becomes an unconscious habit.

Finally, poor dental care may contribute to misaligned teeth in both children and adults. Dental experts stress that the proper care of the deciduous teeth improves the chances that the permanent teeth as well as the gums and jawbone will develop properly. For example, if a baby tooth falls out too soon because of decay or trauma, nearby teeth may move into the vacant space. As a result, the permanent tooth for that space may not be able to erupt properly. Similarly, the loss of a permanent tooth also may cause neighboring teeth to become misaligned.

Bad bites

Malocclusion is the medical term for the failure of the teeth of the upper and lower jaws to meet properly when a person bites. In a normal bite, the upper front teeth slightly overlap the lower front teeth, and the molars line up and meet on both sides of the mouth. The teeth are straight, properly aligned in the mouth, and spaced just enough apart for dental floss to fit easily between them.

There are three main types of malocclusion: Class I, often known as *crowding;* Class II, known as *overbite,* and Class III, known as *underbite.*

Class I malocclusions are the most common form of misalignment. In a Class I malocclusion, the upper and lower jaws meet properly but the teeth do not because they are spaced too far apart or, more often, are crowded together.

When a person with crowding bites down, the lower first molars end up slightly forward of the upper first molars. The upper jaw sits directly above the lower jaw and the lower front teeth rest against the backs of the upper teeth. Crowding may cause teeth to "turn" in their sockets or to flare out of the jaw.

In Class II malocclusions, the top teeth extend farther forward than normal in relation to the lower teeth, usually because the upper jawbone is larger than the lower jawbone. Serious cases of overbite are sometimes called buck teeth.

In Class III malocclusions, a larger lower jaw extends in front of a smaller upper jaw, often creating a jutting jaw and chin. In relatively

Early treatment needed?

The American Association of Orthodontists lists the following conditions that may signal the need for an orthodontic examination by age 7:

- crowded, misplaced, or blocked-out teeth
- protruding teeth
- early or late loss of teeth
- difficulty chewing or breathing
- mouth breathing
- thumb-sucking
- jaws that shift or make sounds
- speech difficulties
- grinding or clenching of teeth
- facial imbalance
- biting the cheek or roof of the mouth while eating
- teeth that meet abnormally or do not meet at all
- a jaw that juts too far forward or recedes too far back

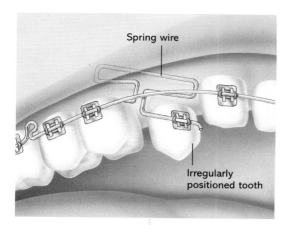
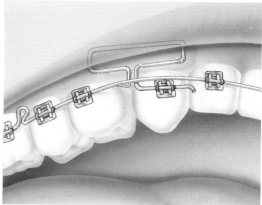

Spring wire

Irregularly
positioned tooth

Braces, the most common device for straightening teeth, consist of a system of brackets, wires, and elastics. Brackets are square platforms that are attached to the surface of the teeth. The brackets have slots to hold the wires (also called archwires), which are gradually tightened to exert pressure on the teeth and which act as guides for their movement. Elastics are rubber bands that connect two teeth or the sides of a jaw to put additional pressure on the teeth and jaws.

Clear plastic brackets, *right*, are one option for orthodontics patients who want their braces to be less noticeable.

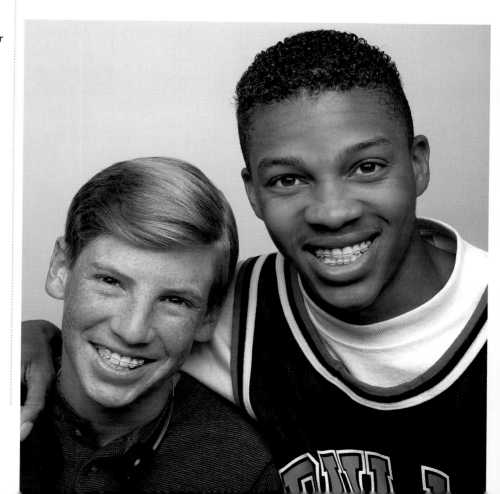

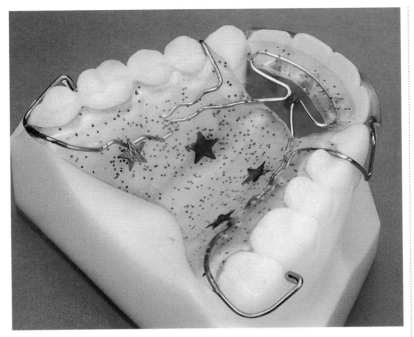

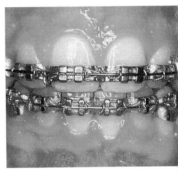

Modern retainers, *left*, come in a variety of colors and may be decorated with designs, images of animals or famous personalities, or even the logo of a patient's favorite sports team. Colorful retainers may encourage patients to wear and care for their appliance properly.

The bulky metal collars formerly used to attach brackets to the teeth, *above*, have been replaced, for the most part, by strong adhesives.

mild cases of underbite, the top front teeth rest on the backs of the lower front teeth. In one type of Class III malocclusion, known as crossbite, however, the upper front teeth actually close behind the lower front teeth. This condition usually causes discomfort, chewing problems, and sometimes difficulty talking. Class III malocclusions are among the most difficult of all dental problems to treat. Patients sometimes must undergo the surgical removal of excess bone in their jawbone so that their lower teeth can be brought into proper alignment.

Effects of a bad bite

Malocclusions may affect a person's physical and psychological health. One of the most common effects is dental disease. When teeth are crooked or twisted out of their correct position, they are more difficult to clean. People with improperly cleaned teeth are more likely to develop cavities and *periodontitis,* a bacterial infection of the gums, which can be painful as well as damaging to teeth, gum tissue, and even the bone of the jaw.

Severe malocclusions, especially severe Class III malocclusions that prevent a person from chewing normally, can affect the digestive process and result in heartburn. In addition, severe malocclusions can make speaking difficult and embarrassing.

People with poorly aligned teeth also are prone to other problems. For example, in cases of serious overbite, the front teeth are not protected by the lips and may be easily chipped or even knocked out

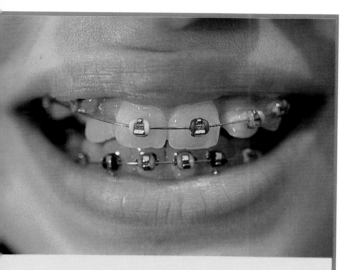

during physical activity.

Malocclusion may also result in the loss of bone in the jaw. The bones of the jaws must be stimulated by chewing to stay healthy. If an individual's teeth are severely out of alignment, parts of the jawbone do not receive the stimulation needed to promote growth, and they begin to resorb. If untreated for a long time, jawbone resorption can eventually cause most of an individual's permanent teeth to weaken and fall out.

Even minor malocclusions often have serious psychological effects. People with misaligned teeth may feel extremely self-conscious in school, social, and professional situations. In such cases, braces can not only improve appearance but also boost self-confidence and self-esteem.

Basics on braces

The most commonly used orthodontic appliances are *braces, headgear, palatal separators,* and *retainers.* Braces consist of a system of brackets, wires (also called archwires), and elastics. Brackets are square, flat platforms that are attached to the surface of the teeth. The brackets have slots to hold the wires, which are gradually tightened to exert pressure on the teeth and which act as guides for their movement. Elastics are removable rubber bands that connect two teeth or the sides of a jaw to put additional pressure on the teeth and jaws.

Headgear is a removable appliance that consists of curved metal rods called a bow and an elastic strap that goes around the back of the head. Both are attached to brackets on metal bands wrapped around the back teeth. Headgear is used to guide the growth of the jawbone as well as the movement of the teeth. It is normally worn along with braces for from 12 to 14 hours daily, including bedtime.

A palatal separator is an orthodontic appliance that spreads the two halves of the roof of the mouth. It is used for people whose upper jaw is much narrower than the lower jaw.

Once these appliances have moved the teeth to their desired posi-

Caring for your braces

- Do not chew gum under any circumstances.
- Cut hard fruits and vegetables, such as carrots and apples, into small pieces to avoid the risk of damaging orthodontic devices.
- Avoid foods with sugar, including most kinds of candy, potato chips, and soda pop. These foods can cause plaque to accumulate on the teeth.
- Avoid crunchy foods like popcorn and nuts that can damage the braces.
- Avoid sticky foods like caramel and candy bars that can loosen brackets and snap wires.
- Avoid hard foods, such as ice, pizza crusts, corn on the cob (slice corn off the cob), barbecued ribs, peaches, and foods with a hard center.
- Always brush after eating.
- Brush immediately after eating sweet foods.

Sources: American Association of Orthodontists; Academy of General Dentistry.

tions, patients usually wear an appliance called a retainer for a period of time. This device, which looks like an athlete's mouth guard, "trains" the teeth and jaw to remain in the correct position.

High-tech changes

Technological innovations in the design and use of orthodontic appliances have brought about many of the changes that have significantly altered modern orthodontic treatment. For example, braces have become lighter and more comfortable. High-tech materials, along with new treatment techniques, also are helping many patients get better results in less time with less pain.

Braces themselves have become streamlined. Brackets are now available in ceramic and clear plastic as well as the traditional stainless steel. Stainless steel brackets are still the most common choice, especially for children, however, because they are the most durable and least expensive of the three types. Ceramics and plastics are more popular among adults, who may be more image-conscious and who are less likely to damage their appliances, by eating forbidden foods, for example.

In the past, brackets were attached to the teeth with bulky metal collars. In the 1990's, strong adhesives allowed orthodontists to bond brackets directly onto the teeth. Metal bands now are generally used only around molars, which are harder to move than front teeth.

Oral fashion

Braces also are a lot more fun than they used to be. Patients can opt for brightly colored wires, elastics, and *ligatures* (the small wires or elastics that hold the wires to the brackets), as well as designs for their retainers, including the logo of their favorite sports team. Although fashionable orthodontic appliances make braces more aesthetically pleasing, they also serve useful functions. They help dispel fear of the experience and encourage cooperation with the orthodontist's directions for caring for the appliances.

Or, instead of flashing their hardware, patients can chose less noticeable options. Among them are clear plastic or tooth-colored brackets. Least noticeable of all are lingual braces, which are attached to the back of the teeth. Although this technique was gaining popularity in the late 1990's, it had several drawbacks. Treatment generally takes longer because lingual braces exert less pressure than do traditional braces. They are also more expensive, frequently irritate the tongue, and are much more difficult to adjust.

Metal with a memory

Orthodontic appointments used to be painful ordeals as orthodontists tightened the steel wires in short bursts, moving the teeth with brute force. Often, patients remained in pain for weeks afterward.

In 1999, this procedure was usually less painful thanks to Nitinol, a nickel-titanium alloy used in wires. Nitinol has been called the "memory metal" because once it is bent into a particular shape then heated and cooled, it will return to that shape no matter how much it is stretched. Within the warm environment of the mouth, the wires, which are stretched to follow the contours of the teeth, gradually return to their original length. In the process, they apply a continuous, more gentle pressure to the teeth.

As a result, many patients need to have their wires tightened only every four weeks instead of the traditional three weeks. Some patients can go even longer. The continual pressure also may result in a shorter treatment time. And because Nitinol is stronger than stainless steel, wires made of this alloy are less likely to break during the tightening process and more likely to withstand everyday wear and tear.

Imaging teeth

Computer imaging has become a common part of the orthodontic evaluation process, especially for adults. Orthodontists still X-ray and make casts of the teeth and visually examine the patient's teeth and jaws.

But in addition, many orthodontists use a special computer program that digitally alters an image of the patient's mouth to give patients a look at how treatment could change the teeth. This information also helps the orthodontist assess the patient's needs. In addition, the "after" images also often encourage patients to wear their headgear and other removable dental appliances and to follow the sometimes inconvenient instructions for keeping their braces undamaged and their teeth clean.

Starting earlier

Years ago, orthodontists generally advised that treatment not begin until most of a child's permanent teeth had erupted. Now, many orthodontists feel that beginning treatment at a younger age can produce great benefits.

The AAO encourages parents to schedule a child's first orthodontic appointment around the age of 7, even before the child has lost all of his or her baby teeth. Orthodontists now believe that misaligned jawbones can cause more serious problems for growing children than crooked teeth do. If treatment begins early enough, orthodontics can encourage the expansion of the jaws. In many cases, diagnosing malocclusions and installing appliances between the ages of 7 and 9, when children's jaws are growing the fastest, can reduce the amount of time spent in braces or prevent crowding of the permanent teeth altogether.

Treatment at an early age also may be less painful—and less expensive—than in older children because teeth need not be moved as far as they would in adolescence. However, dental experts warn, even with early treatment, patients may have to wear braces during the teen years if their teeth drift back toward their original positions.

Starting later

Perhaps the biggest change in orthodontics is the number of adults pursuing a more appealing smile. Propelled by the availability of less conspicuous braces and a new acceptance of braces for adults, increasing numbers of the *baby boom generation* (people born between 1945 and 1964) are seeking orthodontic treatment. In addition to improving their oral health, many adults who get braces report doing it for the increased self-confidence that a better appearance gives them. For many people, crooked teeth are an embarrassing impediment to performing at their best at work and relaxing in social situations. Adults may also be encouraged by the fact that many dental plans cover the cost of orthodontic work, putting less of a strain on the family budget.

Orthodontic treatment is often uncomfortable, inconvenient, expensive, and time-consuming. But even for those with minor malocclusions, the payback in healthier teeth and gums and an improved self-image may be worth the effort.   ●●●

For additional information:

Books
Understanding Orthodontics. Quintessence Publishing, 1997.
The Columbia University School of Dental and Oral Surgery's Guide to Family Dental Care. W. W. Norton & Co., 1997.

Web sites
American Association of Orthodontists—www.aaortho.org

Preventing and Treating Childhood Obesity

Small changes in diet and exercise
habits over time can help obese children
achieve and maintain a healthy weight.

By Pamela Livingston

AFTER SCHOOL, ANDREA, LIKE MANY OF HER SIXTH-GRADE classmates, grabs a snack then checks out a few of her favorite television shows. After dinner, which often consists of take-out or convenience foods, she watches more television or does some homework. Before going to bed, her parents reward her for doing her homework or for cleaning her plate with a big bowl of ice cream.

Andrea gets good grades, gets along well with her parents, and has several close friends. But she is neither happy nor healthy. Andrea suffers from straining mental and physical hardships caused by obesity. Other kids at school tease her about her appearance. She is always picked last for sports teams. She has difficulty finding clothes she likes to wear. Worst of all, she feels ugly and defeated.

Andrea's mother, who is also overweight, tells her daughter that she has "inherited" obesity and will just have to accept it. But Andrea's mother is wrong. According to child health experts, small changes in the daily diet and exercise habits of obese children, continued over time, can have a profound impact on their weight and, ultimately, their physical and emotional well-being.

Andrea is not alone. Obesity now affects 20 percent of U.S. children, according to the National Center for Health Statistics (NCHS), a U.S. government agency. In 1997, the NCHS reported that since the 1970's, obesity among U.S. children ages 6 to 11 has climbed by 54 percent, while obesity among adolescents has risen by 39 percent. And in a March 1998 report, the American Academy of Pediatrics (AAP) ranked obesity first of all nutritional diseases affecting children and adolescents in the United States and predicted that the current generation of children will grow into the most obese generation of adults in U.S. history.

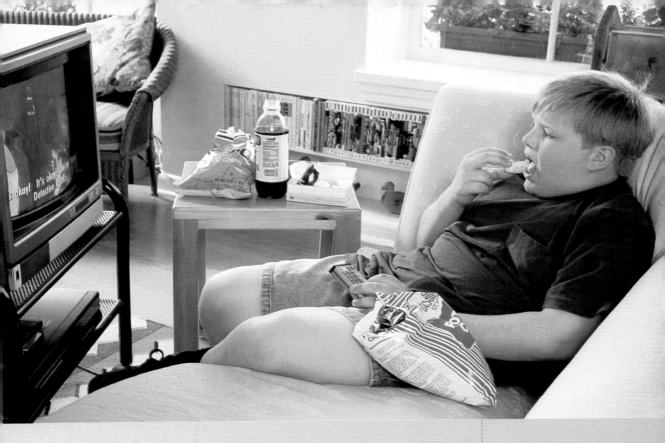

Defining childhood obesity

Obesity occurs when a person takes in more calories in the form of food than he or she burns for energy. Obesity can be calculated in several ways. Many pediatricians use a growth chart, which compares a child's height and weight with those of other children of his or her age. In general, children who are at least 20 percent or more above the average weight for their height are considered obese.

A newer, increasingly popular system for measuring weight is the body mass index, or BMI. BMI is calculated by dividing a person's weight in kilograms by his or her height in meters squared. Children with a BMI at or exceeding the 95th percentile for those of the same age and sex are considered overweight, according to the NCHS's third National Health and Nutritional Examination Survey, conducted from 1988 to 1994. Experts caution, however, that because children normally grow in unpredictable spurts, parents should rely on their pediatrician for a diagnosis of obesity in a child.

Why obesity is increasing among children

Most health experts believe childhood obesity is the result of a combination of genetic, environmental, and psychological factors. (In rare cases, illness or drugs used to treat illness may cause weight

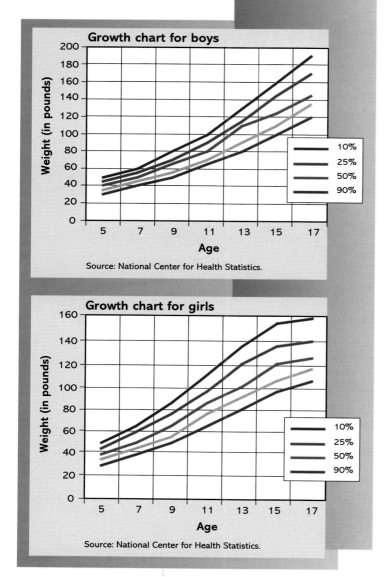

Growth chart for boys

Weight (in pounds)

200
180
160
140
120
100
80
60
40
20
0

Age

5 7 9 11 13 15 17

10%
25%
50%
90%

Source: National Center for Health Statistics.

Growth chart for girls

Weight (in pounds)

160
140
120
100
80
60
40
20
0

Age

5 7 9 11 13 15 17

10%
25%
50%
90%

Source: National Center for Health Statistics.

Measuring size

Growth charts, *left*, compare a child's weight and height to the average weight and height of others of his or her age and gender. Here, rankings are indicated by percentages. For example, 90 percent of boys age 11 weigh more than 65 pounds, while only 10 percent weigh more than 100 pounds. Among 11-year-old girls, 90 percent weigh more than 65 pounds, while only 10 percent weigh more than 110 pounds. In general, children who are at least 20 percent or more above the average weight for their height are considered obese.

The author:

Pamela Livingston is a free-lance medical writer.

gain.) For example, numerous studies have shown that children with at least one obese parent have the greatest risk of becoming obese themselves. However, researchers are still unclear to what extent genetics predetermines obesity, and certainly not all children with obese parents grow up to be obese adults.

Environmental factors that contribute to childhood obesity include activity level, diet, and eating habits. Emotional factors also play a role. Many people, including children, eat in response to negative emotions, such as boredom, sadness, or anger. Most child health experts attribute the jump in childhood obesity since 1980 to two environmental factors: the rise in the consumption of high-fat foods and the decline in leisure- and work-related exercise.

During the first few years of life, children gain fat rapidly—faster, in fact, than they do muscle. As the rate of fat storage increases, so too does the number of fat cells. According to the Mayo Clinic in Rochester, Minnesota, obese children may have three times the number of fat cells as do children of normal weight. Children who become obese before age 6 have a 50 percent likelihood of remaining obese in adulthood. Among obese adolescents, the likelihood rises to 70 to 80 percent. After adolescence, the number of fat cells remains almost constant throughout life.

Lack of adequate physical activity may play a greater role in childhood obesity than eating lots of high-calorie or high-fat foods, however. According to a 1996 report by the U.S. Surgeon General, nearly half of young people ages 12 to 21 are not vigorously active.

A study of more than 4,000 children ages 8 to 16 by a researcher at Johns Hopkins University School of Medicine in Baltimore, Maryland, showed a strong link between childhood obesity and television viewing time. Children in the study who watched more than five hours of television daily were five times more likely to be overweight than children who watched less than two hours per day. Children in the United States watch 17 hours of television a week, according to the American Heart Association. This figure does not include time playing computer and video games.

Unfortunately, school-based physical education programs are not making up for children's exercise shortfall. Although these programs provide both immediate health benefits as well as aid in the development of good health habits, fewer than half of school children receive daily physical education. By 1999, financial problems had forced two-thirds of U.S. schools to eliminate their physical education classes, according to the American College of Sports Medicine.

Effects of childhood obesity

Overweight children face a number of health risks, the greatest of which is that they will grow into obese adults. Obese children who become obese adults are more likely to develop heart disease, diabetes, high blood pressure, high cholesterol, gallbladder disease, arthritis, and certain cancers, according to the Mayo Clinic. These conditions also may appear at a younger age. According to the American Medical Association, more than half of all U.S. adults were overweight in 1999, and obesity-related conditions were second only to smoking as a leading cause of preventable deaths in the United States. One 1993 study calculated that an estimated 300,000 Americans die prematurely each year because of obesity.

Overweight children are more likely to develop high blood pressure and blood cholesterol levels, particularly if there is a family history of these conditions. In young children, excess weight can lead to orthopedic complications such as the bowing of the major leg bones, the tibia and femurs, according to the 1998 report by the AAP.

Often times, however, the most serious and painful problems associated with childhood obesity are emotional. Overweight children are likely to suffer rejection from other children and other forms of social and emotional stress. Several studies have shown that children begin to express a preference for thinness at a young age. In one study, 10- and 11-year-olds ranked overweight children last among those they would like as a friend. Another study found that children ages 6 to 10 associated obesity with a variety of negative characteristics, including laziness and sloppiness. Because of these attitudes, obese children often feel overwhelmed by their weight problem and may suffer from depression.

Treating childhood obesity

Health experts stress that no one weight-control plan works for everyone. But the most successful programs include three common elements: changing the way an overweight person thinks about weight control, improving the diet, and increasing physical activity.

Overweight children who can change the way they think about diet and exercise are much more likely to succeed in any weight-loss or weight-control plan, according to health experts. In this, family support is vital. Parents must be committed to helping their children develop healthy long-term diet and exercise habits.

Children's feelings about themselves are fundamentally affected by their parents' feelings about them. Once a child is aware that a

Between 1970 and 1994, the number of obese children ages 6 to 11 in the United States jumped by 54 percent, *below*, while obesity among adolescents climbed by 39 percent.

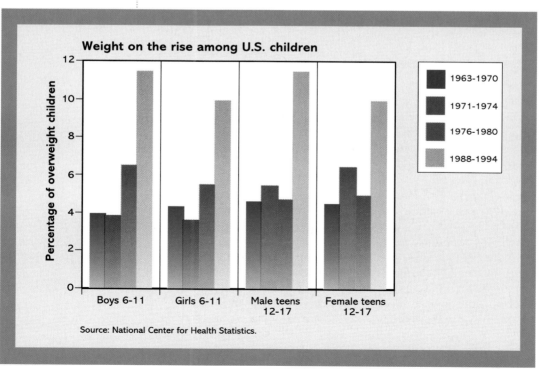

Source: National Center for Health Statistics.

Healthy snacking

Snacks can satisfy appetites and taste without adding unnecessary fat or sugar to the diet. Here are some suggestions.

Chili Popcorn
4 servings, about 1 cup each
Calories: 50; cholesterol: 0; fat: 3; sodium: 42.
Ingredients:
1 quart popped popcorn
1 tablespoon melted margarine
1-1/4 teaspoons chili powder
1/4 teaspoon ground cumin
dash garlic powder
Mix hot popcorn and margarine. Mix seasonings thoroughly and sprinkle over popcorn. Mix well. Serve immediately.

Other healthy snacking suggestions:
Wheat pita bread stuffed with chopped vegetables seasoned with low-fat salad dressing.
Dried fruits
Snack mix made with bite-size wheat, rice, corn, and bran ready-to-eat cereals. (To make: toss each cup of cereal with 1 teaspoon melted margarine. Add flavor with low-sodium seasonings such as garlic, onion, or chili powder. Toast in oven.)
Fresh fruits
Raw vegetables. Dip in cottage cheese or unflavored yogurt with salad dressing herb mix.
Bran muffin
Tangy yogurt cubes or popsicles. (Combine 6 fluid ounces of undiluted frozen fruit juice concentrate with 8 ounces of plain low-fat yogurt and freeze in ice cube trays. Place a popsicle stick in center when mixture is partially frozen.)
Celery stuffed with a peanut butter spread or a low-fat cheese spread.
Whole-grain crackers with a peanut butter and fruit spread.
Low-fat milk (1 cup) and 1/2 cup fresh fruit mixed in blender.

Sources: "The Dietary Guidelines for Americans" developed by the U.S. Departments of Agriculture and Health and Human Services; the Mayo Clinic.

weight problem exists, he or she may feel unhappy or depressed. Health experts stress that parents should help their children feel valued no matter how much they weigh. They should also encourage an overweight child to accept that a problem exists. They should demonstrate a true commitment to the child's success, offering constant support and encouragement. In addition, the entire family should promote healthy living in a way that is fun and inviting to the child. Ideally, parents should teach by example.

Weight-control programs that minimize the sense of deprivation are likely to result in more long-term behavioral changes and a decreased likelihood of a return to unhealthy behaviors, according to health experts. In addition, children who feel they have choices in the plan and are in control of their weight-loss treatment are more likely to succeed.

Figuring out the environmental factors contributing to a child's weight problem is an important first step. To do this, health experts recommend keeping a detailed record of daily food choices and activities. The food diary should include everything the child eats and drinks in a day's time—the type of food, the amount, the place the food was eaten (school, home, restaurant), what time it was eaten,

Risk factors of obesity

Obesity among children results from a combination of genetic and environmental factors. Having at least one obese parent, *right*, greatly increases a child's risk of becoming obese. However, child health experts attribute the rise in childhood obesity chiefly to a decline in the amount of physical exercise children get, *below*, and an increase in the amount of high-fat foods they eat, *below right*.

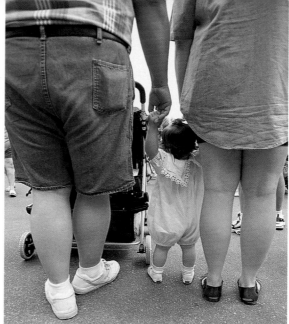

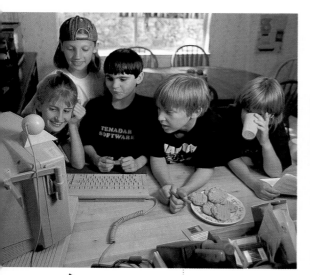

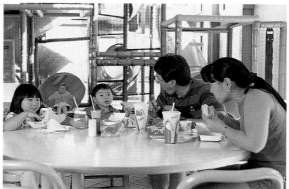

and how the food was prepared. Noting how the child felt when he or she ate is also useful.

Parents and children should then review the food and activity record and identify behaviors that contribute to the child's weight problem. For example, are high-fat snacks more available to the child than healthful snacks? Are second and third helpings at meals a habit? Does the child get at least 30 minutes of exercise daily? Does the child eat because he or she is bored or upset?

A nutritious diet

Child health experts stress that children should not be put on a low-fat diet. Children need a certain amount of fat for normal growth. Those who eat too little fat risk developing nutrient deficiencies and impairing their growth. "The Dietary Guidelines for Americans," issued by the Centers for Disease Control and Prevention in Atlanta,

Georgia, recommend that after age 2, children gradually adopt a diet that, by about age 5, contains no more than 30 percent of calories from fat.

Instead of limiting the total amount of food overweight children eat, child health experts recommended that parents stress eating different types of foods. The government's dietary guidelines include six relevant dietary tips for children: eat a variety of foods; balance the food you eat with physical activity; eat plenty of grain products, vegetables, and fruits; limit the amount of fat, saturated fat, and cholesterol in your diet; limit the amount of sugar in your diet; and limit the amount of salt and sodium in your diet.

One dietary approach that has been successful in treating childhood obesity is known as the "traffic light diet." Designed for preschool and preadolescent children, this diet regulates nutritional and caloric requirements by grouping foods into categories. Green foods (go) may be consumed in unlimited quantities; yellow foods (caution) should be eaten in moderation; and red foods (stop) are to be avoided, if possible. Studies have shown that children who followed the traffic light diet as part of a comprehensive treatment program that also included exercise, behavioral counseling, and family support

Health risks of childhood obesity

- orthopedic complications (bowing of legs)
- high blood pressure
- high cholesterol levels
- social isolation
- depression
- emotional stress
- low self-esteem
- skin disorders
- adult obesity
- higher risk of developing: heart disease, high blood pressure, high cholesterol levels, diabetes, gallbladder disease, arthritis, and certain cancers

Source: The National Center for Health Statistics.

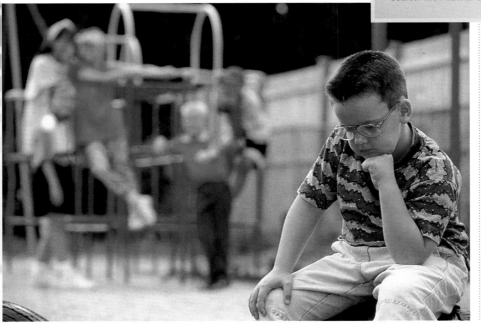

Overweight children often suffer from serious emotional problems. They frequently are teased about their appearance and rejected as teammates or playmates by other children.

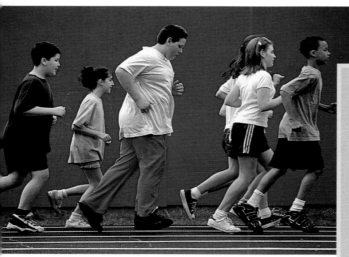

Children should get at least 30 minutes of moderate to vigorous physical exercise daily, according to a 1966 report by the U.S. Surgeon General. However, nearly half of Americans ages 12 to 21 are not vigorously active, the report found.

Managing weight loss

- Set a reasonable goal for weight loss.
- Improve food management:
  - establish a well-balanced diet;
  - keep a food diary; and
  - increase amount of dietary fiber
- Increase physical activity.
- Modify behavior:
  - educate parents and child about food's nutritional content;
  - reduce temptation by limiting the amount of high-calorie food available
  - reduce TV viewing;
  - give rewards for healthy eating and exercise;
  - work to change child's negative attitudes; and
  - involve child in managing weight loss with contracts and goal-setting.

improved their diet and significantly improved their eating habits. In addition to these short-term effects, researchers observed long-term obesity changes extending from 5 to 10 years after the beginning of treatment.

Nutritional experts stress that parents should model good eating themselves and offer a variety of healthful foods. Involving children in menu planning also may encourage the development of good eating habits. In the guidelines, the CDC noted that children and adolescents often understand the importance of limiting fat, cholesterol, and sodium in their diet but are not aware of which foods are high in these substances. In addition, according to the CDC, children and adolescents frequently decide what to eat without adult supervision. "The increase in one-parent families or families having two working parents outside and the greater availability of convenience foods and fast-food restaurants inhibited parents' monitoring of their children's eating habits," the report said.

Getting enough exercise

Physical activity is as important as good eating habits in weight control. In July 1996, the U.S. Department of Health and Human Services issued the first Surgeon General's Report on Physical

Checklist for healthy menus for the family

Write out your family's typical menu for a week and then answer the following questions:

1. Does a day's menu provide at least the lower number of servings from each of the major food groups including:

    6 servings of grain products? (yes/no)
    2 servings of fruit?
    3 servings of vegetables?
    2-3 servings of lean meat or the equivalent (totaling 5 oz. a day)?
    2 servings of milk, yogurt, or cheese?

2. Do the menus have several servings of whole-grain breads or cereals each day?

3. Do the menus for a week include several servings of: dark-green leafy vegetables (spinach, broccoli, romaine lettuce) and dry beans or peas (kidney beans, split peas, lentils)?

4. Do menus include some vegetables and fruits with skins and seeds (baked potatoes with skin, summer squash, berries, apples or pears with peels)?

5. Underline all of the foods in your menus that are high in fat, sugar, or sodium.

Are other foods that are served with them lower in fat, sugars or sodium, so that total intake is moderate?

Are other meals on the same day lower in fat, sugars or sodium, so that total intake is moderate?

6. Are the menus practical for you in time, cost, and family acceptance?

Source: "The Dietary Guidelines for Americans."

Activity and Health. It recommended 30 minutes of moderate to vigorous physical activity per day for children and adults. Although this goal may seem modest, child health experts note that many children fall short.

As with nutrition, parents can be instrumental in discouraging sedentary activities, mainly by reinforcing the positive benefits of physical activity. For example, parents can praise children for playing outside after school. Participating in a sport with a child and organizing family activities, such as a bike hike or even a walk after dinner, can provide children with powerful inducements to modify their behavior.

Experts caution that overweight children may be more prone to injuries of the joints than children of normal weight because of the extra stress on their joints. The Mayo Clinic recommends that overweight children begin an exercise program gradually, starting with lower impact exercises such as swimming and biking rather than high-impact activities like running. Proper warm-up and cool-down exercises are especially important to prevent injuries.

In any weight-control plan for children, gradual change is best. In a five-year study of school-age children, researchers at the Mayo Clinic found that kids who were able to make small, progressive changes in their eating and exercise habits were more likely to lose and control their weight than those who attempted major changes.

To begin, a child can identify a single specific change he or she is willing to make. For instance, rather than vowing to cut down on all snacks, a child may start by substituting a piece of fruit for a cus-

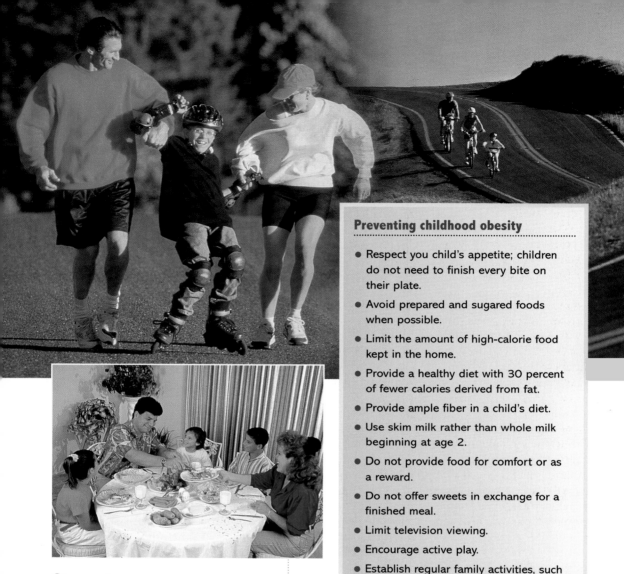

Steps to a healthy lifestyle

Family support is essential for any child who needs to control his or her weight. Parents should promote healthy living, including engaging in frequent physical exercise and eating a well-balanced diet, in ways that are fun and inviting to the child.

tomary bowl of ice cream before bedtime. Or he or she can play outside or ride a bike after school rather than watching television. A child who reduces his or her total caloric intake by just 100 calories a day—a piece of bread, a cookie, or an extra half-bowl of cereal—will lose 10 pounds within a year.

Sometimes, obese children need more than family support, diet, and exercise to help them reach their goal. According to the Mayo Clinic, support groups made up of children of the same age may provide additional encouragement and offer a welcome opportunity to share feelings and discuss problems and possible solutions.

Child health experts note several factors that give them optimism about the chances of reducing obesity in children. First, unhealthy eating and exercise habits are not as ingrained in obese children as they are in obese adults and so are usually easier to change. Second, families are more likely to make fundamental changes in their eating and exercise habits for the sake of an obese child than they are for an obese adult. Finally, few overweight children actually need to lose weight, experts say. Instead, parents should focus on appropriate changes that will bring an obese child's height-weight proportions into balance. In reducing the prevalence of childhood obesity, the primary goals are to get children moving, cut out high-fat foods, and teach healthy fitness habits that will last a lifetime. • • •

For additional information:

Books
Burridge, Keith, and Landy, Joanne M. *50 Simple Things You Can Do to Raise a Child Who Is Physically Fit.* Arco Publishing, 1997.

Fraser, Kate, and Tatchell, Judy. *Food, Fitness and Health.* EDC Publications, 1987.

Levine, Judith, Bine, Linda, and Levine, Judi. *Helping Your Child Lose Weight the Healthy Way: A Family Approach to Weight Control.* Birch Lane Press, 1996.

Pescatore, Fred, and Atkins, Robert. *Feed Your Kids Well: How to Help Your Child Lose Weight and Get Healthy.* John Wiley & Sons, 1999.

Piscatella, Joseph C., Piscatella, Bernie, and Roberts, William C. *Fat-Proof Your Child.* Workman Publishing, 1997.

Web sites
WIN (Weight Control Information)— http://www.niddk.nih.gov/health/nutrit/win.htm

Shape Up America!—http://www.shapeup.org/sua

Dietary Guidelines for Americans— http://www.nal.usda.gov/fnic/dga/dguide95.html

American Obesity Association—http://www.obesity.org

Parents, teachers, and children can learn techniques to combat bullying.

Bullying:
A Silent Nightmare in the Schoolyard

By Dianne Hales

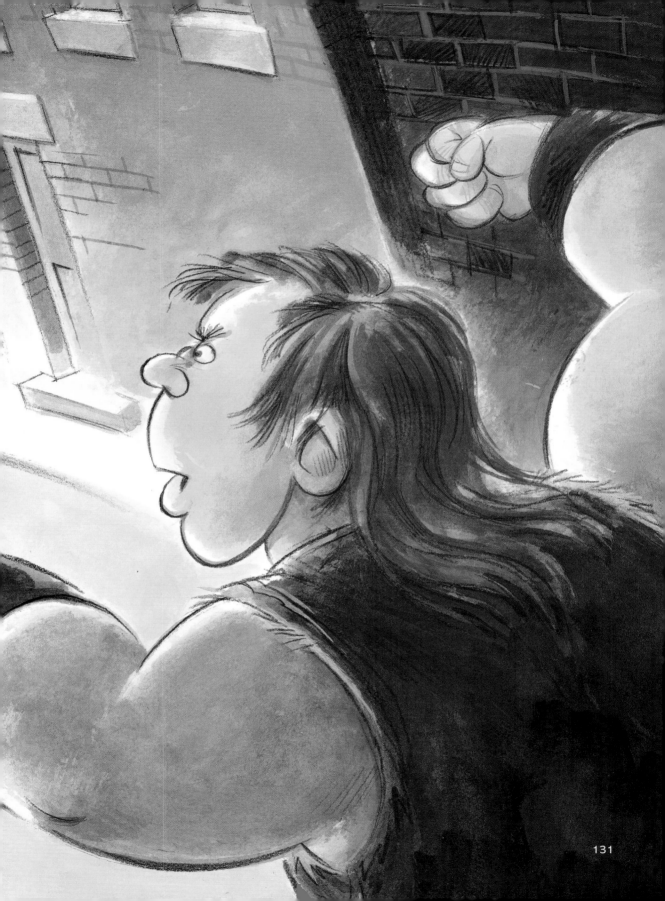

D
AY AFTER DAY A SECOND-GRADER FORCES A KINDERGARTNER
to turn over his lunch. A trio of 10-year-olds pounce on a
smaller classmate, toss his backpack off the school bus, and
throw his jacket in the mud. A sixth-grade girl spreads rumors about
another girl in class. A high school junior pushes a freshman down
the stairs and charges him a daily toll to pass in peace.

For more than 2 million students in schools throughout the
United States, bullying—the use of intimidation or force to assert
power over another person—is a daily reality. For years, many
schoolteachers and counselors dismissed such behavior as a normal
rite of passage. By 1999, however educators recognized bullying as a
"silent nightmare" affecting as many as 20 percent of school-age
children on a regular basis.

Bullying is not only common, but extremely hazardous to everyone involved—bullies, victims, and bystanders. According to a study
of almost 900 U.S. third-graders, a bully has a five times greater risk
of engaging in criminal behavior as other children. The study also
reported that a child who becomes a bully by age 8 has a 25 percent
chance of ending up with a criminal record by age 30.

Problems also exist for children who are the targets of sustained
bullying. These children often suffer long-lasting fear and humiliation as the result of being victimized. In extreme cases, children who
had been relentlessly teased and bullied have committed suicide.
Even bystanders who witness bullying can become victims, as they
are sometimes bothered by feelings of apprehension and guilt for not
having done something to stop the attack.

Shattering myths about bullies

Research conducted in the 1990's shattered many myths about both
bullies and their victims. For example, contrary to some traditional
stereotypes, both boys and girls bully, though in different ways.
Sometimes, bullying trends cross generations, with the children of
bullies becoming bullies themselves while the children of victims
grow up to be victimized. However, psychologists believe that bullying is neither inevitable nor irreversible. It flourishes in settings
where children silently suffer and adults ignore or dismiss aggressive
behavior displayed by some children. By working together, psychologists in 1999 believed that parents and educators can prevent bullying at its earliest onset, establish a zero-tolerance policy against victimization, and take the dread out of going to school for millions of
youngsters.

For years, psychologists theorized that bullies suffer from underlying anxiety and insecurity. But personality and hormonal tests
have shown that this is not the case. Nor do all bullies fit the stereo-
type of being tough kids from high-crime, low-income neighborhoods. Bullies are found in all sorts of families and communities.
However, the parental, physical, and environmental influences that
cause someone to become a bully can vary.

The author:
....
Dianne Hales is a
free-lance writer.

132

Reasons why children become bullies

A theory set by psychologist Dan Olweus of the University of Bergen in Norway links bullying to a combination of too little love and care and too much freedom in childhood. Olweus, a pioneer in the study of bullying, theorizes that children may fail to form a deep, lasting bond with parents who do not show them affection. Because such children feel unloved, they lack empathy for other children and try to coerce them into doing what they want. At the same time, their parents may not set limits and may tolerate aggressive behavior toward siblings or peers.

Inconsistent parental discipline of children may also lead to bullying, according to some psychologists. For example, one day parents may respond to their child's misbehavior with a violent emotional outburst or physical punishment. The next day, the same inappropriate behavior is ignored by the parent. Thus, the child becomes uncertain about what might happen, begins to fear the worst in any situation, and attacks other children because he or she fears being attacked themselves. Boys in particular conclude that "might makes right," especially if their parents are themselves aggressive, encourage their sons to fight, use physical punishment, and admire aggression in others.

Physical characteristics can also make some difference, at least for boys. In general, male bullies pick on children who are shorter, smaller, and younger than they are.

Environmental factors also play a role in making a child a bully. Dorothea M. Ross, a research psychologist at the University of California Medical School in San Francisco and author of the book *Childhood Bullying and Teasing*, believes that negative consequences for bullying are generally rare in American homes and schools. In other words, children bully when they know they can get away with it. Usually, victims of bullying don't tell adults what happened and parents don't ask.

"The contention that bullies often are given the protection that is normally accorded to an endangered species is not an exaggeration," says Ross. She says that young victims are often fearful of snitching on a schoolmate because they are embarrassed about their humiliation and doubtful that anyone will take serious action.

There are other environmental problems, as well. Some parents may dismiss their son's aggressive behavior as being a part of adolescence and following the adage of "boys will be boys." Teachers and school officials traditionally have not considered bullying as serious a problem as other forms of violence, though such beliefs were beginning to change in the late 1990's. And children who watch bullies in action without protesting, often to avoid becoming targets, also contribute to an atmosphere in which bullies survive and thrive.

What is a bully?

Experts define bullying as the use of verbal or physical intimidation or force to assert power over another person. School officials recognize bullying as a "silent nightmare" affecting as many as 20 percent of school-aged children on a regular basis.

Causes of bullying

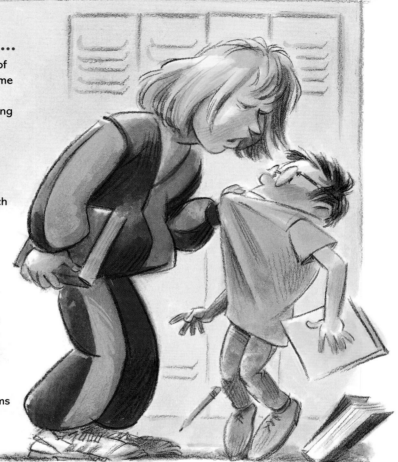

Bullies are found in all sorts of families and communities. Some influences that have been implicated as factors of bullying include:

- Lack of parental affection
- Inconsistency in parental discipline techniques
- Physical characteristics, such as being physically larger than victims
- Imitating the behavior of older children or adults
- Inconsistency in discipline techniques at school
- Belief on the part of adults that aggressive behavior is a part of adolescence
- Belief on the part of some educators that bullying is less serious than other forms of school violence

Finding a role model

Bullies often model themselves after other bullies. These role models can be modern-day heroes, including actors, historical figures, and even teachers. In one study, 2 percent of the bullying that children endured came from teachers who used sarcasm or mockery in the classroom. Another strong influence is television, which often rewards situation-comedy bullies with big laughs. Even when bullies are depicted as cruel, continued exposure to bullying desensitizes child viewers to the pain and misery of being bullied, says Ross. "With this deterrent removed, the way is further cleared for the child to engage in bullying others," Ross says.

Bullying is not a phenomenon of the late 1990's. As the English novelist Charles Dickens recounted in his book *Oliver Twist* (1837-

1839), children have long been subjected to bullying by peers, families, teachers, and employers. According to some surveys, as many as 60 percent of school-aged children have been bothered by bullies. About 15 percent of those children surveyed reported being bullied on a regular basis.

Places where bullying occurs

Bullying usually starts in elementary school, peaks in the middle-school years, and continues at a lower level in high school. It most often takes place in or around schools, but usually out of direct sight or supervision of teachers. In grade school, playgrounds are the prime sites for bullying. In later grades, bullying most often occurs in the hallways, where a bully can sidle next to another student, say something demeaning or disturbing or "accidentally" push or trip the victim.

Some researchers in 1999 believed that bullying was increasing in both frequency and intensity, as teases and taunts gave way to such physical violence as beatings. By the late 1990's, bullying had taken on more violent characteristics, including the use of guns and other dangerous weapons.

The differences between boy and girl bullies

According to Olweus, there are two common types of bullying—direct bullying and indirect bullying. Direct bullying refers to any form of physical or verbal aggression, including hitting, kicking, intimidating, threatening, or mocking. Indirect bullying involves such tactics as telling stories behind someone's back that in turn affect the way others perceive and respond to an individual. Regardless of the method, psychologists say that both forms of bullying have the same purpose: to cause distress to and assert control over someone else.

Girls rely more on indirect bullying than boys. Their victims are almost always girls within their own age range. They often bully them by excluding them from cliques, conversations, or parties; suddenly refusing to be friends; or spreading gossip. One common example of what researchers call "relational aggression" among female bullies in elementary school is accusing a girl of carrying a highly contagious "germ."

Olweus also distinguished between two types of bullies—aggressive and passive. Aggressive bullies are easily frustrated, fearless, and belligerent and are much more inclined to use violence than other children. Such children are often focused on power, are physically strong, and feel a need to dominate others. They often see the world as being full of potential enemies, whom they must either dominate or submit to, and overreact to what they see as slights or hostilities. They also often claim that they are unappreciated by others. However, aggressive bullies are not equally aggressive toward all children; rather they strike out only at select victims. Such bullies are often popular in grade school, but both their popularity and their academic performance plunge by the time they enter middle school.

Passive bullies, also called anxious bullies, rarely go out of their way to victimize others, but they admire and ally themselves with aggressive bullies. Once an episode of bullying begins, they eagerly join in, often as a way of gaining acceptance and approval. Passive bullies, says Ross, are often less popular than aggressive bullies, have few likable qualities, poor self-esteem, and difficulties at home.

Choosing their targets

Bullies choose their targets for a variety of reasons, often picking on someone who is of a different race, ethnicity, economic status, or appearance. In one survey of students in grades 4 through 12, both girls and boys ranked "didn't fit in" as the number one reason for bullying. Among 8th- through 12th-graders, boys said physical weakness, having certain friends, and style of clothing were the primary reasons for bullying. Girls cited facial appearance, crying or being emotional, being overweight, and getting good grades as frequent causes of bullying.

Psychologists note that boys who are bullied most often tend to be more passive and physically weaker than their tormentors. In middle schools, girls who enter puberty early are the most frequent victims of bullying, which usually takes the form of sexual harassment.

Research has shown that in middle and high school, bullying by both sexes frequently takes the form of sexual harassment. In a 1993 survey sponsored by the American Association of University Women, an organization that lobbies for education and equity headquartered in Washington, D.C., 1 in 3 girls and 1 in 5 boys reported frequent sexual harassment, most of it occurring in hallways and classrooms. To boys, taunts about homosexuality were the most disturbing form of sexual harassment. Girls reported feeling upset and embarrassed by comments about their bodies or by being referred to in derogatory terms.

The majority of bully victims are considered to be passive victims. Researchers describe passive victims as being more anxious and insecure than other youngsters, as well as cautious, sensitive, quiet, and serious. They often suffer from low self-esteem and see themselves as unattractive, unintelligent, and unpopular. Boys are physically weaker than their tormentors, and both sexes tend to lack humor and basic social skills that would help them deflect a bully's taunts. Many also suffer from unrecognized and untreated depression. According to many psychologists, everything about passive victims, including posture and facial expression, signals that they would be unlikely to retaliate either physically or psychologically to an attack. Their typical responses to bullying include crying and feelings of helplessness. A passive victim may avoid a potential confrontation by walking several miles to school rather than taking the bus with a bully.

Where does bullying take place?

Bullying usually occurs where there is a group of children, most commonly in or around schools. In elementary schools, playgrounds are often the site of bullying. In middle schools and high schools, bullying often takes place in hallways.

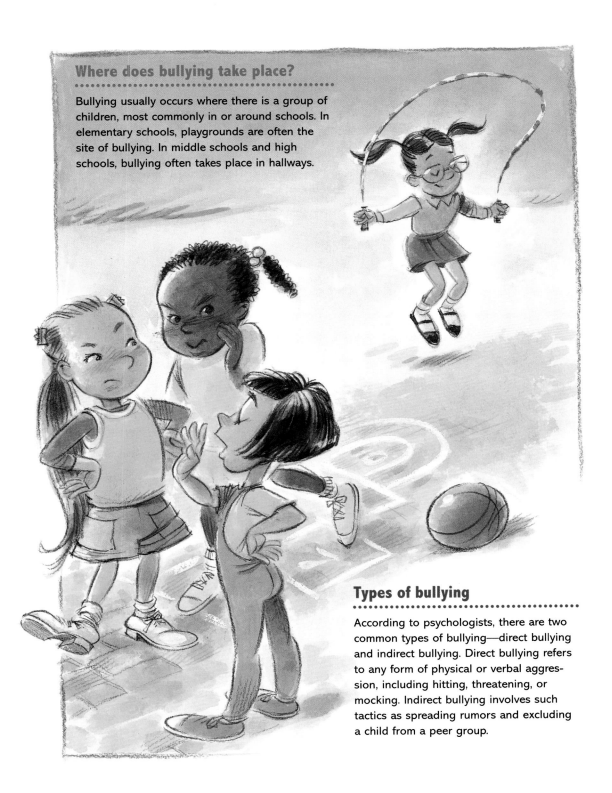

Types of bullying

According to psychologists, there are two common types of bullying—direct bullying and indirect bullying. Direct bullying refers to any form of physical or verbal aggression, including hitting, threatening, or mocking. Indirect bullying involves such tactics as spreading rumors and excluding a child from a peer group.

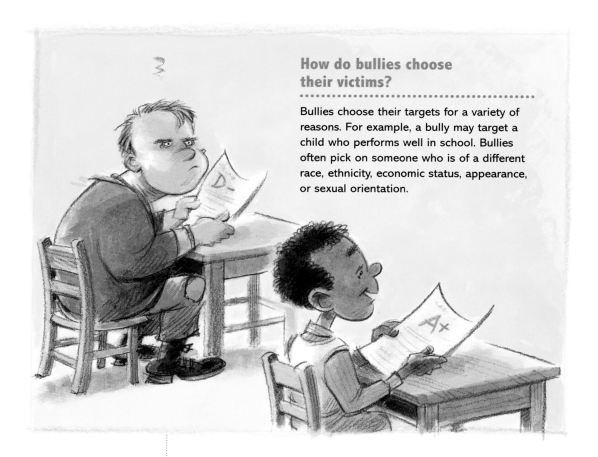

How do bullies choose their victims?

Bullies choose their targets for a variety of reasons. For example, a bully may target a child who performs well in school. Bullies often pick on someone who is of a different race, ethnicity, economic status, appearance, or sexual orientation.

Provocative victims are more active and assertive, and fewer in numbers than passive victims. They often behave in ways that irritate others. When attacked, they fight back, though usually ineffectively, and end up prolonging the confrontation. Because provocative victims tend to be hot-tempered and easily aroused, bullies justify their attacks on them by claiming that they "asked for it" or that they "had it coming."

A small subgroup of victims are referred to by psychologists as bully-victims. These are youngsters who are bullied—usually by someone bigger than themselves—and then bully someone else, usually smaller than themselves. Like provocative victims, they are easily agitated and often goad a bully into attacking. They often go to great lengths to be accepted, and may play class clown and try to laugh off a bully's show of force. However, they often end up unpopular and rejected.

Just as the children of bullies often become bullies, research has shown that victimization also crosses generations. A study that spanned 24 years reported that men who had been bullied between the ages of 8 and 14 were more likely to have children who were bullied.

The effects of bullying

Bullying may have other very different effects—both immediate and long-term—on bullies, victims, and bystanders. Experts had once believed that the victims of bullies were the ones to suffer significant psychological effects. Later studies, however, have shown that both bullies and their victims will often suffer in silence, sometimes becoming suicidal or homicidal.

For many children who bully, their primary gain is a sense of being in control. "This feeling overrides any possibility of empathy for the victims or anyone else and reduces any anxiety they may be experiencing," says Ross, noting that bullies often feel pleased with what they do to their victims. Forcing a child into obedience is even more gratifying, for example, then having a youngster give them money or a new sweatshirt. Bullies also enjoy the deference with which they are treated by other kids, especially in grade school.

As children enter higher grades, some bullies outgrow such behavior, while others become leaders of a group of kids who want a chance to succeed at something. Researchers note that such children typically do not do well at school. Some shift to shoplifting and other crimes. In one study of bullies conducted in Norway, about 60 percent of boys identified as bullies in grades six through nine had at least one criminal conviction by age 24, and 40 percent had three or more arrests.

Research has also shown that bullies are also more likely to drop out of high school, be arrested for drunken driving, and abuse their spouses and children. Their children are also more likely to become bullies themselves.

For victims, the immediate impact of repeated bullying is fear. Children may become so terrified that they live like fugitives and try avoiding the bully at all costs. This tactic, which researchers agree is the most common response among victims, can lead to social and academic problems. In one study, 90 percent of the victims of bullying had a

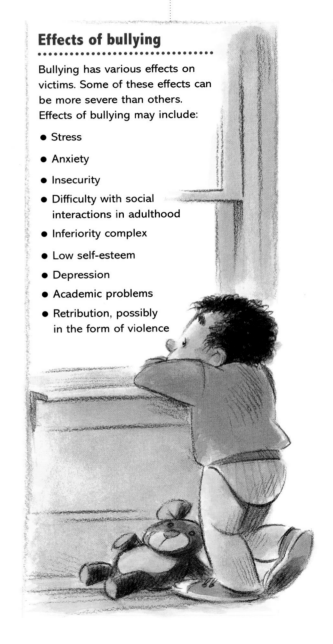

Effects of bullying

Bullying has various effects on victims. Some of these effects can be more severe than others. Effects of bullying may include:

- Stress
- Anxiety
- Insecurity
- Difficulty with social interactions in adulthood
- Inferiority complex
- Low self-esteem
- Depression
- Academic problems
- Retribution, possibly in the form of violence

significant drop in grades. Other youngsters, including those who were friends or at least friendly in the past, may reject them to avoid becoming targets as well.

Over time, the victims of bullies may come to see themselves as unworthy, inferior, even deserving of abuse. Some begin skipping school or run away, while others develop physical symptoms. Some have been so overwhelmed by the effects of being victimized that they have committed suicide.

Even those who survive seemingly intact may carry permanent scars. Psychologists theorize that some childhood victims may have greater difficulty with social interactions as adults. One study of two groups of Swedish boys reported that by age 23, those boys who had been victimized in middle school were well-adjusted adults in many respects, but had poorer self-esteem and were more likely to be depressed than those who had never been bullied.

Psychologists believe that even bystanders can be affected by bullying. Because fear can be viewed as being contagious, children may worry that they may also become the bully's targets if they try to help or tell anyone about an incident. Feeling helpless and guilty for not intervening, children may then have nightmares or feel stress. If repeated bullying goes unpunished over time, an atmosphere of fear and apprehension can fill an entire school and interfere with the students' ability to concentrate and learn. Such an atmosphere may also fill a time like recess with tension and anxiety.

Techniques to combat bullying

Although victims of bullies may feel alone in their fight, experts agree that there are effective techniques that teachers, parents, and children can use to combat bullying. In school, close supervision is critical. Psychologists stress that school officials should also actively watch for aggressive behavior and hand out consistent, nonphysical punishment. The judicial system in the United States has also taken a stand on the issue. For example, in 1996, a federal judge ruled that school districts have a responsibility to protect a student from physical and emotional harm while on school property. The case stemmed from a homosexual student in Wisconsin who had been harassed. And in May 1999, the U.S. Supreme Court ruled that educators who fail to stop students from sexually harassing other students may be forced to pay the victims.

Some schools in Great Britain have attempted to reduce bullying by encouraging all students to report any aggressive or inappropriate behavior. In what they call a "telling school," officials remind students that they have a right to come to school without being afraid, that silence protects bullies, and that they will get in trouble only if they don't report a bully. Other schools have established bully courts in which students and faculty advisers convene to consider charges of bullying behavior and determine punishments, such as after-school detention.

Coping with bullying

Experts say that there are certain measures that schools, parents, and children can take to combat or reduce the effects of bullying.

Parents
- Sympathize with a child and ensure that appropriate action will be taken against the bully.
- Do not blame a child for being victimized.
- Do not promise to keep quiet about the incident.
- Meet with school officials to discuss any incident of bullying.
- Discuss the incident with the parents of the bully.
- Work at uncovering the underlying cause of the bullying behavior.

Schools
- Encourage students to report aggressive or inappropriate behavior.
- Closely supervise children and administer consistent punishment for inappropriate behavior.
- Establish student-watch programs.

Children
- Stay close to a group of friends.
- Report any incidents of bullying to an adult.

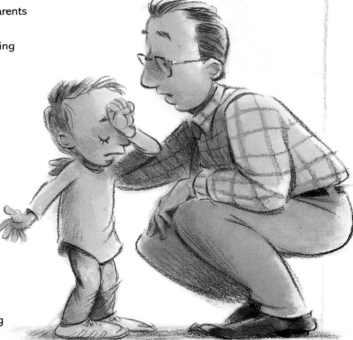

For additional information

A number of books are available to help parents and their children cope with childhood bullying.

- Cohen-Posey, Kate. *How to Handle Bullies, Teasers and Other Meanies: A Book That Takes the Nuisance Out of Name Calling and Other Nonsense.* Rainbow Books, 1995.

- Fried, SuEllen, and Fried, Paula. *Bullies & Victims: Helping Your Child Through the Schoolyard Battlefield.* M. Evans and Company, 1996.

- McNamara, Barry E. *Keys to Dealing With Bullies.* Barrons Educational Series, 1997.

- Olweus, Dan. *Bullying at School: What We Know and What We Can Do.* Blackwell Publishers, 1993.

- Ross, Dorothea M. *Childhood Bullying and Teasing: What School Personnel, Other Professionals, and Parents Can Do.* American Counseling Association, 1996.

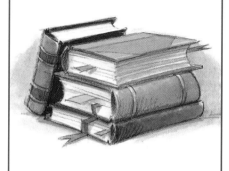

Still other approaches include the use of video cameras to monitor student behavior in playgrounds and hallways, student-watch programs in which student volunteers patrol the school grounds and report any incidents of bullying, and big brother programs in which students in upper grades pair with those in lower grades to make them feel safer and to deter older bullies. Some communities have set up toll-free hotlines that children who are being bullied can call for advice and support.

While different schools emphasize specific types of interventions, the most successful programs share several common elements. For example, the school condemns bullying and acknowledges it as a serious problem. Parents, teachers, and students commit themselves to banning bullying. And students refuse to remain silent.

What parents can do

Experts agree that parents should take steps to prevent bullying, starting in the home. For example, parents should establish rules of behavior at home and commend the child for following those rules. Such actions help build self-esteem, according to many experts. Spending time with a child who also may have a tendency to bully can also create positive experiences for that child, as well as provide them with a positive role model.

According to experts, there are a number of actions that a parent can also take to help stop bullying. For example, if your child is being bullied, sympathize and let your child know that you are angry about the bullying and will take appropriate action. Don't blame your child for being victimized or suggest nothing can be done. Also, don't promise your child that you will keep silent about the incident. Parents should explain that secrecy protects bullies so they can hurt more people.

Find out as much as you can about exactly what happened during a bullying incident, including when and where it took place, who was involved, and if others witnessed the scene. Parents should ask if this was the first incident and how the child responded.

Parents should also consider making an appointment to see the school official who handles parental complaints and bring a written report of the incident. They should also consider contacting the parents of the bully. Although some parents will be concerned and address the problem, others will not. If they dismiss the incident, explain that what happened was an assault, has been reported to the school, and that could become a police matter.

If you discover that your child has been a bully, listen to what others are saying about your child's behavior. Get as much information as you can from your child's peers and teachers, including a description of the incidents that led to the complaint.

In either situation, psychologists urge parents to think of bullying as a symptom and try to determine its underlying cause. If handling the situation on your own proves to be unsuccessful, experts recommend parents seek professional help from a school counselor, psychologist, or local social services personnel. Before the first appointment, write descriptions of your child's behavior at home and at school. Both parents and children should be ready to participate in family and perhaps also marital counseling. These sessions may be crucial in building healthier relationships within your family and with others.

How kids can help themselves

Similar guidelines exist for children who are bullying victims. Experts encourage children to understand that they have the right to feel safe. To prevent attack, stick close to your friends, since studies have shown that bullies rarely pick on an entire group of youngsters. If someone bullies you, always tell an adult, even if you think you've solved the problem on your own. If you find it difficult to talk about what happened, write down what has been happening and give it to a parent, teacher, a friend's parent, or a school counselor.

Psychologists recommend that children who witness bullying take some type of action. If you see someone else being bullied, don't just stand by. Alert an adult to what is going on. If you do nothing, you send the message that bullying is okay with you.

If you've ever bullied someone else, think about why you did it and how you were feeling at the time. Try to think of other ways that you can act to feel good about yourself. Make it a rule to treat others the way you would like to be treated.

The good news for both parents and their children is that bullying does not have to be a constant problem. Experts view open lines of communication between bullies, victims, and their parents as one of the first steps in ending the situation. ●●●

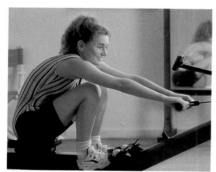

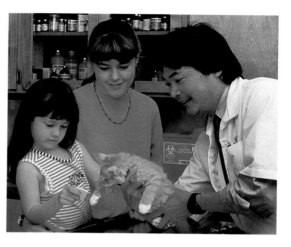

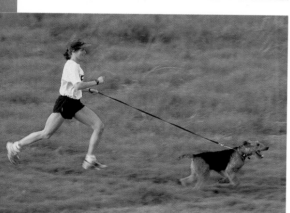

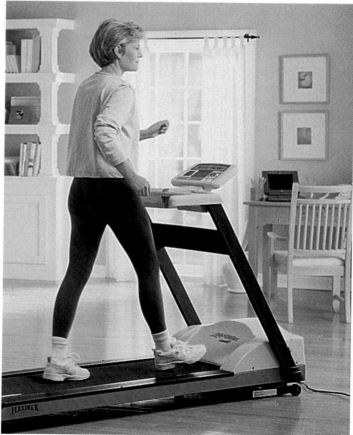

CONSUMER HEALTH

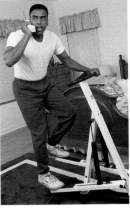

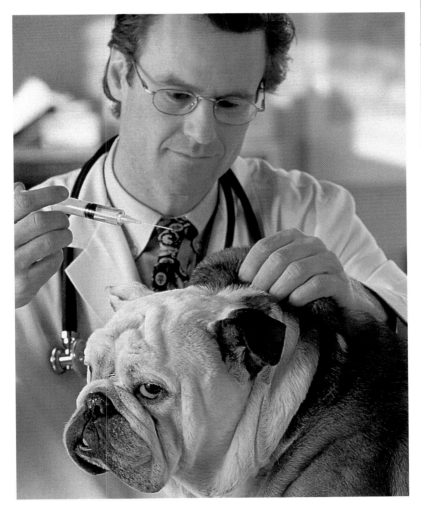

Home Exercise Equipment

By Lauren Love

The author:

Lauren Love is a freelance writer.

UNTIL THE 1990'S, THE PHRASE "HOME EXERCISE EQUIPMENT" meant little more than a stack of weights in a basement or bedroom. By 1999, however, a number of exercise machines were available that allowed people to huff, puff, and stretch their way to fitness in their own homes. In 1998, adults in the United States spent approximately $5 billion on home exercise machines, more than double the $1.9 billion spent in 1990, according to the Fitness Products Council, a trade association that manufactures and distributes fitness equipment.

Approximately one-third of all households in the United States have some type of fitness equipment, according to a study released in 1998 by the Fitness Products Council. Some 50 million adults exercise on home equipment at least once a week, according to the council's survey of more than 1,600 people.

Most people purchase home exercise machines for the sake of convenience and to avoid long waits for equipment at fitness centers, the survey found. Although machines in health clubs are typically more sophisticated—and expensive—than equipment purchased for home use, many home machines offer gadgetry similar to their fitness-center counterparts. For example, one type of stationary bike used in both homes and health clubs in 1999 allowed riders to surf the Internet while peddling. Many home-use machines also have computer technology that allows users to program workout routines geared toward specific goals, such as burning fat, building cardiovascular fitness, or endurance training.

Machines in health clubs and home gyms offer similar health benefits. Machines such as treadmills, stationary bicycles, stair climbers, cross-country ski machines, and rowing machines, primarily offer aerobic exercise. Studies have shown that regular aerobic exercise, which increases the use of oxygen by the body, can help prevent high blood pressure and heart disease or reduce the severity of these life-threatening problems. These machines also help strengthen and tone muscles. Resistance machines are another way to strengthen muscles. *Resistance exercise* (working your muscles against your own body weight, elastic bands, air pressure, or weighted objects) and weight training also are recommended by the American College of Sports Medicine as a way to stave off bone thinning disease.

Individuals need a combination of aerobic and strengthening exercise to maintain physical fitness, according to the President's Council on Physical Fitness and Sports. There are four components to fitness: aerobic endurance; muscular strength; muscular endurance; and flexibility, according to the council. Aerobic endurance is the body's ability to exercise whole muscle groups over an extended period of time using aerobic energy. Muscular strength is the capacity of muscles to generate extreme amounts of force in a short period utilizing *anaerobic* (does not require oxygen) energy. Muscular endurance is the measure of how well muscles can repeatedly generate force and the amount of time they can maintain activity. Flexibility is the ability to stretch muscles and the tendons and ligaments that connect them to bones.

Many machines allow users to gauge their level of fitness by offering such features as highly accurate heart-rate monitors and controls. There are two types of heart-rate monitors—contact monitors and transmitters. Contact monitors, which a person holds in their hand while exercising, detect your heart-rate and display it on the machine's console. They are less accurate than transmitters, which are worn in a belt around the chest, and transmit the heart rate either to a watchlike monitor on the wrist or the machine's console.

Individuals can use heart-rate monitors to keep within their tar-

Home Gym Tips

The President's Council on Physical Fitness and Sports established guidelines for personal exercise programs in 1998 to help people recognize the four components of physical fitness. Following are the council's suggestions on using exercise to build aerobic endurance, muscular strength, muscular endurance, and increase flexibility.

Building aerobic endurance
- Maintain your workout for at least 15 to 30 minutes at your target heart rate.
- If you have trouble maintaining 30 minute workouts, try staggering three 10 minute shifts throughout the day.
- Slowly improve performance. Generally, the more aerobic demands you make on your body, the stronger it will become.
- The body needs time to recover and grow. Alternating days and staggering intensity of your workout can aid in your overall development and prevent injury. Paying attention to your body's messages, such as soreness, tension, and aches, can help you figure out when to workout and when to rest.

Building muscular strength
- Stagger your exercises. Concentrate on activities that work specific muscle groups. Work slowly with concentration on form and resistance to gravity. Directed energy provides the best effect, while lessening the risk of injury.

- Anaerobic activity produces lactic acid build-up in muscle tissue, which can be painful. Stretching before and after workouts can prevent this condition.
- Moderation is key to avoiding injury and realizing benefits. A gradual progression of stress on muscles will increase muscular strength. A one or two day recovery time is necessary for maximum effect and injury prevention.

Building muscular endurance
- Overworking muscles makes them stronger and gives them more endurance. But don't overdo it. Moderate increases in levels of resistance achieve the same result with lower risk of injury.
- When weight lifting, averaging three sets of 10 to 12 lift repetitions is an excellent way to build endurance.

Increasing flexibility
- Always stretch before a workout. Stretched muscles will be more limber and less at risk for rips and pulls.
- Stretching should never be painful. Stretch gently so you feel it, but not so much that you feel it hurt.
- Stagger stretching different body parts throughout the day.
- For maximum results, stretch regularly, several times a day, at least five days a week.

get zone, or optimum heart rate. According to the American Heart Association, an individual's optimum heart rate is between 50 percent and 75 percent of their maximum heart rate. Maximum heart rate is approximately 220 minus a person's age. Some machines use heart-rate information to control the intensity of the workout to keep users within their target zone. A treadmill with heart-rate controls, for example, makes constant, small adjustments in speed or incline to keep the user in his or her target zone.

Target heart rates are effective in measuring initial fitness level and monitoring progress after you begin a fitness program. For example, when an individual begins an exercise program they should aim at the lowest part of their target zone (50 percent of maximum heart rate) and then gradually build up to the higher part of your target zone (75 percent percent of maximum heart rate), according to the American Heart Association. After six months or more of regular exercise, a person might be able to exercise comfortably up to 85 percent of his or her maximum heart rate.

The following profiles of popular types of exercise machines are based on information provided by the President's Council on Physical Fitness and Sports, the American Heart Association, and the Fitness Products Council.

Treadmills

Treadmills are the fastest-growing category of exercise machines. Individuals spend more money on treadmills (about $1.5 billion in 1998) than on any other major piece of exercise equipment. Studies show that treadmills are most likely to be used by all family members. The newest models have shock-absorbing decks that are easier on the joints and preset programs and features to hold the user's attention while they are exercising.

How they work

There are two types of treadmills, motorized and manual. Most motorized treadmills have two motors. One drives the belt, maintaining a constant pace. The other—the lift motor—raises and lowers the running bed to create an incline. The motor that drives the belt should be at least 1.5 horsepower, and most fitness experts recommend that it be a continuous duty motor. The motor should drive the belt at a slow start speed—from 0.1

miles per hour (mph) to 0.5 mph. Top speed depends on your intended use. Some go as fast as 12 mph.

Manual treadmills do not have motors. They tend to have steep inclines that force the user to work hard to drive the belt and maintain the pace.

Many treadmills feature a console that displays your speed, distance, and the time expended. Machines with more sophisticated technology allow users to create an exercise routine to fit personal specifications.

Fitness benefits

Several studies have shown that the treadmill provides one of the best cardiovascular workouts offered by any aerobic exercise machine. Most people can reach their target heart rate at a relatively low exertion level. Brisk walking and running on a treadmill also is a good way to improve lower body muscle tone. Holding small weights can provide a light upper body toning while the exerciser is walking or running.

Health risks or cautions

Mounting and dismounting the moving belt are the chief hazards of treadmill use. To avoid injury, do not stand on the belt when starting the machine. Set the machine at a slow speed and then step onto the belt. Gradually increase the speed.

After mounting the moving belt, the principal challenge is getting used to the belt length and width. At the end of a session, gradually slow the speed and step off the belt before turning off the motor.

Most machines have an emergency switch that immediately stops the belt. Some machines can be started only by special safety keys.

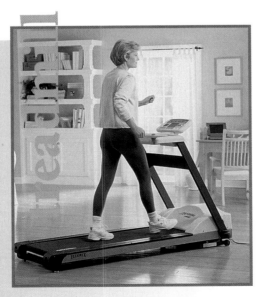

Treadmills provide one of the best cardiovascular workouts offered by any aerobic exercise machine.

How it compares with alternatives

Properly cushioned treadmills reduce impact on knees, legs, and joints—an advantage over walking and running outdoors.

Cost

Treadmill prices range anywhere from $500 to more than $6,000. The major difference between a lower-priced treadmill and more expensive models is durability. Manual treadmills cost less than motorized ones.

Stationary bicycles

About 35 million people ride stationary bicycles, making them the second most popular type of aerobic exercise machines, just behind treadmills. Stationary bicycles are popular because cycling is a familiar and easy-to-learn form of exercise. In addition, these machines take up a small amount of space—usually no more than 4 feet of floor space. Some people like stationary bikes because their hands are kept free to read or engage in other activities while exercising. The newest models feature comfortable designs, smoother pedaling, and more computerized programming options to ensure variety.

How they work

There are four basic types of stationary bicycles: upright; semi-recumbent; recumbent; and dual action. Upright bikes are the most popular type of stationary bike. They are similar in form to traditional bicycles, where the person sits upright and the pedals are located straight beneath the seat.

Semirecumbent bikes, the second most popular type, have a chairlike or bucket seat that provides more comfort and lower-back support than upright varieties. The pedals are located in front of the user. Recumbent bikes are built close to the ground and allow the user to sit back in a reclined position in a loungelike seat. Pedals are located well in front of the user, almost level with the user's chest. People who use these bikes can exercise without raising their blood pressure as high as it would go if they exercised on other types of stationary bicycles. Dual-action bikes are upright bikes with movable handle bars or arm handles that move the arms in

synchronization with the legs.

Most bikes provide resistance training using a flywheel or fan system. Flywheels enable the user to increase resistance without increasing speed, and fan systems require users to pedal faster for a harder workout.

Most bikes include at least 10 difficulty settings (some of the more sophisticated models have more than 20 settings). Computerized bikes may typically track distance and allow you to preset a workout routine, such as simulating going uphill at varying difficulty levels. More elaborate models include video screens that stimulate outdoor scenery or allow users to play video games.

Fitness benefits

Upright stationary bikes provide users with a thorough low-impact aerobic workout and are especially good for toning quadriceps muscles. Dual-action bikes tone the upper body, as well. Semirecumbent and recum-

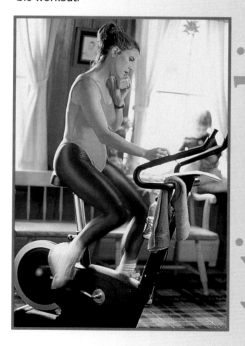

Stationary bicycles provide users with a thorough low-impact aerobic workout.

stationary bicycle

bent bikes provide all the benefits of upright bikes, plus they tone the gluteal and hamstring muscles. They also place less strain on the knees than upright bikes.

Health risks or cautions

Exercising on a stationary bike, especially upright models, can be uncomfortable. Some bikes allow the user to change the angle of the seat as well as it's height; sometimes a seat tilted forward provides more comfort to the rider. Similarly, some models offer interchangeable seat posts, offering a selection of seat styles for different users. Individuals with back problems should use semirecumbent or recumbent bikes, rather than upright models.

Bicycles should be equipped with pedal straps. The straps reduce risk of injury, provide more stability, and make the leg muscles work on both the upstroke and downstroke.

How it compares with alternatives

Riding a stationary bicycle does not replicate the feeling of biking outdoors, but it does offer similar fitness benefits. It is also safer in that the user will not be riding in car or pedestrian traffic.

Cost

Stationary bicycles cost between $200 and $2,000. Semirecumbent and recumbent models are more expensive than upright models. A stationary bike can be made by attaching a regular bike to a stand designed for that purpose. The stands cost less than $200.

Stair Climbers

Approximately 16 million people regularly exercise on a stair climber, or steppers, making them the third most popular aerobics machine on the market. Once used predominately by women, the modern stair climber,

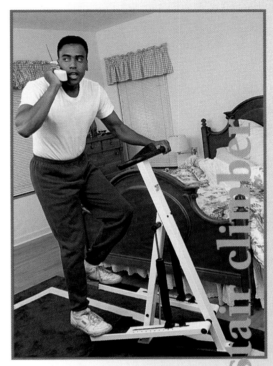

Stair climbers provide excellent aerobic exercise and build and tone muscles in the legs and buttocks.

with its high-tech programming features, is now just as popular with men. Many people like them because the feet never leave the steps during a workout. Thus, the user remains securely positioned on the machine and can easily watch television or read while exercising with little fear of slipping or falling.

How they work

There are two types of stair climbers, hydraulic and electric. Hydraulic, or manual, steppers use pistons under air pressure to regulate the stepping movement. Electric stair climbers use motorized controls to regulate the movement of the steps. In each type of stepper, the foot panels operate as resistance devices, providing a low-impact workout.

Some stair climbers have steps that move independently of each other, which means the user controls the height of each individual stepping movement; on others, the steps are linked to ensure full stepping range. Some models allow alternating between the two modes at the flip of a switch.

Fitness benefits

Individuals who use stair climbers achieve greater cardiovascular benefits than people who use stationary bicycles, rowers, or cross-country ski machines, according to a study of several types of exercise machines conducted at the Medical College of Wisconsin in Milwaukee. Stair climbers provide excellent aerobic exercise and build and tone muscles in the legs and buttocks.

Health risks or cautions

Good posture is essential to a successful work out. Standing on tiptoe or leaning too heavily on the handrails, for example, will cheat the user of the benefits of the exercise. Newer models feature handles that are designed to keep users from supporting themselves on the handrails. They allow users to hold on for balance, but force them to stand up straight.

Make sure step platforms are sturdy. The steps should operate parallel to the floor at all times. They should be covered with a nonslip material and should be wide enough so the foot does not slip off.

The machines provide a steady rate of intensity, and some people may find the exercise too strenuous. People with bad knees should not use these machines.

How it compares with alternatives

Most stair climbers are designed to take the monotony out of climbing stairs, but provide the same health benefits. Most models feature consoles that constantly display feedback, including the number of stairs climbed and the calories burned. Exercising on a machine is much easier on the legs, knees, and joints than climbing flights of stairs.

Cost

Hydraulic stair climbers range in price from $200 to $1,200. Motorized steppers cost more than $1,500.

Cross-Country Ski Machines

There has been a dramatic growth in cross-country ski machines since the late 1980's. Approximately 7 million people used a cross-country ski machine in 1997. They have a reputation as excellent aerobic conditioners and calorie burners, but some people find them awkward to use. A popular feature of ski machines is that most will fold for easy storage.

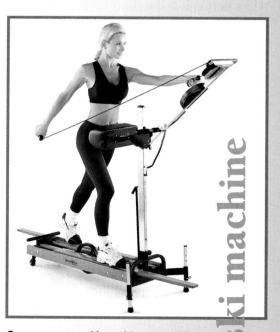

ski machine

Cross-country ski machines provide one of the most effective exercises for burning calories.

How they work

The benefits of cross-country skiing come from repetitive movement with minimal resistance. Cross-country ski machines simulate the kicking and gliding motions of cross-country skiing. The skis are operated by a flywheel and belt mechanism. Cords and pulleys or moveable handles are used for upper body movement. In place of skis, ski machines have long, narrow boards or foot pads that glide on rollers.

The machines come with either independent or dependent leg motion. Independent machines use unlinked skis, which can be hard for beginners to use. But they provide a more intense workout because they require a more natural leg motion that simulates actual skiing. Dependent models have linked skis so that when one foot slides forward, the other automatically slides back, and vice versa. These machines can help beginners from sliding their legs too far, but they also can force a stiff shuffling movement.

Some machines have programmable resistance settings that allow the user to repeat the same difficulty level during subsequent workouts. This feature is useful if several people will be using the machine at different levels. Machines with variable-incline features simulate uphill skiing and provide a more rigorous workout for the front thigh muscles.

Fitness benefits

Studies have shown that cross-country skiing is one of the most effective exercises for burning calories. It also improves cardiovascular fitness. The poling motion builds all-over upper body strength, while the leg movement builds the leg muscles and tones the lower back.

Health risks and cautions

Some individuals may never master the complex motion required by the cross-country ski machine. People who are not comfortable on the machine are at risk of injury, such as hyperextending a knee, or falling off the machine.

How it compares with alternatives

The machines' goal is to provide a nonimpact workout that is easy on the knees and joints and feels just like skiing—minus the cold weather. The machines can not re-create the experience of skiing in a natural setting. More sophisticated machines attempt to compensate by allowing users to choose resistance level by snow type, everything from power to wet snow conditions.

Cost

Ski machines start as low as $200 and are priced as high as $3,500. The most popular models for home use cost between $600 and $750.

Rowing machines

Rowing machines offer the benefit of a full-body workout with little impact on the joints. However, using a rowing machine is not as easy as using some other exercise machines, such as treadmills and stationary bicycles. Individuals usually must practice before they learn how to row properly. Many people find rowing too strenuous, which may be the reason why only 8 million people used the machines in 1997.

How they work

A good rowing machine simulates the experience of rowing a scull in open water. The rower glides back and forth on a seat while pulling back oars or pulleys. You can change the resistance and rowing speed according to your fitness level and ability.

Rowing machines once were made only with hydraulic pistons, which produced a dragging rather than gliding feel. New rowing machines, called wind-resistance pulley models, use flexible graphite composite and

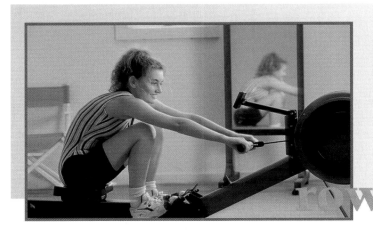

Rowing machines, which provide a strenuous aerobic workout, work muscles in the arms, legs, back, and chest.

rowing

water-filled flywheel tanks in place of pistons. This technology simulates the feel of actual rowing on water. Electronic control panels on computerized models offer a number of preset program options and display elapsed time, stroke count, strokes per minute, calories burned, and tempo.

Fitness benefits

Vigorous rowing is one of the most effective calorie burners, potentially using up more than 800 calories per hour, according to a study conducted at the Medical College of Wisconsin in Milwaukee. In addition to the cardiovascular benefits these machines provide, they are also excellent for strengthening arm, shoulder, back, and abdomen muscles. To maximize strengthening benefits to the arms, it is important to keep elbows tight to the body.

Risks and cautions

Rowing causes little to no impact on the joints, but users should be alert to strain on the knees and lower back. Hyperextension of the back is a common mistake made by rowers.

Rowing is a very strenuous exercise. People who use rowing machines as their main exercise equipment should be in good physical condition.

How it compares with alternatives

Wind-resistance pulley models provide a realistic rowing experience. As in pulling against water with oars, the harder the user draws back on the machine's pulleys, the greater the resistance created and the exertion required.

Cost

Piston models cost approximately $200. Wind-resistance pulley models cost from $600 to $2,000.

Resistance Machines

Approximately 43 million Americans exercise with *free weights* (barbells and dumbbells), making it the single most popular fitness activity in the United States. Home resistance machines are designed to mimic free-weight exercises, only with more safety and less strain.

How they work

A typical resistance machine has a number of cables, pulleys, levers, straps, and bars configured around a metal frame with at least one padded seat or bench. The pulleys are attached to a device, such as a stack of weights, elastic bands, or a piston filled with

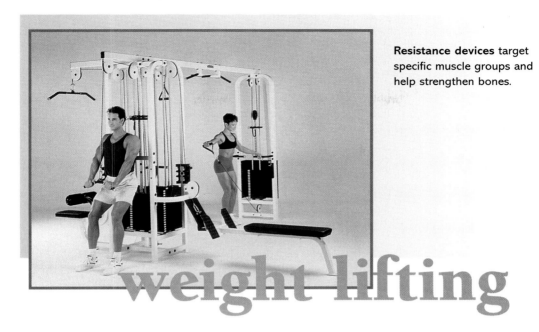

Resistance devices target specific muscle groups and help strengthen bones.

weight lifting

compressed air, that resists lifting, pushing, and pulling.

Lifting, pushing, and pulling exercises on weight machines are designed to build and tone different muscle groups. Adding more resistance (more weight) will build muscle, while doing more repetitions of an exercise will tone muscles without bulking them up. Typical exercises include leg extension and curl, chest press, biceps curl, and triceps extension.

Fitness Benefits

A number of medical studies cite weight training as the single most important factor for people over age 30 in maintaining muscle mass. *Circuit training,* performing a continuous series of different strengthening exercises in quick succession for a set amount of time, can provide the added benefit of a mild aerobic workout.

Health risks and cautions

Machines should include instructions for performing exercises properly. Beginners should test each muscle's level of fitness before using the machine to lessen risk of in-jury. Start out with a light weight or level of resistance and perform at least 10 repetitions before moving to a heavier weight. If the muscle feels tired after the set of repetitions, do not advance to the next weight level.

How it compares with alternatives

Exercising with free weights requires more control to achieve proper form than weight machines. There is also a greater risk of injury with free weights. Machines target individual muscles better than free weights, and they also are better at working all muscle groups.

Free weights take up less space in the home than resistance machines. However, newer machines are small enough to fit in a corner and have more simplified cable systems so they don't have to be repositioned for different exercises. They are more adjustable than they once were, so they can accommodate people of different sizes, gender, and fitness levels.

Cost

Resistance machines cost between $1,500 and $5,000.

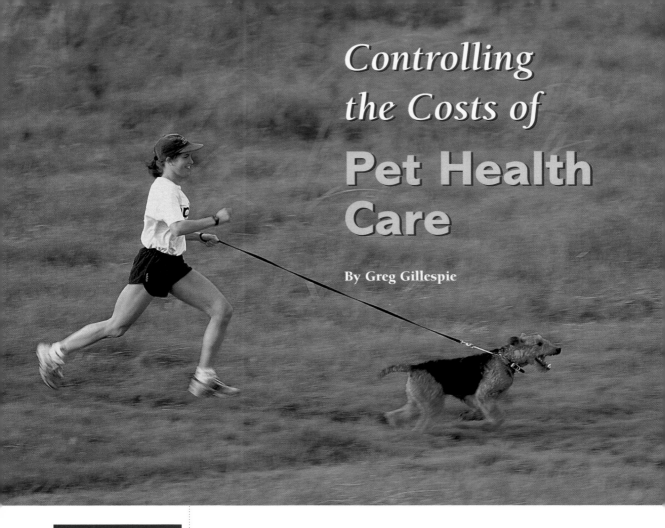

Controlling the Costs of Pet Health Care

By Greg Gillespie

Pet owners can prevent many forms of illness—and their associated costs—through simple preventive measures.

AFTER PERFORMING A SERIES OF TESTS, A VETERINARIAN determines that your family cat has a severe kidney disease. The cat will die within six months without immediate treatment, the veterinarian explains. One of the treatments he suggests is a kidney transplant, a procedure once available only to human patients.

By 1999, almost every medical treatment available to humans was also available to pets. Veterinarians had the tools and the training to perform complicated procedures and surgeries, such as cardiovascular surgery, organ transplant, and joint replacement. They also had a wide array of drugs, including chemotherapy, to treat disease, and improved methods to diagnose illness. For example, veterinarians had access to the same sophisticated imaging devices as those found in hospitals.

These advances in veterinary care come at a price, however. Pet owners spent more than $10 billion annually on health care for their pets in 1998, according to the American Veterinary Medical Association (AVMA). A large portion of that money was spent on treating serious illness and on emergency care.

In 1998, dog owners spent an average of $130 per dog on veterinary care, according to the AVMA. Cat owners spent about $80 per pet. But costs can skyrocket if a pet is treated for a serious medical condition. For example, a kidney transplant for a cat in 1999 cost between $3,500 and $4,500, according to the Veterinary Medical Teaching Hospital of the University of California, Davis. In addition, the cat would need to be given drugs for the rest of its life to ensure that the new kidney functioned properly. These drugs cost between $30 and $60 per month.

Pet owners can prevent many forms of illness—and their associated costs—through simple preventive measures, such as taking their pets to veterinarians for routine checkups and vaccinations, and providing a healthy diet and regular exercise.

The cost of treatment

Pets are susceptible to many of the same illnesses as humans. Cancer, for example, accounts for almost half the deaths of cats and dogs over 10 years of age. Dogs, in fact, get cancer at approximately the same rate as humans. Two of the most deadly cancers in dogs and cats are breast and bone cancer. Pets rarely develop lung and colon cancer, which are associated with such risk factors as smoking and a low-fiber diet.

Skin tumors are a common condition in older dogs, and a somewhat less common condition in cats. These tumors, which appear as unusual lumps or sores under the animal's coat, are often *benign* (not dangerous) in dogs. Cats, however, are at greater risk of *malignant* (threatening to health) tumors.

Cancers produce varied symptoms depending upon the type of tumor. In general, appetite loss, weight loss, fatigue, behavior changes, breathing difficulty, or any persistent change in normal body habits might be symptoms of cancer, according to the AVMA. Lameness in older, large-breed dogs may be a symptom of bone cancer.

Medical treatments for dogs and cats with cancer vary depending on the type and severity of the cancer. By the late 1990's, chemotherapy had become a widely available cancer treatment for pets. Chemotherapy is the treatment of disease through the use of medications that destroy malignant cells. Chemotherapy often causes severe side effects in humans. Animals suffer fewer side effects than humans, according to the AVMA. Chemotherapy can be an expensive treatment. Costs range from $50 to $4,000 or more depending on the type of drug, the animal's size, and the number of treatments.

Other cancer treatments available to dogs and cats include surgery, *radiotherapy* (the use of radiation to destroy cancer cells), and *cryosurgery* (the freezing of a tumor). These treatments can cost several hundred dollars, according to the AVMA.

Heart disease: a growing problem

Cardiovascular disease is a growing problem among pets, and among dogs in particular. The increase in heart problems can be attributed to longer life span and diets that include more fatty table scraps, according to the AVMA.

Heart valve problems are the most common cause of heart disease in dogs. This condition occurs when heart valves thicken and leak blood. Another common heart condition in pets is *myocarditis,* an inflammation of the heart muscle. This may result from one of a number of infections that affect the heart muscle. Coronary artery disease, the major cause of heart disease in humans, is not common in pets.

Cats and dogs with heart disease may experience labored breathing, frequent coughing, fainting, and abdominal swelling. Veterinarians may treat heart disease with drugs or surgery.

In some cases, a veterinarian may recommend a pacemaker, an electronic device that produces an electrical current to stimulate regular contractions of the heart muscle. The pacemaker's generator and batteries are placed under the skin, and wires are passed to the heart. In 1998, approximately 200 animals in the United States received pacemakers. This procedure can cost as much as $2,500, but the use of recycled pacemakers can reduce that cost.

Other common illnesses

Diabetes is another condition common in dogs and cats. Diabetes is a disorder in which the body cannot make use of sugars and starches in a normal way. A key element in the proper use of sugar and starches is the hormone *insulin,* which is secreted by cells within the pancreas. Diabetes results from either a lack of insulin or an inability of the body to use the insulin properly. In pets, as in humans, one cause of diabetes is poor diet. Symptoms of diabetes include increased frequency of urination and persistent thirst, accompanied by increased appetite.

In some cases, diabetes can be controlled through diet alone. In more severe cases, however, a veterinarian might recommend daily insulin injections. The cost of this medication ranges from $500 to $1,000 per year, according to the AVMA.

Dogs are more prone to bone and joint disorders than cats. For example, *hip dysplasia* (abnormal development of the hip) is a genetic disorder that commonly affects dogs. Dogs with this condition often develop arthritis and related joint pain as they age. The condition mainly affects large-breed dogs. In severe cases, dogs with hip dysplasia may be lame by age 2. In most cases, however, a dog will not experience symptoms until age 6 or older.

This condition can be treated only by surgery. Veterinarians can improve the hip joints in young dogs by changing the shape of the thighbone or pelvis. Another option for dogs is hip-replacement surgery. In this procedure, the joint is replaced with a stainless steel

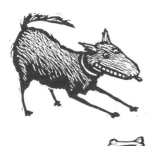

The author:

Greg Gillespie is a free-lance writer.

ball-and-socket joint. In 1999, hip-replacement surgery cost approximately $3,000, according to the AVMA.

Cats are particularly susceptible to infections of the urinary tract. *Feline urological syndrome (FUS),* a common ailment among cats, is a group of disorders that can result in *uremia,* a life-threatening accumulation of toxic wastes in the kidney and bloodstream. Infections of the bladder and blockage of the *urethra* (the tube that conducts urine out of the body from the bladder) are the most common FUS disorders. Veterinarians treat these infections with medications, which costs approximately $50, according to the AVMA.

Trauma and emergency care

Every year, thousands of pets are struck by automobiles, poisoned by pesticides, or attacked by sick or unfriendly animals. These conditions are often treated in an emergency room. Visits to an emergency room start at $50 or more, with costs mounting depending on the treatment, according to the AVMA.

Poisoning is one of the most common reasons owners seek emergency care for their pets. Many substances in the home are toxic to animals. Animals may be attracted to certain poisons because they smell or taste good. For example, dogs are particularly attracted to antifreeze, which tastes sweet. Certain houseplants, such as ivy and philodendron, are poisonous to cats.

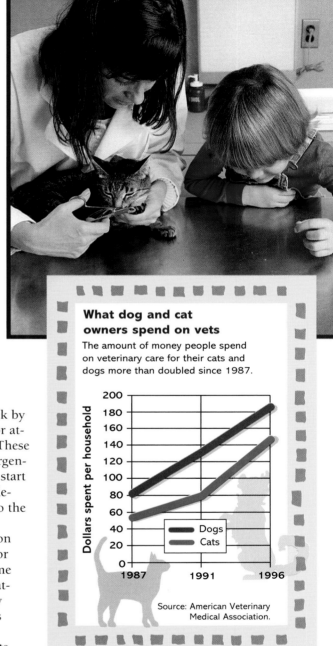

What dog and cat owners spend on vets

The amount of money people spend on veterinary care for their cats and dogs more than doubled since 1987.

Dollars spent per household

Dogs
Cats

1987   1991   1996

Source: American Veterinary Medical Association.

Choking is another common emergency among pets. Bones in food—particularly chicken and fish—that lodge in a pet's throat are most often the cause of choking. Treatments for a choking emergency range from manual retrieval of the bone to surgery.

Bloat is a life-threatening condition that lands hundreds of dogs in an emergency room every year. Bloat is a twist or kink in an intestine that can become fatal within hours—or even minutes—of appearance of the first symptoms. It typically occurs in large dogs that

159

Costs of some medical treatments for pets

	Average cost
Routine office visit	$40-45
Routine spaying	
cat	$65
dog	$130
Vaccination	$15-20
Emergency room visit	$50
After-hours rate	$80
X ray	$30-60
Ultrasound	$150
Routine blood tests	$20-35
Dermatology consultation	$25
Acupuncture treatment	$45-65
CT scan	$290
Pacemaker implant	$2,300-2,500
(or $1,000 to implant recycled pacemaker)	
Heart surgery	$1,000
(balloon valvectomy)	
Surgical removal of	
brain tumor	$2,600-3,600
Reconstructive facial	
surgery	$1,200-1,700
(skin graft)	
Knee surgery to	
repair ligaments	$800-1,100
Radiation treatment	$2,500-2,700
Total hip-replacement surgery,	
dog	$3,100-3,200
Kidney transplant,	
cat	$3,500-4,500
(including surgery and post-operative care)	

Sources: Angell Memorial Animal Hospital, Boston; Veterinary Teaching Hospital of the University of California, Davis.

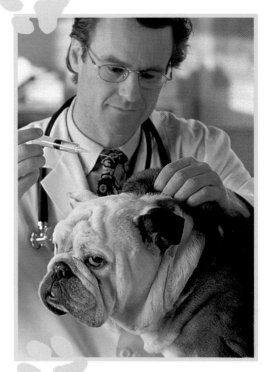

During a regular checkup, a veterinarian will make sure a pet's vaccinations are up to date. Pets are susceptible to a variety of highly contagious diseases. Many of these diseases can be prevented through immunization.

have swallowed an excessive amount of water or exercised strenuously after a meal. Symptoms include a *distended* (swollen) abdomen, belching, dry heaves, increased salivation, restlessness, and whimpering. The only treatment for bloat is emergency abdominal surgery.

Alternative therapies

In additional to conventional treatments, pet health-care specialists in 1999 were frequently turning to alternative methods to treat disease and injury. For example, many veterinarians regard acupuncture as an integral part of veterinary medicine. Acupuncture is an ancient Chinese therapy that uses tiny needles inserted into the skin at specific places on the body in order to relieve pain and disease. Researchers have determined that acupuncture somehow boosts the production of chemicals that lower the brain's ability to perceive pain. Veterinarians use acupuncture to relieve pain in pets with chronic arthritis, for example. Another use of acupuncture is in post-operative recovery. Cost ranges from about $45 to $65 per session.

Growing demand for health insurance

In response to the growing cost of pet health care, many insurance companies offer plans to cover pets. By 1999, only 1 percent of the U.S. population carried health insurance on pets, but insurance experts expected that number to grow rapidly.

Pet health insurance typically covers the cost of accidents and injuries. Most policies also cover diagnostic procedures. Policies typically do not cover the costs of routine procedures such as vaccinations, checkups, and elective surgeries. The plans rarely cover preexisting or genetic conditions. Yearly premiums range from approximately $100 to more than $300.

How pet owners can control costs

The best way to control costs, however, is to practice preventive care. Pet owners who maintain their pet's health protect the animal against catastrophic illness and protect themselves against enormous veterinary bills.

A routine physical examination is an essential step in preventing illness and in controlling costs of pet health care. A physical examination allows a veterinarian to monitor the health of a pet and to treat health problems before they become serious—and costly. Adult dogs and cats under age 10 should get a checkup once a year, according to the AVMA. Pets age 10 and older should visit a veterinarian twice a year. Veterinarians recommend that puppies and kittens receive their first physical examination a few weeks after birth.

A physical exam typically includes measures of body temperature, pulse, respiration rate, and body weight. Blood and stool samples are also typically part of the exam. A veterinarian will also check the animal for lumps or other abnormalities.

Physical exams can cost between $40 and $45, according to the AVMA. Physical checkups also include examination of the animal's teeth and gums. Many veterinarians offer complete dental exams and teeth cleaning, which cost between $50 and $100, according to the pet health care experts.

A dog's annual checkup should include examinations for parasitic worms. Heartworm may cause serious illness or even death. Adult heartworms live in the dog's heart, but young forms of the worm are found in the blood. Mosquitoes transmit the infection after feeding on the blood of an infected dog. All dogs should receive medicine to prevent heartworm.

Many puppies are born with roundworms. A dog may acquire tapeworms by swallowing an infected flea or by eating raw fish or

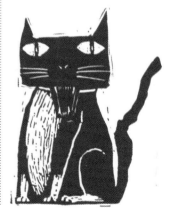

meat. To prevent spreading the parasites to other dogs and people, veterinarians recommend deworming pups with medication every two to three weeks until they are 3 to 4 months old.

Vaccinations: an important tool in prevention

During a regular checkup, a veterinarian will also make sure a pet's vaccinations are up to date. Pets, like humans, are susceptible to a variety of highly contagious diseases. Many of these diseases can be prevented through immunization. Vaccinations cost between $15 and $20.

All dogs, cats, and other mammals should be vaccinated against *rabies,* a viral infection of the nervous system. Rabies primarily affects animals, but it can be transmitted from a rabid animal to a human by a bite or by a lick over a break in the skin. The United States requires that all dogs be vaccinated against rabies. Puppies and kittens should receive their first rabies shot at about 3 months of age, followed by another shot in one year. Dogs and cats

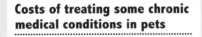

Costs of treating some chronic medical conditions in pets

Cost estimates are for one year of medical care.

Allergy treatments..........................$300

Arthritis medication $180-330

Cancer chemotherapy
   cat..$25-1,700
   large dog $50-4,200
      Cost varies widely according to
      drug and size of animal.

Heartworm disease (preventive)
   dog $30-90

Immunosuppressive
drugs/kidney transplant
   cat..$360-720

Insulin for treatment
of diabetes..........................$500-1,000
      Cost varies widely according to
      severity and pet's response
      to treatment program.

Sources: Angell Memorial Animal Hospital, Boston; Veterinary Teaching Hospital of the University of California, Davis.

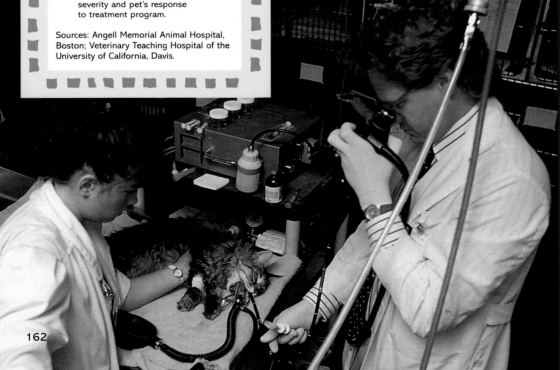

A veterinarian, *below,* examines a cat using a medical scope. In recent years, medical technology for pets has become almost as sophisticated as the technology used in human health care.

should receive a booster shot every three years thereafter, according to the AVMA.

Another important vaccination for dogs is the DHLP-P vaccine. This vaccine immunizes dogs against several diseases, including *distemper* (a viral disease characterized by fever, reddened eyes, loss of appetite, and discharges containing pus from the nose and eyes); two forms of *hepatitis* (a viral disease that causes inflammation of the liver); *parainfluenza* (a respiratory illness similar to influenza); *parovirus* (a gastrointestinal disease caused by a virus); and *leptospirosis* (a bacterial disease that damages the kidneys and liver). A puppy should receive its first DHLP-P vaccine at about 6 weeks old. It will then need several more doses three to four weeks apart. Adult dogs require a booster shot annually.

Some veterinarians recommend the vaccine against Lyme disease for dogs living in the Northeastern and Midwestern United States. By 1999, however, research had not yet established whether the vaccine protected dogs against the disease. Lyme disease is caused by bacteria and spread to animals by ticks. The disease is characterized by joint inflammation.

A panel of feline veterinarians recommended in 1998 that all cats receive three vaccinations in addition to a rabies shot. These include vaccines against *feline panleukopenia* (a viral gastrointestinal disease, also called feline distemper); *feline viral rhinotracheitis* (a viral upper-respiratory disease); and *feline calicivirus* (a viral upper-respiratory disease). Cats should be vaccinated against these diseases as kittens and then receive boosters at three-year intervals, according to the panel.

The panel also recommended that cats allowed to roam outside be vaccinated against three additional diseases: *chlamydiosis,* a bacterial upper-respiratory disease; *feline leukemia,* a viral disease that affects the feline immune system and causes tumors; and feline *infectious peritonitis,* a viral disease that causes either fluid build-up or dry deposits in body organs. Cats should be vaccinated as kittens and then receive booster shots annually, according to the panel.

Spaying or *neutering* (the surgical removal of sex organs) cats and dogs is another essential step in preventive health care, according to the AVMA. In addition to reducing the overpopulation of cats and dogs, spaying or neutering reduce the risk of certain forms of cancer. For example, studies have shown that spaying a female dog before its first *heat cycle* (reproductive cycle) reduces its risk of breast cancer. Spaying or neutering costs between $100 and $150 for dogs and $50 to $75 for cats, according to the AVMA.

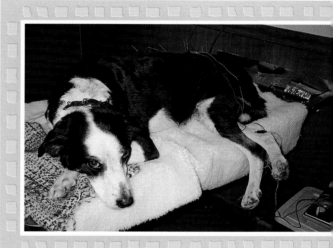

A dog, *above*, relaxes during a session of acupuncture, a therapy that uses tiny needles inserted into the skin to relieve pain and disease. According to the American Veterinary Medical Association, acupuncture is effective in treating pain and behavioral problems in pets.

Good grooming and pet health

Pet owners can also adopt healthful practices at home to prevent illness in animals. For example, the AVMA recommends that owners groom their pets regularly. Grooming prevents skin problems by keeping a pet's coat clean and free from fleas and ticks.

The kind and amount of grooming a dog needs is determined by the animal's fur type and length and by the animal's lifestyle. In general, dogs with longer fur need more frequent combing and brushing than those with short coats. Dogs who spend a lot of time outdoors usually need more frequent grooming than those who live mostly indoors. Dogs also need regular ear inspection and cleaning, toenail trimming, and tooth inspection and cleaning.

Owners should brush or comb a cat's fur daily to clean it and to remove loose hairs. In the case of long-haired cats, such care is essential to prevent the coat from tangling and matting. Daily brushing or combing also reduces the amount of loose hairs that cats swallow when they clean themselves. Swallowed hair may wad up and form a hairball in the cat's stomach. Hairballs can cause gagging, vomiting, and loss of appetite. If a cat cannot spit up a hairball, surgery may be required to remove it. Owners may feed their cat a small amount of petroleum jelly or a commercial preparation once a week to prevent hairball formation. A veterinarian can suggest safe methods of using such products. If necessary, owners may clean their cat's ears with a soft cloth and brush their teeth with a cotton-tipped swab or a small toothbrush. Owners may also trim the tips of a cat's claws.

Cats instinctively clean themselves. They do so by licking their fur with their tongue. They also rub and scratch their fur with their paws. At least once a day, a cat licks a paw and washes its face and head with the wet paw. But not all cats groom themselves well. Some cats—especially those allowed outdoors—become so soiled that they need a bath. Most cats dislike bathing. But if cats are bathed about once a month when they are kittens, they will become accustomed to water. Kittens also should be brushed or combed so that they will be easier to care for when they grow older.

Many pet owners mistakenly believe that a dog should be bathed as seldom as possible. In fact, pet owners may wash their dogs often—in many cases, once a week, according to the AVMA. Owners must, however, use a special shampoo that does not strip the oils from the dog's coat.

When giving a dog a bath, carefully pour warm—not hot—water over the pet. The temperature of the water should feel comfortable to your own skin. Apply a gentle shampoo and lather well. Be careful not to get any shampoo in the dog's eyes. Rinse thoroughly because any soap that remains on the skin may cause itching. After the bath, apply a flea dip, spray, or powder as recommended by your veterinarian.

Like human beings, pets need exercise to remain physically fit and mentally healthy. Excess weight and a *sedentary* (inactive) lifestyle in dogs and cats may lead to many health problems, including obesity, heart disease, diabetes, and joint deterioration, among other conditions. The easiest way to exercise a dog is to release it in an enclosed space with another friendly dog. Dogs left alone may not remain active long enough to stay in shape. A dog will also benefit from daily brisk walks or jogs with its owner. Owners should confine their dog to a leash if they walk or jog where there is traffic or if the city they live in has a leash requirement.

Choosing a healthy diet for your pet

A balanced diet is necessary for a pet's health. Owners can buy prepared food for most kinds of pets. Scientists plan these foods so that they contain the right amounts of vitamins, minerals, and proteins for each type of animal. By using these foods, owners can be sure that their pets receive the right nourishment.

Dogs require different kinds of foods during the various stages of

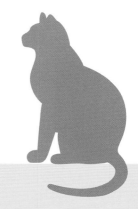

Health care for pets that slither or fly

The most common pets in the United States are dogs and cats. But many people keep exotic or unusual pets, such as reptiles and tropical birds.

Exotic pets—like their nonexotic counterparts—need regular examinations to stay in good health. In general, veterinary fees for treating reptiles and birds are comparable with those for cats and dogs.

A common disease in reptiles is metabolic bone disease, which is caused by a lack of vitamin D in the diet. The disease causes bones to become fragile and fracture easily. It also results in swelling of limbs and joints. The disease can be treated with vitamin injections.

Infectious stomatitis, or mouth rot, is another common illness in reptiles. It is caused by bacteria and results in bleeding in the mouth and gums. It can be treated with antibiotics.

Birds are particularly susceptible to psittacosis, a disease caused by the parasite chlamydia. Symptoms of this condition include eye and nasal discharge. Infected birds can pass the disease onto humans. Veterinarians treat the condition with oral medications.

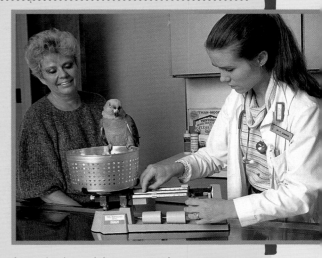

A veterinarian weighs a parrot, *above*, on a specialized scale during a physical exam. Exotic animals require regular checkups to stay in good health.

their lives. At about 3 to 4 weeks of age, puppies need to supplement their mother's milk with solid food. Provide a good-quality commercial product, either dry or canned, that is labeled as food for puppies. Soften dry food by moistening it with water or a puppy milk-replacement formula, or by mixing it with canned food, to make it easier for young pups to chew. Owners may also give a puppy cooked eggs and cottage cheese, but these foods should make up no more than 10 to 20 percent of the dry weight of the puppy's diet, according to the AVMA.

A puppy should be fed four times a day until it is about 3 months old. The pup should then eat three times a day until it is 6 months old, and then twice a day until it is fully grown. Adult dogs need only one meal a day, but many dogs prefer two smaller meals, one in the morning and one at night, according to the AVMA.

Avoid feeding large amounts of meat and table scraps to dogs. Dogs who are given these foods quickly develop a preference for them and may develop dietary imbalances and deficiencies. Vitamin and mineral supplements are unnecessary for healthy dogs who eat a complete, balanced diet.

Bone chewing is natural for dogs, but it can cause broken teeth, and splinters of bone may cause digestive upsets or internal injuries. For these reasons, many veterinarians recommend offering rawhide strips or special chew toys instead of bones. Old dogs and dogs with certain medical conditions such as heart or kidney disease may require special diets. A veterinarian can advise you when special food is needed.

Cats are not naturally finicky eaters. But owners should give them a variety of commercial foods to prevent them from developing fussy appetites. Cats may occasionally be fed small amounts of such cooked foods as beef liver, eggs, fish, and vegetables, according to the AVMA. Many cats also enjoy milk, cheese, and other dairy products. However, such foods cause diarrhea in some cats.

Kittens that have been *weaned* (taken off mother's milk) should be fed small amounts of food four times a day until they are 3 months old. They should eat three times daily until they are 6 months old, and then twice a day until they are full grown. Adult cats require only one meal a day, but many seem happier with two smaller meals. Food may be kept available at all times for a healthy cat that does not overeat. Sick cats, pregnant and nursing cats, and old cats often need special diets, according to the AVMA.

Hygiene and its role in health care

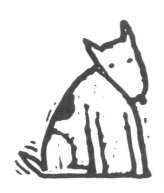

Proper hygiene is an essential part of preventive health care. Keep animal's food dishes clean and provide pets with a warm, clean sleeping area. Indoor cats should learn to use a litter box. Cats instinctively bury their body wastes, so training them to use a litter box is easy. Kittens raised with a mother that uses a litter box will usually begin to use it themselves before they are 5 or 6 weeks old.

Guidelines for choosing a veterinarian

- Choose a vet *before* you adopt a pet or before moving, if possible.
- Ask neighbors, coworkers, or friends for recommendations.
- If you have any connection with a breed club, seek a recommendation from someone in the club.
- You can find a vet by locating an animal hospital nearby. For a local listing, phone the American Animal Hospital Association (AAHA) at 1-800-883-6301 or visit the AAHA web site at www.healthypet.com.
- When you've narrowed the search, verify the vet's credentials. He or she should have a degree from an accredited veterinary school of a college or university and should be licensed by the state.
- Talk with the prospective vet. You'll want to feel at ease with him or her.

- Visit the clinic with which the vet is associated. Check that it is clean, well run, and odor-free.
- Ask if there are any other vets on staff. Coverage should be provided when your vet is unavailable.
- Ask if the clinic uses gas anesthesia. Gas is safer than an injectable anesthetic.
- Ask for a schedule of fees. Find out about the clinic's payment policy.
- Make sure that office hours are compatible with your schedule.
- Find out about availability of emergency care. How does the clinic deal with emergencies outside of regular office hours?

Sources: American Animal Hospital Association; American Veterinary Medical Association; Kimberly Meenen, University of Illinois College of Veterinary Medicine: "Consider More Than Proximity When Choosing a Veterinarian."

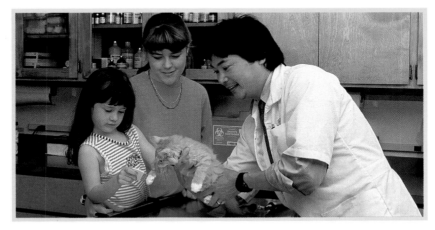

A veterinarian might encourage pet owners to become involved in their pet's health care by educating them on common examination procedures, *above*.

Good grooming practices, such as regular bathing, *right*, prevent skin problems by keeping a pet's coat clean and free from fleas and ticks.

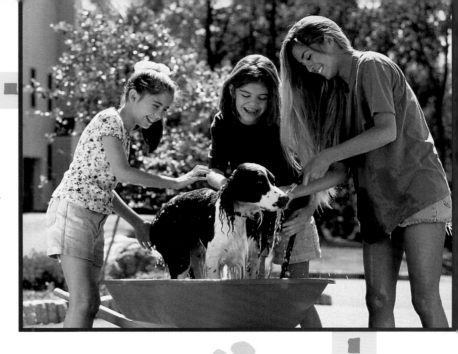

How owners can help their pets

- Choose a veterinarian who can provide regular care for your pet.
- Arrange annual checkups for your pet. For dogs and cats 10 and older, plan six-month checkups.
- Make sure that your pet receives a full range of appropriate immunizations, as your vet advises.
- Spay or neuter dogs and cats. These procedures reduce pets' risks of reproductive cancers.
- Provide a proper diet. Don't overfeed, and don't feed your pet table scraps. Ask your vet to recommend an appropriate diet.
- Exercise your pet. Consult your vet about a proper exercise regimen.
- Carefully observe your pet. If it exhibits a change in behavior or appetite, weight loss, fatigue, coughing, or a skin problem, visit the vet.

- Brush your pet's teeth. Visit the vet if you detect signs of gum disease: swollen, bleeding gums; pus; or loose teeth.
- Keep pet cages and sleeping areas clean. Keep cat litter boxes clean.
- Protect your pet from toxins. Keep poisons and medications—even aspirin—out of reach. Don't let pets nibble poisonous houseplants, and don't give pets chocolate, which is toxic to many animals.
- Make your home safe. Keep harmful objects from pets. Don't allow chewing pets near electrical cords.
- Never leave your pet in a car unattended, even on a mild day with windows opened.

Sources: American Animal Hospital Association; American Veterinary Medical Association; University of Illinois College of Veterinary Medicine.

Any smooth-surfaced plastic or enamel pan can be used as a litter box. Put the pan in a quiet spot. Place a layer of commercial clay litter, sand, sawdust, or sterilized soil in the bottom. Sift the litter clean with a strainer each day. Clean the pan and change the litter whenever a third of the litter is damp or, at least, every fourth day.

Most pets will enjoy good health with proper food, housing, and grooming. If a pet gets hurt, swallows something harmful, or otherwise becomes ill, it should be taken to a veterinarian. Don't try to treat your pet's illness yourself, unless you know exactly what is wrong and what to do. Home treatment may seriously delay finding out what is wrong with your pet, and may even harm the animal.

Common signs of illness in dogs include a change in behavior, a change in appetite, and fever. Most animals become less active when they are sick or injured. Any change of appetite that lasts for more than a few days calls for a veterinary examination. If there are other signs of illness such as vomiting, diarrhea, sneezing, or coughing, take your pet to a veterinarian as soon as possible.

Many pet illnesses—and their associated costs—can be prevented through good pet care. By providing pets with healthful diets, plenty of exercise, and regular visits to the veterinarian, owners will protect their pets as well as their pocketbooks. ●●●

For additional information:

Web sites

American Animal Hospital Association (AAHA)—
http://www.healthypet.com.

American Holistic Veterinary Medical Association (AHVMA)—
http://www.altvetmed.com.

American Veterinary Medical Association (AVMA)—
http://www.avma.org.

University of Illinois Veterinary Extension "Pet Columns"—
http://www.cvm.uiuc.edu/CEPS/index.html.

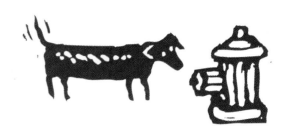

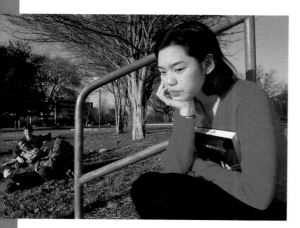

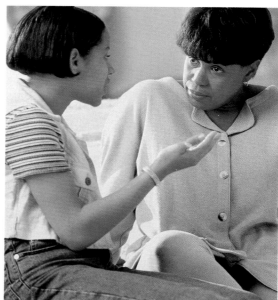

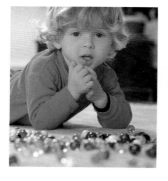

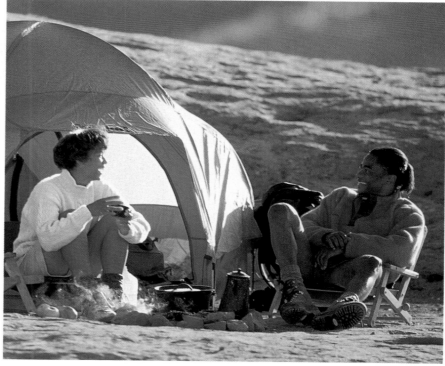

MEDICAL AND SAFETY ALERTS

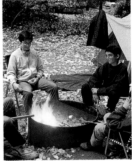

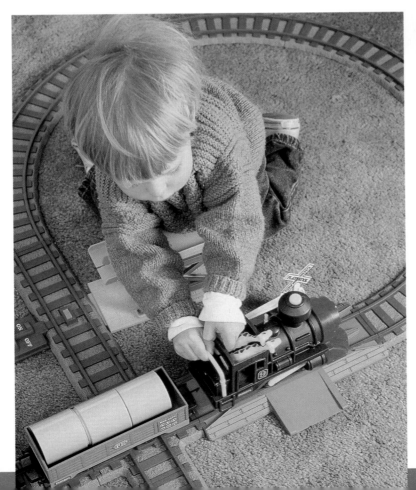

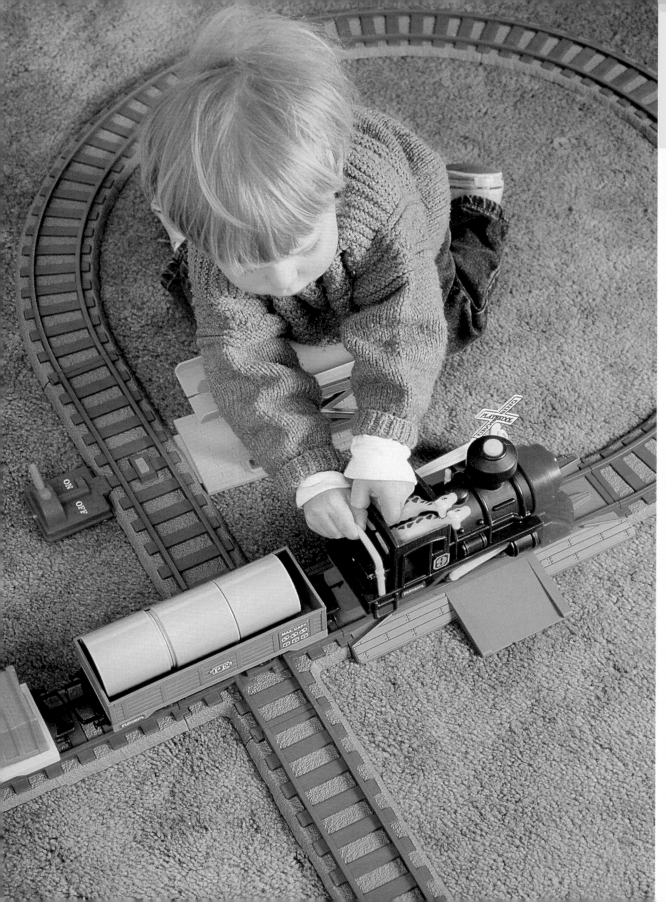

Selecting

SAFE TOYS

By Lorna Luebbers

More than 100,000
children are injured
in toy-related
accidents annually.
Parents can take
steps to prevent
most toy injuries.

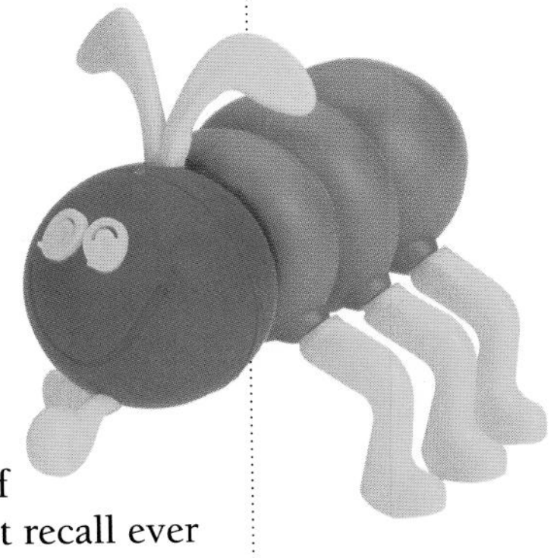

I N OCTOBER 1998, FISHER-PRICE, A TOY MAKER IN
East Aurora, New York, recalled almost 10 million of
its Power Wheel ride-on cars and trucks—the largest recall ever
involving a toy sold in stores. The Consumer Product Safety
Commission (CPSC) said the flawed electrical systems in the child-
sized roadsters sparked 150 fires that burned nine children and
caused $300,000 in property damage to 22 houses and garages. The
safety agency also received another 700 reports of electrical components failing or overheating, causing smoke or melted parts, and
complaints about the toys failing to stop when the foot pedal was
released.

Approximately 2 billion toys are sold annually in the United
States. Although most of these toys are safe, manufacturers recall
dozens of defective toys every year for causing injury to children.
Toys with no defects also can become dangerous if misused or
played with by children who are too young to use them safely.

More than 100,000 children are injured in toy-related accidents
every year, according to the CPSC, the federal agency that enforces
government regulations concerning the safety of all consumer products including toys. Falls and choking account for the majority of

toy-related injuries. Children also suffer strangulation, burns, drowning, and poisoning while playing with toys.

Most toy-related injuries are not life-threatening. Only 1 percent of children sustaining toy-related injuries are hospitalized, according to the CPSC. Occasionally, however, a toy maims or kills a child. In 1997, 13 children died in toy-related incidents.

The leading cause of toy-related death is choking. In 1997, 85 percent of toy-related deaths were due to choking, according to the CPSC. Riding toys, mostly tricycles, also have been involved in toy-related deaths. These deaths occurred when a child was hit by a motor vehicle while riding a toy or when a child rode a toy into a swimming pool, pond, or other body of water.

Children ages 4 and under are at highest risk for toy injury. In 1997, children ages 4 and under accounted for nearly 85 percent of toy-related fatalities and nearly 60 percent of all toy-related injuries, according to the CPSC. Small children are especially susceptible to choking on toys because of the small size of their upper airways and their natural desire to put everything in their mouths.

Why toys cause injury

Toy injuries occur for a number of reasons. Some toys cause injury because the product is defective. For example, in December 1998, Newell Rubbermaid Inc., of Wooster, Ohio, recalled 60,800 toboggans following reports that the sleds broke apart during use, causing injury. And in September 1998, Tara Toy Corporation of Hauppauge, New York, recalled 670,000 Flying Warrior dolls after the dolls broke off in mid-flight, causing serious eye injuries in two children.

In some cases, a toy is harmful not because it is defective, but because it is inherently unsafe. The most famous example of this type of toy is the lawn dart—a sharply pointed projectile that annually injured some 650 people, mostly children, until the CPSC banned its sale and manufacture in 1988. Another such toy is the aluminized polyester film kite, banned by the CPSC after some users were electrocuted when their kites tangled in power lines.

Most toys that harm children, however, do not cause injury through malfunction or unsafe design. They cause injury when used by children who are too young or inexperienced to play with them in the manner intended by the manufacturer. The toys are, in fact, perfectly safe when used properly. Balloons, for example, pose almost no health risk to children when used appropriately. Yet, balloons that are misused by children cause almost half of all choking deaths from toys. Nearly 50 children choked to death in the 1990's after stuffing balloons in their mouths, according to the National Safe Kids Campaign, a nonprofit organization that attempts to prevent childhood injury.

Some toys that are safe for older children may pose a health hazard to younger children. Toys that contain small balls or parts are unsafe for small children, who could choke on the tiny pieces. Even

The author:

Lorna Luebbers is a free-lance writer.

button eyes on stuffed toys can choke a small child to death. Yet, the same toy may pose no choking danger to older children, who have larger throats and are less likely to mouth objects.

Other toys may pose an invisible threat to children. Government studies show that hazardous chemicals can be found in or on some toys. As recently as 1994, for example, the CPSC discovered that certain brands of imported crayons contained hazardous levels of lead. Children who chewed on the crayons were at risk of developing lead poisoning, a condition that can cause damage to the brain, nerves, red blood cells, and digestive system.

Research released in November 1998 by the nonprofit environmental groups Greenpeace and the National Environment Trust stated that numerous toys used by children contain a chemical that caused cancer in laboratory animals. The studies' figures proved that up to 20 percent of toys in the United States contain *phthalates*, a widely used plastic additive that gives plastic toys a softer, more pliable feel. By 1999, most large toy companies had stopped using phthalate additives.

Pesticides (insect-killing substances) are another toxic risk. A study released in January

Thousands of children are injured every year while playing with toys. The majority of injuries occur when children are allowed to play without adult supervision.

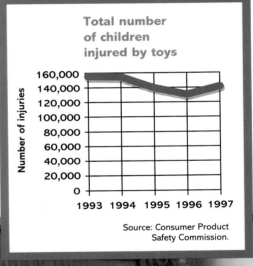

Total number of children injured by toys

Number of injuries

160,000
140,000
120,000
100,000
80,000
60,000
40,000
20,000
0

1993 1994 1995 1996 1997

Source: Consumer Product Safety Commission.

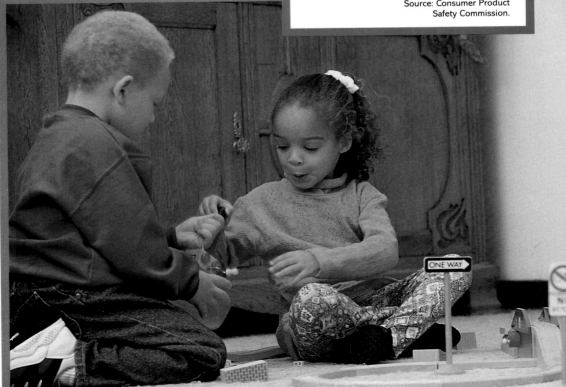

1998 showed that pesticides tend to stick to toys at dangerously high levels. Researchers at Rutgers University in New Jersey sprayed an apartment with pesticide. An hour later, they placed toys throughout the apartment. Two weeks after spraying, the researchers examined the pesticide residue on the toys. They concluded that children playing with the toys would be exposed to 20 times the government-recommended daily amount of pesticide.

Industry safety controls

The toy manufacturing industry is the first line of defense against toy injury. The Toy Manufacturers of America (TMA), an association that includes the producers of 85 percent of all toys sold in the United States, is the industry's most powerful regulatory arm. Safety experts rank the standards set by the TMA as the most comprehensive in the world. For example, the TMA requires that toy makers perform rigorous safety testing on products, sometimes requiring more than 100 safety tests on a single toy. Among other safety factors, manufacturers evaluate a toy based on a child's age and skill level. They then label the product with an age designation to help parents and other adults choose safe and suitable toys.

In 1997, more 1-year-olds were killed in toy-related accidents than any other age group. A total of 13 children under age 7 died that year from accidents involving toys.

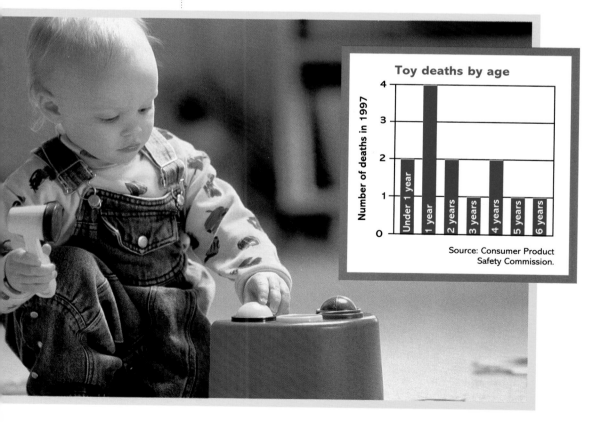

Toy deaths by age

Number of deaths in 1997

Under 1 year · 1 year · 2 years · 3 years · 4 years · 5 years · 6 years

Source: Consumer Product Safety Commission.

Industry standards are sometimes tougher than safety laws. For example, in 1998, the TMA prohibited its members from using any lead in toy production. In contrast, the Federal Hazardous Substance Act prohibits only hazardous amounts of poisonous material, such as lead, in toy manufacturing.

Government's role in toy safety

In addition to voluntary industry standards, toy makers must also meet safety requirements set by the federal government. For example, federal law mandates that toys for children under 8 years of age contain no glass or metal edges. In addition, the Child Safety Protection Act of 1994 regulates safety labeling on toys and games. The act requires that toy makers post hazard labels on toys containing small parts, such as balls or marbles, that may cause choking in children aged 6 and under. It also bans the use of balls smaller than 1.75 inches (4.4 centimeters) in toys for children under age 3. Congress enacted these strict labeling requirements in 1994 after looser regulations set in 1979 proved to have too many loopholes for toy manufacturers to abuse.

Companies that do not adhere to federal safety standards can be investigated and prosecuted by the CPSC. In December 1998, for example, the CPSC charged that Small World Toys Inc. of Culver City, California, imported and sold toys that violated the Federal Hazardous Substances Act. The CPSC fined the company $225,000.

Federal law requires that toy makers report any product defects to the CPSC. Companies that fail to do so can be fined up to $1.5 million. Laws also require toy makers to report any toy-related injuries to the CPSC.

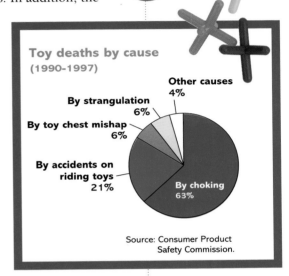

Toy deaths by cause (1990-1997)

- Other causes 4%
- By strangulation 6%
- By toy chest mishap 6%
- By accidents on riding toys 21%
- By choking 63%

Source: Consumer Product Safety Commission.

Choking is the leading cause of toy-related fatalities, followed by riding toy accidents.

Toy recalls

In the event that a toy causes injury to a child, the CPSC may demand that the toy maker recall the product. In October 1998, for example, the CPSC announced that a xylophone made by Playwell Toy Inc. of Lake Forest, California, included parts smaller than allowed by the Child Safety Protection Act of 1994. According to the CPSC, the rounded ends of the xylophone mallets could become lodged in the throats of small children and block their airways. The CPSC asked the toy maker to recall xylophones after a six-month-old girl suffered severe brain damage as a result of choking on one of the mallets.

Selecting safe toys

- Read and heed age recommendations and any hazard labels on toy packaging.

- Reject toys or parts that could fit in mouths of children 3 years or younger. Avoid marbles, balls, or pieces less than 1.75 inches (4.4 cm) in diameter. If an item can fit through the hollow tube of a toilet tissue roll, it's a hazard.

- Don't buy toys with strings, cords, or necklaces for children under 3. Such items could pose strangulation hazards.

- Look for well-made toys with tightly secured eyes, noses, and other parts. Such parts could pose choking hazards if they pull off.

- Don't buy toys made of thin, brittle plastic, or glass that might break, creating sharp edges.

- Avoid old, recycled toys that are painted; they might contain unsafe levels of lead.

- Buy child-safe toy chests or boxes. Look for a box with ventilation holes and with a removable lid or lid with spring-loaded support.

- Reject loud toys, which could cause hearing damage. Use this rule: if noise made by the toy hurts an adult's ear, don't buy it.

- Avoid toys that might contain toxic substances. Be wary of art supplies, nail polish, and makeup sets. Reject anything containing toulene. Look for the following designation, indicating review by a toxicologist: *ASTM D-4236.*

Sources: Consumer Product Safety Commission (CFSC); Toy Manufacturer's Association (TMA); U.S. Public Interest Research Groups (PIRG).

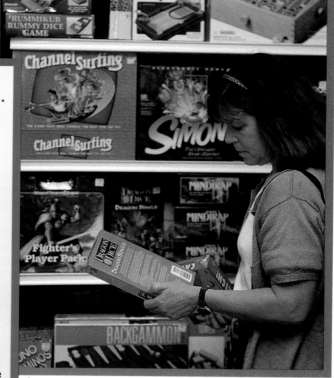

Selecting toys is an important responsibility of parents and other adults. Determining age-appropriateness and checking for hazard labels are key steps in the process.

The manufacturer is responsible for repairing, replacing, or refunding the cost of recalled toys. Toy makers almost always cooperate with the CPSC in product recalls. If a company refuses to recall a toy, however, the CPSC can force them to recall the toy with a court order.

The most difficult part of a recall is informing the public. The CPSC and the toy maker attempt to publicize a recall through press releases, advertisements, store postings, and announcements on web sites. The most effective way to notify toy owners is through product registration or warranty cards. However, only a small percent of individuals bother to submit this important information to manufacturers after purchasing a product. In many cases, recalled toys remain in children's hands because their parents either never learned of the recall or never bothered to send the toy back to the manufacturer. In 1997, for example, a 7-year-old Indiana boy suffered a brain injury after his skull was pierced with a lawn dart, which the CPSC had recalled nearly 10 years before.

Several citizen action groups also monitor toy safety. Public Interest Research Groups (PIRG), a leading citizen action association with local branches in most states, conducts its own toy safety studies. PIRG annually publishes a report on toy safety and maintains a web site offering toy safety information.

How adults can prevent toy-related injuries

Government and industry regulation does much to protect children from toy-related injuries, but parents and other adults are chiefly responsible for toy safety. By reading labels on toys, examining toys before giving them to children, teaching children how to use toys correctly, and supervising play, adults can prevent most toy injuries.

Safety begins with selection of an appropriate toy. The National Safe Kids Campaign advises adults to buy age-appropriate toys and

Toys and choking: hazard labels

Federal law requires that toy manufacturers post hazard labels on certain toys. For example, the Child Safety Protection Act of 1994 requires that toy makers post hazard labels on toys containing small parts that may cause choking in children ages 6 and under. Many manufacturers also label toys with an age designation to help adults choose safe toys. Safety labels contain a triangular hazard icon, a warning heading, and a description of the choking hazard. Safety labels commonly found on toy packaging include:

- This toy is a small ball. Not for children under 3.
- This toy contains a small ball. Not for children under 3.
- Small parts. Not for children under 3.
- Children under 8 can choke or suffocate on uninflated or broken balloons. Adult supervision required. Keep uninflated balloons from children. Discard broken balloons at once.
- Toy contains a marble. Not for children under 3.

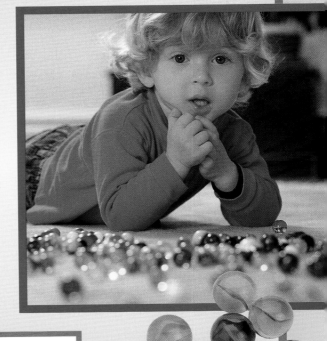

**WARNING:
CHOKING HAZARD:**
This toy is a marble.
Not For Children Under 3.

to keep toys designed for older children away from younger siblings. When purchasing a toy for a child under 6 years of age, carefully check for choking hazard labels. Make sure the toy's package has not been opened before purchase.

After purchasing the toy, examine it for cracks, sharp edges, and loose pieces that could end up in a child's mouth. Strings longer than 12 inches (30.5 centimeters) pose a strangulation hazard for young children. If a toy or toy part fits inside a cardboard toilet paper tube, then it poses a choking danger for children under age 3, according to the CPSC. Check stuffed animals for loose eyes and other sewn-on objects. Do not let children under age 8 play with balloons.

Once you bring the toy home, discard any plastic packaging immediately to prevent a child from choking on it. Before you allow a child to play with a toy, read the instructions, and explain its proper use to the child.

The CPSC recommends that toys requiring the use of fire or heat, such as wood-burning kits, toy ovens, and chemistry sets, never be given to children under age 12. Older children using these toys require adult supervision.

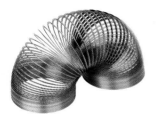

Parents should also closely supervise children playing with projectile toys or toys with flying parts, such as darts or rockets. Also, check the noise level of each toy to prevent hearing damage to the children who play with it.

Maintenance is another important safety factor. Adults should regularly check the working condition of toys. Wooden toys may develop sharp edges and splinters, for example, and metal toys may rust. Repair or dispose of worn or broken toys. Never repaint a toy using older paint; it may contain lead.

Instruct older children to keep their toys out of reach of younger siblings. And, finally, require that children put their toys away in a safe place after play.

Selecting age-appropriate toys

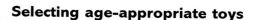

In addition to safety factors, adults should also consider a child's intellectual and physical development when choosing a toy. The American Academy of Pediatrics has established guidelines to help adults select toys that provide stimulation for children in different age groups. According to these guidelines, appropriate toys for infants (newborn to 1 year old) include those that stimulate senses of sight, hearing, and touch. Large wood or plastic blocks, rattles, soft washable animals or dolls, and squeeze toys are suitable toys for infants. Rattles should be new, sturdy, and not subject to breakage.

Toys appropriate for toddlers, ages 1 to 2 years, help them begin their exploration of the world around them. Appropriate toys include picture books of cloth or plastic, sturdy dolls, kid-sized vehi-

Some toys recalled in 1998-1999

Toy and manufacturer	Hazard	Any injuries reported?	Action taken in recall
Plastic toy storage chest (IRIS U.S.A., Inc.)	Lid could close, entrapping child; because chest lacks ventilation holes, child could suffocate.	no	Manufacturer offers refund; remarkets product with "not for use by children" hazard label.
VeggieTales' Dave and the Giant Pickle playset (Chariot Victor Publishing)	Plastic plug in base of some figurines can detach, creating a choking hazard.	no	Manufacturer offers refund or replacement with safe figurines.
Toy basketball set (Ohio Art; Little Tikes; Today's Kids; Fisher-Price)	Net cords that become unhooked from hoop rim present strangulation hazard for small children.	yes	Manufacturers will replace net with reengineered net that does not pose hazard.
Stuffed crab toy (Great American Toy Co. Inc.)	Crab antennas have sharp points that present puncture hazard.	no	Manufacturer offers refund or safe replacement toy.
Child's jewelry set (Almar Sales Co. Inc.)	Detachable plastic beads from necklace and bracelet pose choking hazard.	no	Manufacturer offers refund.
Bubble Beauties floating balls (K•B Toys)	Ball contains a toxic petroleum substance that could be harmful or fatal if swallowed.	no	Manufacturer offers refund.
Hot dog-shaped pedal car decorated with decals (Oscar Mayer Foods Corp.)	Decals contain high levels of lead, presenting toxic hazard.	no	Manufacturer offers safe replacement decals.
Mascot Plushes animal toy (Sanrio Inc.)	Small bell can detach, presenting a choking hazard.	no	Manufacturer offers refund.

Source: U. S. Consumer Product Safety Commission (CPSC).

Safe use and maintenance of toys

- Discard all packaging in a new toy. Plastic wrapping poses a suffocation hazard, and plastic peanuts pose a choking hazard in young children.

- Keep product literature and send in warranty cards. If the toy is recalled, the product registration will help the manufacturer locate you.

- Read and keep toy instructions. Make sure that children who will play with the toy understand how to use it.

- Keep balloons from children under 8 years old. Uninflated or broken balloons are the number one choking hazard.

- Remove *crib gyms* (toys that are stretched across an infant's crib) when the child is old enough to pull up on its hands and knees. Some children have strangled when they fell across their crib gyms.

- Never hang toys with string, cord, necklaces, or bead strings, particularly if the toys are used by children under age 3.

- Wash stuffed and cloth toys frequently. Soiled fabrics can become breeding grounds for germs.

- Teach older children to keep their toys from younger siblings. Toys that are safe for the designated age may be unsafe for younger children.

- Supervise play with projectile toys, which have the potential to blind or deafen a child. Teach children never to aim darts, arrows, or other projectile objects at others.

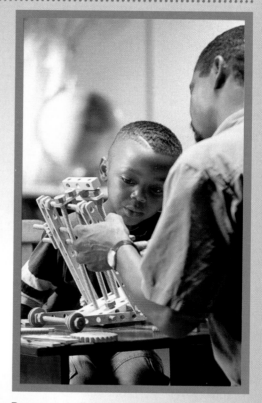

Parents can eliminate most toy-related injuries by teaching their children how to properly use a toy and by supervising play.

- Inspect toys frequently for breakage and potential hazards, such as loose parts, sharp points, or splintered edges. Especially check outdoor toys for corrosion or rust. Repair or discard damaged toys immediately.

Sources: Consumer Product Safety Commission (CPSC); Toy Manufacturer's Association (TMA); U.S. Public Interest Research Groups (PIRG).

cles that are foot-powered, nesting blocks, push-pull toys (with strings no longer than 12 inches), and toy telephones (avoid phones that accept coins or those that ring loudly).

Toys for preschoolers, aged 3 to 5, should allow for experimentation and also imitation of older children and adults. These toys include books, simple puzzles with large pieces, nontoxic crayons or finger paints, and nontoxic clays. Outdoor toys include sandbox (with lid), slide, swing, and transportation toys, such as tricycles and wagons.

Toys for school-age children, aged 6 to 9, should promote skill development and creativity. Children in this age group enjoy making things out of paper, and toys that involve drawing, cutting, and pasting are appropriate. Other toys that children in this age group might enjoy include hand puppets, card and table games, jump ropes, and bicycles.

The guidelines recommend crafts and science-based toys for preteens and young teens, aged 10 through 14. These toys include computer games; sewing, knitting, and needlework kits; microscopes and telescopes; and hobby equipment. Sporting equipment, with the appropriate safety accessories, such as a helmet for bike riding, is also an appropriate choice.

Parents and other adults share responsibility with toy manufacturers in protecting children from toy injury, safety experts point out. With wise, careful selection of age-appropriate toys and instruction on their proper use in play, parents can help prevent almost all toy-related accidents. ●●●

For additional information:

Recall information
U.S. Consumer Product Safety Commission Recall Roundup phone line: 1-800-638-2772.

Web sites
Public Interest Research Groups (PIRG)— http://www.pirg.org/consumer/

Toy Manufacturers of America (TMA)— http://www.toy-tma.com.

U.S. Consumer Product Safety Commission (CPSC)—http://www.cpsc.gov

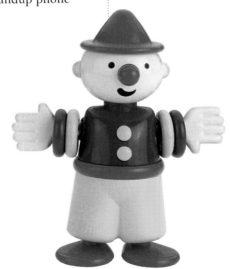

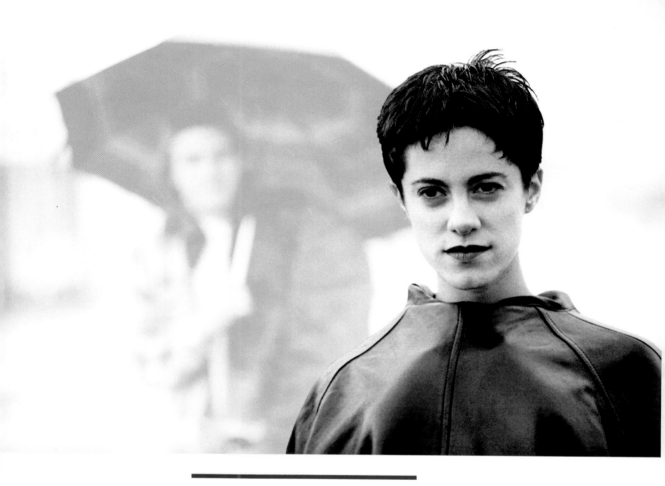

The number of teen suicides
increased throughout the 1990's.
But there are steps parents can take
to reduce the risk for their child.

Teen Suicide:
A Growing Concern

By Vivian Auerbach

P AUL, A LONELY HIGH-SCHOOL DROP-OUT, gives his favorite leather jacket to a younger brother. Sarah, a gifted student, fails three classes in one semester. Michael, a 13-year-old with a history of aggressive and delinquent behavior, suddenly becomes quiet and withdrawn. What do these teen-agers have in common? All exhibit behaviors that are warning signs of suicide. In the 1990's, teens turned to suicide with alarming frequency as a tragic "solution" to their adolescent problems.

Suicide is the third leading cause of death among adolescents (individuals between 10 and 19 years old) and young adults (ages 20 to 24). Only accidents and homicides killed more teens in the 1990's. According to a report by the U.S. Centers for Health Statistics (NCHS) in Hyattsville, Maryland, the rate of suicide in the 15- to 24-year-old age group almost tripled since 1960. More than 4,300 young people took their own lives in 1996 (the most recent year for which statistics were available) compared with 1,500 in 1960.

Unfortunately, the situation is probably much worse than the statistics suggest, because suicides may be grossly underreported for many reasons. In some cases, a suicide may look like an accident. Coroners often fail to record a death as a suicide if a suicide note has not been found. Families may also attempt to classify a suicide as an accident because of the shame and guilt associated with suicide.

NCHS estimates that 8 to 25 adolescents try unsuccessfully to commit suicide for every one that succeeds. In fact, many teen-agers try to commit suicide at least once before they succeed. A 1998 study by the Centers for Disease Control and Prevention in Atlanta (CDC) reported that 10 percent of teen-agers have attempted suicide. In a survey of high school students, about 65 percent of the students revealed that they had thought about suicide or engaged in suicidal behavior. As many as 13 percent of the teens reported that they had attempted suicide at least once. More than 60 percent of the teens said they knew someone who had attempted suicide.

Boys are at greater risk

Most teen-agers who commit suicide are white males. However, during the 1980's and 1990's, the suicide rates of African American and Native American teen-age boys rose significantly as well. A 1998 study by the CDC found that the rate of suicide among black male teen-agers more than doubled since 1980. Researchers also found that the gap between black and white teen-age suicides was narrowing—in 1980, the rate for white males ages 10 to 19 was more than twice the rate for black males, but in 1995, the rate for white males was only 42 percent higher. Suicides among black teen-age girls increased also, but those rates were much lower than for boys.

Although teen-age boys are nearly five times as likely as girls to commit suicide, according to NCHS figures, girls are much more likely to attempt suicide. Boys succeed more often, in large part, because they tend to choose more deadly means. In the mid-1990's, suicide by gunshot accounted for more than 60 percent of all deaths from suicide. Nearly three-fourths of male teen-agers who killed themselves used guns. Individuals who try to commit suicide but do not succeed are more likely to ingest poison or take overdoses of medication, particularly pain relievers, such as aspirin or acetaminophen. In some cases, teens misjudge the dangers of over-the-counter medications, unintentionally taking an overdose that results in death or disability.

Researchers cite no conclusive cause for the rise in teen suicides. Some believe that the rise can be blamed on the increasing availability of deadly weapons. They point to a 1998 study by the CDC that reported that roughly 1 in 5 teen-agers carries a weapon. According to psychologists, other leading factors include the splintering of community and family support networks, the rise in alcohol and drug use, and the adoption of coping behaviors in which suicide is more commonly used in response to depression and hopelessness.

Why do some teens attempt suicide?

For many teens, presuicidal behavior represents a cry for help. If that cry is left unanswered, the teen-ager could seek a deadly solution to what he or she sees as an insolvable problem. Many factors can place an adolescent at risk for a suicide attempt. Teens may be impulsive or may abuse substances, which further limit their judgment. They may experience low self-esteem or an emotional problem, such as depression. Having a history of suicide in the family or a friend who has committed suicide makes depression more likely and can demonstrate that suicide is an option for escaping a painful situation. Family disruption or family conflict may add to a teen's isolation and reduce sources of support. When such problems exist, additional stress in school or a personal disappointment may be the "last straw," precipitating a suicidal act.

According to psychologists, suicidal thoughts and behaviors arise from problems in coping that are often associated with one or more psychological conditions such as depression, anxiety, *bipolar disorder* (manic depression), and schizophrenia. Such disorders are often overlooked and undiagnosed, particularly early in life. As a result, most teens who kill themselves have never been diagnosed with a mental illness and have never received mental health treatment.

Depression is the emotional disorder most commonly associated with suicidal behavior. While all teen-agers experience sadness, grief, frustration, and disappointment from time to time, sometimes sadness becomes so intense and severe that it interferes with a person's ability to lead a normal, productive life. When such sadness persists for weeks and months, the problem has progressed to the emotional disorder of depression and should be treated.

Depression is an illness with both emotional and physical symptoms. In fact, many of the behavioral changes that are considered warning signs of suicide are actually symptoms of depression. These

The author:

Vivian Auerbach is a consulting neuropsychologist in Atlanta, Georgia, and an adjunct associate professor of psychology at Emory University.

Young adults face a greater risk for committing suicide than any other age group. The suicide rate for teens and young adults has increased significantly since the 1960's.

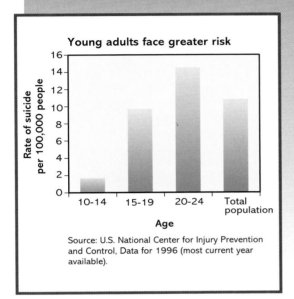

Young adults face greater risk

Source: U.S. National Center for Injury Prevention and Control, Data for 1996 (most current year available).

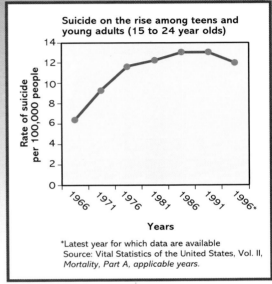

Suicide on the rise among teens and young adults (15 to 24 year olds)

*Latest year for which data are available
Source: Vital Statistics of the United States, Vol. II, *Mortality, Part A, applicable years.*

include changes in eating and sleeping habits, anxiety, inability to concentrate, a tendency to be uncommunicative, and a pervasive sense of hopelessness. In addition, recent research has demonstrated alterations in brain chemistry in people with psychiatric illnesses such as depression and schizophrenia. Medications to treat these disorders act to alter the abnormal brain chemistry, resulting in improved mood or thinking.

Researchers studying the link between heredity and depression have found that the rate of depression is higher among people who have relatives who are depressed than among those who do not. This finding suggests that the tendency to develop the condition may be inherited. For example, studies have shown that identical twins—who have an identical genetic makeup—have higher rates of suicidal behavior than *fraternal* (nonidentical) twins, who do not have identical genes. This genetic factor may help explain why suicides are more common in some families than in others.

The role that families play

In addition to depression, other psychological problems are more often present in the families of suicidal adolescents than in the families of other teen-agers. These problems include addictive and abu-

Males at greater risk

Males aged 15 to 24 in all ethnic or racial groups are more likely to commit suicide than females.

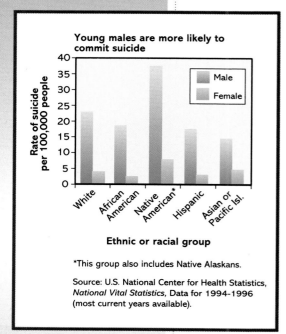

Young males are more likely to commit suicide

Rate of suicide per 100,000 people

Ethnic or racial group

White / African American / Native American* / Hispanic / Asian or Pacific Isl.

*This group also includes Native Alaskans.

Source: U.S. National Center for Health Statistics, *National Vital Statistics,* Data for 1994-1996 (most current years available).

sive behaviors. One result of such a family situation is that the teen receives little parental care or support. Dysfunctional families may teach the wrong lessons about how to cope and may fail to provide necessary security and emotional support. Consequently, the teen is deficient in just those coping and problem-solving skills necessary for dealing with the challenges of growing up.

In addition, factors such as poor self-esteem, depression, and behavioral problems often lead to withdrawal and social isolation from family and peers. Lack of peer acceptance further isolates the troubled teen and contributes to his or her despair. A young person in such a situation may feel unwanted by family and friends. Lacking the skills needed to cope with his or her problems, the teen may feel more hopeless and depressed. Such feelings can lead to a vicious cycle in which the teen alienates others and withdraws, becoming more and more isolated from possible sources of support. Many suicidal teens run away from home and have a history of delinquency and problems with the law. Studies have shown that teen-agers in prison are at particularly high risk for suicide.

Teen-agers who have strong emotional attachments to their parents, on the other hand, are much less likely to attempt suicide. A 1997 study published in the *Journal of the American Medical Association* found that teens who feel loved, understood, and paid attention to by their parents were more likely to avoid high-risk behaviors regardless of whether they came from a one- or two-parent household.

Other factors involved in teen suicide

Researchers have found that a least a third of adolescents who committed suicide were intoxicated at the time and many more were under the influence of drugs. According to experts, all teen-agers who abuse drugs or alcohol are at increased risk of suicidal behavior. Some teens who drink alcohol or take drugs may be attempting to mask their feelings of hopelessness and despondency. These substances also heighten impulsivity and aggression and weaken an individual's ability to make good judgements and cope with everyday life. Ironically, some substances that are abused may heighten depression. Alcohol or other drug use can therefore promote risky or self-destructive behaviors or may be a symptom of underlying emotional problems. Thus, in either case, substance use significantly adds to a teen's risk of suicide.

Both the academic and social aspects of school play a major role in the lives of most adolescents, and many suicidal teen-agers have

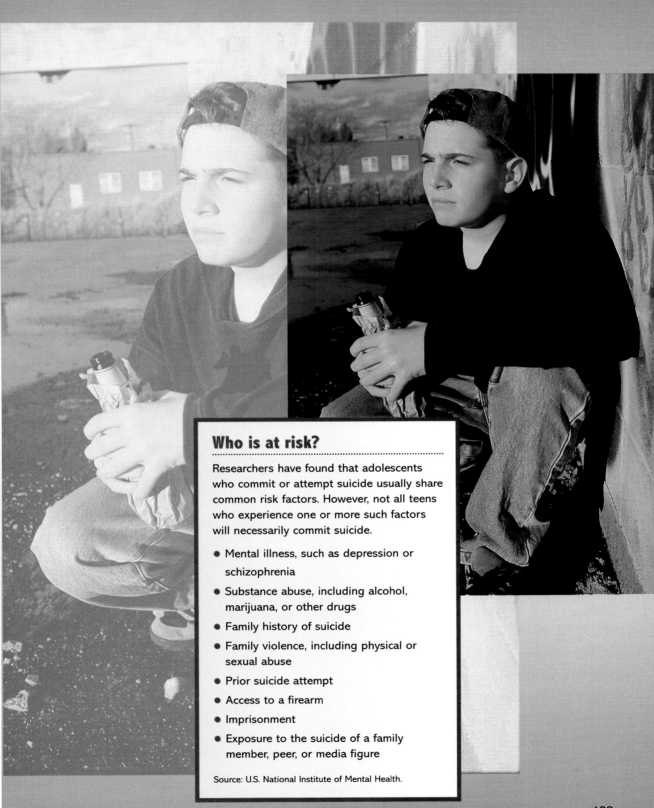

Who is at risk?

Researchers have found that adolescents who commit or attempt suicide usually share common risk factors. However, not all teens who experience one or more such factors will necessarily commit suicide.

- Mental illness, such as depression or schizophrenia
- Substance abuse, including alcohol, marijuana, or other drugs
- Family history of suicide
- Family violence, including physical or sexual abuse
- Prior suicide attempt
- Access to a firearm
- Imprisonment
- Exposure to the suicide of a family member, peer, or media figure

Source: U.S. National Institute of Mental Health.

189

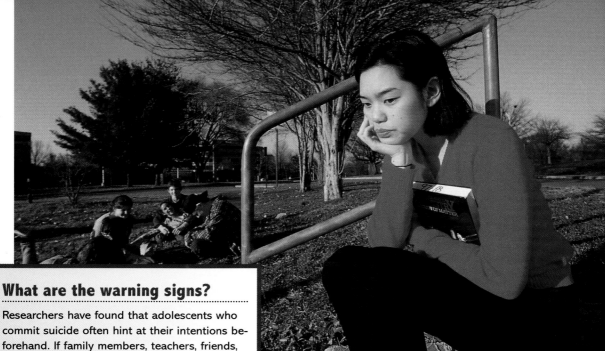

What are the warning signs?

Researchers have found that adolescents who commit suicide often hint at their intentions beforehand. If family members, teachers, friends, or others learn to recognize the warning signs, they may be able to prevent the suicide.

- Verbal hints (statements such as "My family would be better off without me" and "I wish I were dead")
- Preoccupation with themes of death or suicide in own writing or in literature, art, or music
- Giving away possessions
- Drop in grades
- Loss of interest in usual activities
- Withdrawal from friends and family
- Change in eating patterns (either sudden weight loss or gain)
- Change in sleeping patterns (either insomnia or oversleeping)
- Neglecting personal appearance
- Reckless behavior

Sources: Vivian Auerbach; Capuzzi, Dave, and Golden, Larry. *Preventing Adolescent Suicide.* Accelerated Development Inc., 1988.

trouble in school. They tend to be emotionally withdrawn from their classmates, with under-achievement and poor scholastic performance characterizing their presuicidal behavior. Some of these teens may have experienced academic problems early in life because of a learning disability, attention-deficit disorder, or a behavioral problem. Early academic frustrations can evolve into more serious conduct and delinquency problems when the child reaches adolescence.

Other suicidal young people feel highly pressured to do well in school. They set unrealistic expectations for themselves and sink into despair when they fail to meet these goals. Even if they are academically capable, such depressed and potentially suicidal adolescents are rarely pleased with their performance. This ill-perceived sense of failure often increases despair and hopelessness and may lead the adolescent to fear further loss of recognition from parents or others who expect excellence.

The suicide of a family member or friend can serve as a trigger to a troubled teen who had been contemplating suicide. Adolescents are often highly suggestible and eager to imitate others as they search to establish their own identity. So for vulnerable adolescents, who lack positive role models and tend to have low self-esteem, the influence of another person's suicide can be profound. Studies of teens who have experienced the suicide of a family member or friend have shown that adolescents may develop depressive psychiatric disorders that result in recurrent, longstanding depression and presuicidal behavior. Some theorists have suggested that adolescents who experience the suicide of a family member or friend are at double the risk of suicide. These teens are not only burdened with the disturbing emotional effect of the death, but they have also witnessed a graphic demonstration that suicide is an option.

Some researchers claim that celebrity suicides trigger suicidal behavior in teens. These experts say that sensationalistic or romanticized presentations in the media—particularly if the reports include details about the method the celebrity used to commit suicide—can provoke vulnerable teens to kill themselves. For example, several copy-cat suicides followed the 1994 suicide of Kurt Cobain of the rock group Nirvana. In 1997, two teen-age girls in France told friends that they planned to commit suicide like Cobain. The girls shot themselves in the head while listening to a Nirvana tape. Media reports are not thought to provoke suicide in people who are not already at risk, but they may suggest means or encourage imitation in teens who are already disturbed.

Doctors emphasize that possession of one of the risk factors for suicide does not mean that a teen-ager will attempt suicide. In fact, many individuals with one or more risk factors never exhibit suicidal behavior. Generally, doctors believe that suicidal risk accumulates with the number of risk factors. Thus, depression combined with substance abuse, a conduct disorder, and family problems poses a far greater threat than any one of these factors alone.

The warning signs of suicide

Prediction and intervention have become important goals in suicide prevention. According to the American Academy of Child and Adolescent Psychiatry, approximately three-fourths of all teen-agers who consider suicide give verbal or behavioral clues to a family member or friend before committing suicide. Some teen-agers directly threaten to kill themselves by saying such things as "You won't have to worry about me much longer." Others may be more vague, saying that they are tired of being a burden to their family and friends. They may talk about life as "hopeless" or complain of feeling "helpless." Still others may express their intent in poetry, essays, or art.

In addition, major behavioral changes may indicate an individual is considering suicide. The teen's grades may fall, or he or she may lose interest in sports or other extracurricular activities. The teen may withdraw from friends and family and eat or sleep much more or much less than normal. Friends and family members may notice that the teen no longer cares about personal appearance. The teen may suddenly become more rebellious, angry, or violent. He or she may also engage in risk-taking behavior, such as reckless driving or drug and alcohol abuse.

Making final arrangements is another behavioral clue that a teen is considering suicide. For example, a teen-ager may give away his or her treasured possessions or write drafts of a suicide note.

Previous suicide attempts are, perhaps, the most important warning of suicidal risk. Studies have found that 4 out of 5 people who kill themselves have previously attempted suicide.

Help and treatment for suicidal teens

Doctors recommend that any sign of suicide be taken seriously. Psychologists warn against offering simple solutions to a seriously depressed person. Pat advice to "snap out of it" is not helpful and trivializes the distress and hopelessness the teen is experiencing.

Parents or teachers who recognize warning signs of suicidal behavior in a teen should express support and concern. Through sympathetic discussion, a parent or friend may convince the troubled teen that someone cares. Limiting the teen's isolation may open avenues for additional support and treatment.

Friends of the troubled teen may pick up on suicidal signs before parents and teachers. Suicide prevention programs advise teens not to be afraid to talk to a friend who may be contemplating suicide. Experts say that friends should listen, ask questions, and find out how their friend feels and why those feelings persist.

Friends and family, however, are limited in their abilities to alter self-destructive behavior. When the risk of suicide exists, doctors emphasize that a teen needs the professional help available at a suicide-prevention center or a mental health clinic. Parents, teachers, or friends who recognize suicidal behavior should never leave the troubled teen alone until they receive medical treatment. The person trying to help the teen can call a crisis hotline, a local mental health association, or the teen's family doctor. A friend of the suicidal teen should also alert a parent, school counselor, or other trusted adult.

For teen-agers in the throes of a suicidal crisis and for those suffering from serious depression that could lead to suicide, there are a number of medications and therapies that are effective in relieving symptoms. Antidepressant medications help regulate mood, sleep, and appetite symptoms. Other medications can stabilize mood in bipolar disorders or treat the disturbed thinking and perceptions in psychotic conditions such as schizophrenia. Drug therapy, however, may take several weeks to be effective and must therefore be combined with other immediate mental health treatments.

Doctors have found that short-term crisis intervention is sometimes helpful in dealing with troubled teens. A single intervention, however, is usually inadequate to treat the underlying problems that put a person at risk for suicide. Therefore, suicidal teens need consistent, ongoing mental health support. When a teen-ager's life is at risk, hospitalization may be necessary.

What are the treatment options?

While certain intervention measures may save a teen's life, longer treatment is critical in preventing the adolescent from making another suicide attempt.

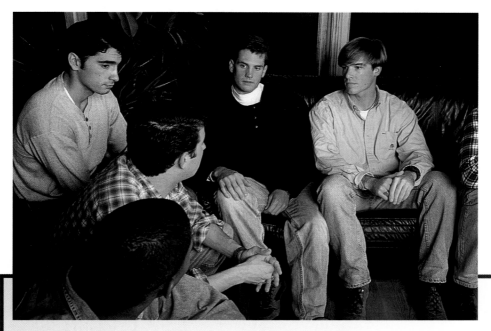

Intervention

- Take every suicide threat seriously.
- Listen to the teen without being judgmental or offering quick solutions to problems.
- Express your concern.
- Do not be afraid to ask directly whether the teen is considering suicide.
- Do not leave the teen alone.
- Make sure the teen does not have access to firearms or other weapons.
- Contact someone who can help, such as a suicide hotline, a local mental health organization, the teen's family doctor, or a school counselor.

Source: Capuzzi, Dave, and Golden, Larry. *Preventing Adolescent Suicide.* Accelerated Development, Inc., 1988.

Treatment

- Group therapy, through which teens can learn that others share similar problems and explore possible solutions.
- Individual therapy, which provides support and permits teens to unlearn destructive patterns of thinking and behaving.
- Social skills training, which can help teens increase their confidence and social competence.
- Programs that gradually help increase activity levels, for teens who have become socially isolated.
- Medication, for teens with such mental illnesses as depression and schizophrenia.
- Substance abuse programs, for teens who have become dependent on alcohol, marijuana, or other drugs in an effort to deal with their underlying problems.

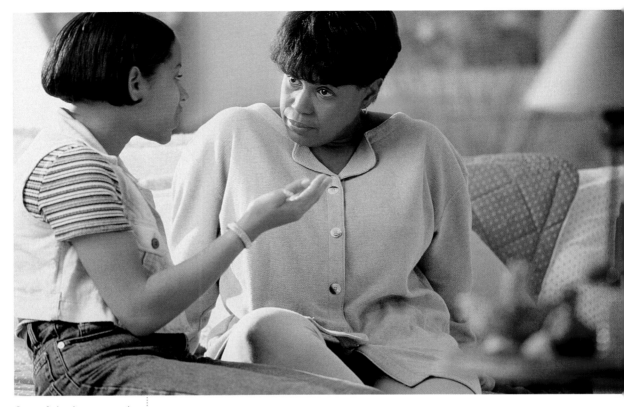

One of the best ways in which parents can help their teen-agers avoid suicide is by talking with them frequently and listening to them attentively. Parents who cope well with their own problems can also serve as role models for teens and reassure them that they are loved and valued members of the family.

Therapists design a treatment program depending on the nature of the problem and the situation or setting in which the adolescent lives. Teens diagnosed with depression, for example, may take antidepressant medication and attend an individual or a group counseling session. Group counseling helps teens realize that they are not alone in their situation. It also allows them to practice new coping strategies and problem solving skills with their peers. Some teens require social skills training to increase their confidence or to reduce inappropriate behaviors. Lonely, withdrawn teens are often helped by a program that gradually increases their participation in activities. Suicidal teens who also have a drug or alcohol abuse problem may need to enter a drug rehabilitation program.

Unfortunately, not all interventions succeed. Some teens commit suicide even in places such as psychiatric hospitals that are designed to provide intensive treatment and supervision. A person who is determined to commit suicide may find a way to do so despite the best efforts of the people who try to help.

When a teen does commit suicide, friends, family members, and other people who were close to the teen will likely suffer intense feelings of grief and guilt. Some survivors blame themselves for not recognizing the teen's despair or for failing to help. Others may feel guilty because the teen's suicide appeared to have been caused by a specific event, such as a humiliation or disappointment, in which the survivor played a part. However, doctors agree that most suicides cannot be linked to a single occurrence, but rather take place only after an individual loses his or her ability to cope with everyday problems.

Mental health experts agree that the best way to prevent suicide is to prevent the problems that lead to suicidal behavior. Parents and other adults can act as role models, teaching young children effective ways to solve life's problems and cope with stress. Adults should become familiar with the stresses in their teen's lives and be certain that parental and personal expectations are realistic. Adults should also know the warning signs of suicidal behavior, so that they can identify problems early, when treatment may be most effective.

Most importantly, doctors say, parents need to communicate openly with their teen-agers. Parents should encourage their teens to talk about the problems in their lives and listen attentively and empathetically when their children speak. •••

For additional information:

Books
Garland, E. J., Garland, J. E., and Garland, B. S. *Depression Is the Pits, But I'm Getting Better: A Guide for Adolescents.* Magination, 1997.

Oster, Gerald D., and Montgomery, Sarah S. *Helping Your Depressed Teenager: A Guide for Parents and Caregivers.* John Wiley and Sons, 1994.

Web sites
American Foundation for Suicide Prevention—www.afsp.org

National Institute of Mental Health—www.nimh.nih.gov

Other ways to help

Researchers have learned that not all teens who attempt suicide actually want to end their lives. Rather, they feel overwhelmed by their problems and convinced that there are no solutions. The best way to prevent teen suicide, doctors say, is to prevent such feelings of hopelessness and helplessness from developing in the first place. They recommend that parents do the following:

- Teach children from an early age how to deal with problems.
- Show children that they are valued members of the family.
- Reassure children that they will always be loved.
- Be aware of the stresses in your adolescent's life and make sure you are not adding to them with unrealistic expectations.
- Teach your teen to talk about the things that worry him or her.
- Listen attentively and empathetically.
- Discuss some of your own concerns, modeling for the teen how to talk about problems and feelings and how to resolve them.

Source: Capuzzi, Dave, and Golden, Larry. *Preventing Adolescent Suicide.* Accelerated Development, Inc., 1988.

Camping is a popular and rewarding pastime for millions of people—especially for those who do it safely.

The Great (and Safe) Outdoors

by Renée Despres

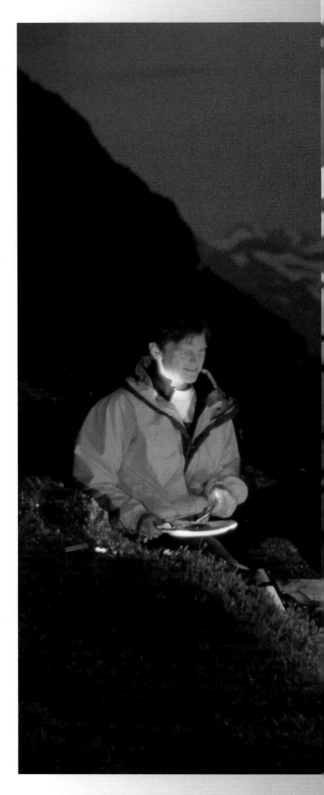

O N THE SECOND NIGHT OF A THREE-DAY hike through the Gila Wilderness, Jessica set up camp and went to sleep under a star-filled sky. It rarely rains in southern New Mexico in late September, so Jessica, who knew the region well, had decided to leave her tent and rain gear at home. She intended to travel far and fast, and decided that the extra weight would only slow her down. So far, she thought as she drifted off, she was almost five miles ahead of schedule.

A few hours later, Jessica awoke. Her feet and hands were numb, and she was shivering violently. Her sleeping bag had been soaked by a passing shower and could no longer protect her from the cold. Jessica struggled out of the bag and changed into dry clothes. She sat for an hour under a tree, eating nuts and raisins before she finally had the strength to walk to a nearby town. She found one house with its lights on, and asked the people inside for help. It took Jessica three days to recover.

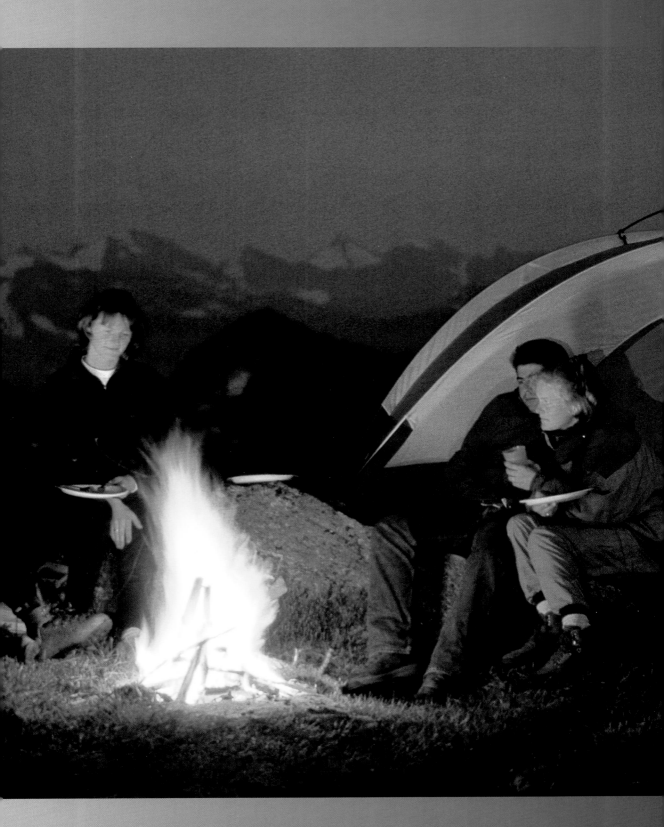

Some people would never consider spending the night out in the wilderness. They fear getting lost, seriously injured, or encountering a wild animal. But outdoor enthusiasts believe that camping can be a safe, rewarding experience. With proper preparation, a few skills, and some common sense, most potential camping hazards can be foreseen and avoided.

Choosing the right gear

Camping can mean different things to different people. For some, camping means driving a fully equipped recreational vehicle (RV) to a developed campground with running water and flush toilets. For others, it means hiking into the *back country* (rural, thinly settled area) with little more than a sleeping bag, a waterproof poncho, and a canteen. But most campers fall somewhere in between those two extremes. Whether you choose to drive or walk to your campsite, your basic needs remain the same—shelter, warmth, food, and water. By carefully choosing your gear, clothing, food, and campsite, you can fulfill those needs safely and comfortably.

Some campers spend thousands of dollars on high-tech, state-of-the-art equipment. But in most cases a few hundred dollars will get you durable, lightweight gear that won't let you down when you need it most. When choosing camping gear, take into consideration the nature and length of your trip, the time of year, weather conditions in the area, facilities available, and your experience level.

One of the first things most people consider when purchasing camping gear is a tent. This important piece of equipment can mean the difference between a comfortable sleep and a miserable night in the rain. In extreme conditions, however, it can also mean the difference between life and death. Tents fall into one of two basic design categories: freestanding tents and tents that need to be secured to the ground with stakes. Staked tents weigh slightly less and are therefore more popular among hikers, but driving stakes into rocky or sandy ground can pose a problem. Freestanding tents, on the other hand, set up easily on almost any type of terrain. The choice of material is also important. Nylon tents generally weigh less—an important factor for hikers. Polyester fabrics hold up better than nylon in the long run under exposure to ultraviolet rays from the sun.

Before using a new tent, it is extremely important to waterproof the seams to prevent leaks. Apply a seam sealer, which comes in a spray can, along all of the tent's seams according to the manufacturer's directions. Practice setting the tent up at home to make sure it meets your needs and to identify problems, such as a torn seam.

Next, look for the right sleeping bag. The insulating ability of sleeping bags is rated in degrees Fahrenheit, from 40 °F (4 °C) to −50 °F (−45 °C). The most efficient bags, called "mummy bags," are cut to be narrower at the bottom than at the top. This helps the bag to conserve heat because it fits more snugly around the legs, thus minimizing the space between you and the bag. Sleeping bags are

The author:

Renée Despres is a free-lance writer.

Camping first aid kit

Proper camping preparation involves planning for illness or injury. A well-stocked first aid kit takes into account the duration, location, and nature of your trip, as well as the terrain, the needs of individuals making the trip, their ages, and the activities you plan. There is no such thing as the perfect first-aid kit, but many camping outfitters sell prepackaged kits that contain some essentials. The least expensive kits, which sell for as little as $20, are designed for one-day hikes or casual weekend trips and feature a few of the essentials. More sophisticated kits, which can cost several hundred dollars, are also available. Some kits also include a basic first-aid manual. A well-stocked kit may include:

- Alcohol swabs
- Sterile gauze pads (4 inches by 4 inches)
- 2 individually wrapped sanitary napkins (to control heavy bleeding)
- Povidone-iodine (sold as Betadine) for cleaning wounds
- Moleskin for treating and preventing blisters
- Elastic bandage wrap
- Burn ointment
- Butterfly wound closures
- Antibacterial ointment
- Hydrocortisone cream for itches
- Finger splint
- Adhesive bandages (assorted sizes and types)
- Emergency blanket
- Antihistamine tablets for allergies and insect bites
- Loperamide (sold as Imodium A-D) or bismuth subsalicylate (sold as Pepto-Bismol) to treat or prevent diarrhea
- Thermometers
- Disposable razors
- Safety pins

- Painkiller (such as aspirin or acetaminophen)
- Medicine dropper
- Scissors and tweezers
- Disposable gloves (to prevent transmission of disease)

For novice campers, purchasing prepackaged first-aid kit, *below,* is a simple way to help prevent most minor illnesses or injuries from spoiling the trip.

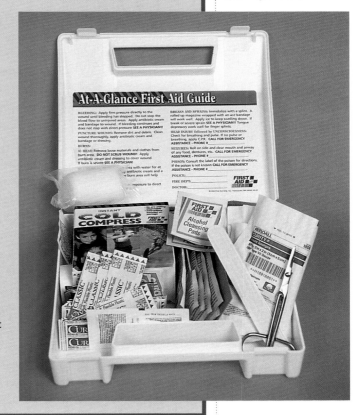

Tips on Choosing Camping Gear

Tent

- Tents come in two basic types: freestanding tents and tents that need to be secured to the ground with stakes. Staked tents weigh slightly less and are more popular among hikers, but driving stakes into rocky or sandy ground can pose a problem. Freestanding tents, on the other hand, set up easily on almost any type of terrain.

- The choice of material is also important. Nylon tents generally weigh less—an important factor for hikers. Polyester fabrics, on the other hand, hold up better than nylon in the long run under exposure to ultraviolet rays from the sun.

- A small, lightweight ground cloth helps protect the bottom of the tent from dirt, punctures, and condensation. A ground cloth, cut to the size of your tent floor, allows moisture to roll away from—not under—the tent on a rainy night.

Sleeping bag

- Sleeping bags are filled with either synthetic materials or *down* (soft feathers). Synthetic bags weigh more, take up more space, and can break down when exposed to heat. Down bags are lighter and more durable, but, unlike down bags, they are useless if they get wet and take a long time to dry.

filled with either synthetic materials or *down* (soft feathers). Synthetic bags weigh more, take up more space, and can break down when exposed to heat. But they are the better choice for camping in rainy or snowy conditions because they provide insulation even if they get wet. Down bags are lighter and more durable, but they are useless if they get wet and take a long time to dry. A sleeping pad—either a self-inflating air mattress or a closed-cell foam cushion—provides an extra layer of insulation between your body and the ground, which robs the body of heat.

Back-country campers and hikers should purchase a high-quality backpack with an internal or external frame. Internal-frame packs have rigid structures, called stays, that run the vertical length of the pack. These fit snugly against the body, ride smoothly, and work well in brushy or rough terrain. External-frame packs have strapping systems on the outside for attaching a sleeping bag, tent, and other gear. External-frame packs also permit the load to ride a few inches away from your body, so they offer better air circulation between your back and the pack.

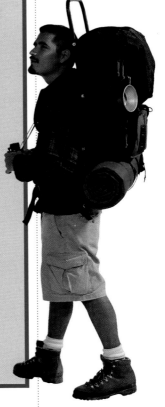

Cooking and eating utensils

- When camping in the United States and Canada, a camp stove fueled by white gasoline is the best choice.
- When selecting cooking and eating utensils, look for a set of lightweight, nesting pots and pans. To conserve space, nesting containers fit inside one another and double as dinner bowls. Utensils made of lightweight, heat-resistant, unbreakable plastic both reduce weight and decrease the risk of burns from hot metal.

Water purification

- Filtering is the fastest method and results in the best-tasting water because it removes many impurities as well as harmful organisms. However, to be effective against harmful microorganisms, choose a filter whose pores are no more than 0.4 microns in diameter.

Clothing

- Avoid cotton, which absorbs moisture. Instead, wear synthetic fabrics, like polypropylene, which provide some insulation but is "breathable" enough to permit air to reach your skin to evaporate moisture. Always dress in layers. Remove layers before you begin to perspire to help keep you dry. Add layers before you become cold. In colder conditions, start with a layer of polypropylene and add insulating layers, and top it off with a water-repellent windbreaker.
- Always pack rain gear to keep you as dry as possible in a downpour. Bring two hats: one to protect you from sun and rain, and one to sleep in at night to help conserve heat.

Dress for the wilderness

As you pack your trip attire, bear in mind that clothing can be considered equipment—especially in the back country. Avoid cotton, which absorbs moisture. Instead, wear synthetic fabrics, like polypropylene, which "breathe" to help evaporate perspiration from the skin but still provide some insulation. Regardless of the temperature, always dress in layers. Add or remove layers before you begin perspiring or get too cold. In wet weather, top it off with a water-repellent windbreaker. It's also a good idea to bring plenty of spare socks.

Rain gear should have a permanent home among your camping supplies. Wear sunglasses to protect your eyes from damaging ultraviolet rays, especially at high elevations where the atmosphere is thinner. Hikers should invest in a pair of sturdy boots, which help prevent ankle twists and slips on rocky ground, and protect you from snakes, insects, and thorny plants. Break in new boots at home. Pack a pair of tennis or water shoes for nighttime wear.

Toiletry items to pack include toothbrushes and toothpaste, biodegradable soap, shampoo, a camp mirror (which includes a hook

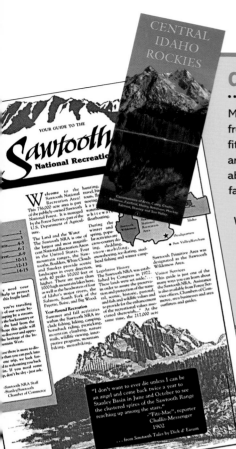

YOUR GUIDE TO THE

Sawtooth
National Recreation

Welcome to the hunting, Recreation Area! travel, big This 756,000 acre area is part tours, hiking, of the publicly-owned Sawtooth moose, kayaking, National Forest. It is managed by the Forest Service, part of the whitewater U.S. Department of Agricul- boating. ture.

"I don't want to ever die unless I can be an angel and come back twice a year to Stanley Basin in June and October to see the clustered spires of the Sawtooth Range reaching up among the stars."

—"Fitz-Mac", reporter
Challis-Messenger
1902

... from *Sawtooth Tales* by Dick d' Easum

Choosing a place to camp

Maps and other camping information are readily available from local forest or park offices, bookstores, or camping out-fitters. Most maps will show areas where camping is permitted and feasible. Local offices are also the best source to ask about local weather conditions, river or lake levels, and other factors that could affect your safety.

Many camping information resources are available on the World Wide Web. Two of the more extensive sources are:

- **Great Outdoors Recreation Pages**
  http://www.gorp.com/

- **Parknet (U. S. National Park Service)**
  http://www.nps.gov/

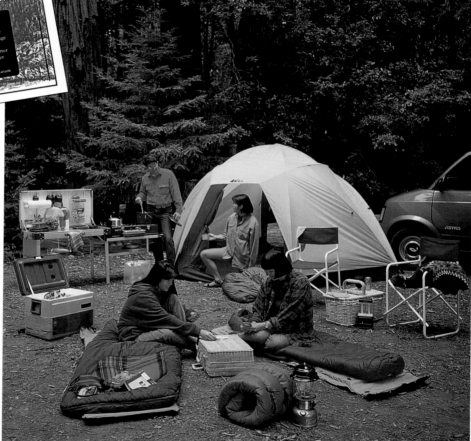

When planning a camp-ing trip, request an in-formation packet from the areas you are inter-ested in visiting. Many camping areas have sites equipped with water and electrical hookups and have recre-ational facilities nearby. If you intend to take ad-vantage of these ameni-ties, plan accordingly.

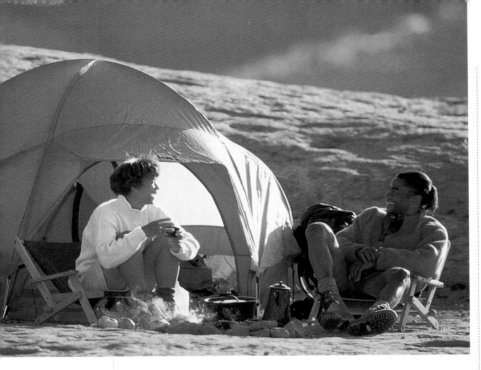

Many so-called primitive camping areas offer little more than a clear area in which to set up camp. Many more experienced campers prefer "backcountry" camping, which means setting up camping in a remote area far from civilization that is usually accessible only by a trail.

for hanging it), deodorant, shaving gear, towels and washcloths, and a laundry bag. Other essential items include sunscreen, a folding pocketknife, flashlight and spare batteries, an eyeglass repair kit or spare contact lenses, duct tape, a whistle, a compass with a built-in (or a separate) signal mirror, and some lightweight nylon rope.

Eating out—*way* out

A camp stove is another piece of essential gear. Cooking over a campfire is romantic, but it requires a fair amount of skill—not to mention a reliable supply of dry wood and a lot of time. "The pioneers burned wood to cook on the trail because they had to," says Jim Capossela, author of *Camp & Trail Cooking Techniques,* "You have better choices." Furthermore, campfires are not permitted in many areas because of wildfire hazard or other environmental considerations. Camp stoves are also more reliable, environmentally friendly, faster, and easier to use. Most can boil a quart of water in about a minute, and require only minutes to set up, prime, and light.

Camp stoves are designed to run on one or more of three fuels, usually white gasoline, kerosene or unleaded gasoline. When camping in the United States and Canada, white gasoline is the best choice. White gasoline (sold under such brand names as Coleman or Blazo) is readily available, burns cleaner, and is the safest and most efficient choice. Campers in other countries, however, may find themselves using the heavier fuels, such as kerosene or unleaded gasoline. These fuels produce noxious fumes, cause stoves to behave unpredictably, and can clog up the stove. Camp stoves that use canister fuel, such as propane or butane, pose less of a fire hazard, but

"The 5 W's"

When setting up your campsite, abide by the rule of the "five w's"—width, water, weather, wind, and widowmakers.

Width. The campsite should be wide and flat, to allow you to safely pitch your tent.

Water. The site should be near a source of water, but not too close. Pitch your tent and do all your cooking and cleaning at least 200 feet (60 meters) away from water sources.

Wind. Choose a site that is out of the wind, generally on the eastern side of a slope, which will allow you to avoid a prevailing westerly wind and also give you early morning sun.

Weather. Keep the weather in mind as you select a campsite. Do not camp on a high, exposed plateau in thunderstorm season. A higher spot may be warmer, however, since cold air tends to settle in low-lying spots at night.

Widowmakers are dangers like overhanging tree limbs that could break off and fall on you, a nearby cliff you might accidentally step off in the middle of the night, and other hazards. Avoid camping in areas subject to water runoff or rockfall, and never camp in a slot canyon or dry riverbed during flood season.

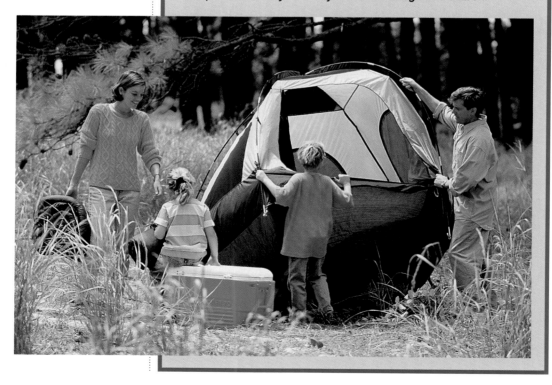

propane is sold in heavy, metal cylinders—a problem for hikers—and butane stoves are sometimes unreliable in colder climates. Another factor in choosing a fuel is the type of lantern you purchase, assuming you decide you need one. To help eliminate confusion and simplify your equipment needs, choose a camp stove and lantern that use the same type of fuel.

You'll also need something in which to cook meals. When selecting cooking and eating utensils, look for a set of pots and pans that nest inside each other and can double as dinner bowls. Utensils made of lightweight, heat-resistant plastic both reduce weight and decrease the risk of burns from hot metal.

When it comes to cooking, most campers prefer to keep things simple. Meal preparation and cleanup can use up a lot of recreation time, so many campers cook just one meal a day—limiting other meals to sandwiches or other simple fare like pasta or prepackaged noodle soups. These foods also clean up easily, leaving no scraps or residue behind to attract hungry creatures during the night.

Back-country campers must plan meals carefully, or run the risk of running out of food. Pack an extra day's worth of food just in case. Dehydrated foods save weight and room. Jerky, hard cheese, peanut butter, and sturdy crackers make easy meals. To conserve fuel, look for items that cook in about five minutes, such as pasta. Most camping outfitters carry a wide variety of prepackaged meals.

Plan light, frequent meals that are high in carbohydrates during the day, and a hot meal at night. Breakfast is essential—you burn calories just sleeping outside in the cold. Although carbohydrates are the mainstay of any camper's diet, don't skimp on the fats and proteins—they'll keep your energy levels up during the day and help you stay warm at night.

Safeguarding your health

Good camping preparation is not complete without planning for illness or injury. There is no such thing as the perfect first-aid kit, says Buck Tilton, founder of the Wilderness Medicine Institute in Pitken, Colorado. But a well-stocked first aid kit takes into account the duration, location, and nature of your trip, as well as the terrain, the needs of individuals in the group, their ages, and the activities you plan. For example, pack antiseptic ointment and adhesive bandages, but also be sure to bring along things like prescription medicines.

Many camping outfitters sell prepackaged first-aid kits that contain some essentials. The least expensive kits, which sell for as little as $20, are designed for one-day hikes or casual weekend trips and feature a few of the essentials. More sophisticated kits, which can cost several hundred dollars, are also available.

Another vital health-preservation measure, especially for hikers, is ensuring the availability of *potable* (fit for drinking) water. Campers should never drink untreated water. Even in remote areas, water in lakes and streams may be contaminated with microorganisms such

Most designated camping areas post signs to indicate available facilities. For example, the icons below stand for a designated campfire area; hiking trail; shower facilities; and a dump station for recreational vehicles.

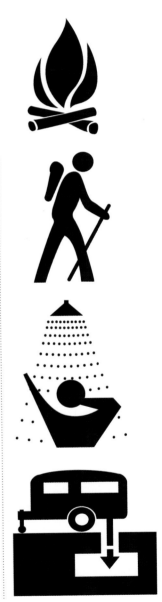

as *Giardia lamblia,* which can cause nausea, diarrhea, and vomiting. Giardia is introduced into streams by infected animals or people. Symptoms usually appear about 10 days after exposure and can persist for two weeks or more without medical attention.

The three most common ways to purify water are boiling, chemical treatment, and filtering. Most organisms are killed when water reaches the boiling point—100 °C (212 °F)—and an additional five minutes of boiling ensures purity. However, boiling requires fuel and time and can therefore be impractical. Chemical purification also takes time, but it involves much less hassle than boiling. Iodine-based purification tablets, such as Potable Aqua, are easy for hikers to carry. Simply drop a tablet in the water and wait 20 minutes. The slight iodine taste can be neutralized by adding a bit of vitamin C. (Do not use iodine tablets if you are allergic to iodine or shellfish.) Filtering is the fastest option and results in the best-tasting water because it removes many impurities as well as harmful organisms. However, to be effective against harmful microorganisms, check to make sure the filter pores are no more than 0.4 microns in diameter.

Choosing a destination and selecting a campsite

A wealth of camping information is available from local bookstores and camping outfitters, and from individual forest or park service offices. You can find important trip-planning information in guidebooks as well. Maps will help you plan your trip by showing, among other things, areas where camping is permitted and feasible. Ask locally about weather conditions, river or lake levels, and other factors that could affect your safety.

Hikers should plan their route according to conditioning level, the type of terrain, and water availability. When plotting out daily mileage estimates, allow a half-hour for each mile (1.6 kilometers) plus another half-hour for every 1,000 feet (305 meters) of rise in elevation. Allow time for breaks and always err on the side of caution.

So you've planned and packed, driven or walked to camp, and you're ready to set up and enjoy your night in the great outdoors. What now? When setting up your campsite, abide by the rule of the "Five W's"—width, water, weather, wind, and widowmakers.

The campsite should be wide and flat, to allow you to safely pitch your tent. It should be near a source of water, but not too close. Pitch your tent and do all your cooking and cleaning at least 200 feet (60 meters) away from water sources. Not only does the distance prevent contamination of the water, it removes you from the path of animals that drink from the stream at night.

Keep the weather in mind as you select a campsite. As frightening as an encounter with a bear might be, *hypothermia* (a drop in body temperature) is a far more likely threat. People can become hypothermic even in the summer, especially if they get wet. But the danger can be minimized by staying dry, wearing appropriate clothing, eating often, and drinking plenty of water. In cold, wet, conditions,

Making a safe campsite

All campers should familiarize themselves with the basic camping safety practices—such as using a fire pit, *right,* to contain a campfire and keeping food away from scavenging animals, *below.* With simple common sense and a sense of respect for the ways of the wilderness, almost anyone can safely enjoy the experience of living in close contact with nature.

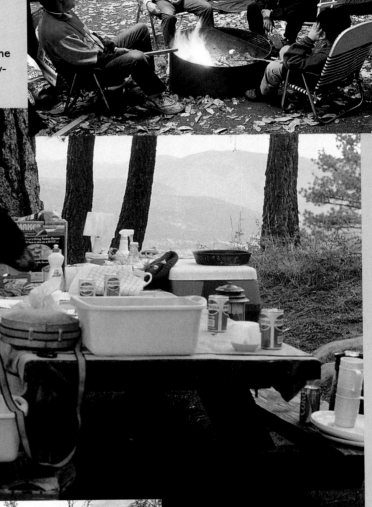

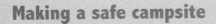

During your stay at a camping area, familiarize yourself with resources for local information, *left.* Paying attention to local developments can help keep you safe and can also help add to your enjoyment of the area.

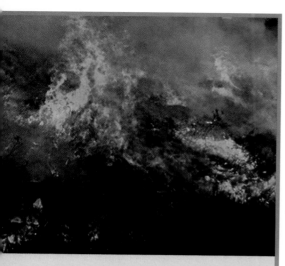

Fire safety

Your own campfire is one of the most dangerous things you'll encounter in the woods. Every campfire has the potential to turn into a raging wildfire that eats up thousands of acres and endangers people and wildlife.

Wildfires are part of a natural cycle that maintains the ecological balance of the forest. But many fires are set due to human error. If you start a forest fire, you are financially responsible for the cost of fighting it. Always check with the local forest or park service to see if campfires are allowed or if you need a permit. Fires are often prohibited at very high elevations and in heavily used areas.

If there is an established rock ring at your campsite, use it. If not, don't build a new ring—you'll only char the rock. Clear out an area large enough so that flying sparks won't land on dry fuels, like grass. Scrape down to the dirt. Never start a fire with gasoline or any other volatile substance. Put the fire out before you go to sleep. Before you leave, douse the ashes with water—they should be cool enough for you to touch them with your bare hand. Scatter the ashes and mix them thoroughly with dirt.

seek or create shelter, even if it means pitching your tent in the middle of the day. Extremely hot conditions can lead to a rise in body temperature, called hyperthermia. In hot weather, drink plenty of water, take frequent rest breaks, and douse or spray yourself with water, which will remove heat from your body as it evaporates. Do not camp on a high, exposed plateau in thunderstorm season. (A higher spot may be warmer, however, since cold air tends to settle in low-lying spots at night.) Choose a site that is out of the wind, generally on the eastern side of a slope.

Finally, look around the site for "widowmakers"—a tongue-in-cheek term used to describe such dangers as overhanging tree limbs that could break off and fall on you, a nearby ledge you might accidentally step off in the middle of the night, or other hazards. Avoid camping in areas that are subject to water runoff or rockfall, and never camp in a slot canyon or dry riverbed during flood season.

Common dangers: wild animals and plants

For most people, the presence of wildlife one is one of the most appealing aspects of camping. Most wild animals are shy and avoid humans, and animal attacks on people are rare. There's really not much to worry about as long as you remember that you are visiting their home and to be respectful. For instance, if you are camping in bear country, ask for information from local offices. Be extra aware when choosing a campsite. Look around for signs of bear scat, overturned rocks, or other indications that a bear frequents the location. If you see any of these signs, move to a safer place. Sleep in a tent, and always cook downwind of your campsite when in bear country.

When camping in the deep wilderness, remember than items like food, garbage, film, and toiletries give off odors that can attract animals. It is important, therefore, to store these materials properly. Along with a fire pit and cooking grate, most developed campgrounds in bear country have a lockable bear box for this purpose. Do not keep food inside a car or trailer, because a hungry bear may be tempted to go after it. Many bears and raccoons that live near campgrounds also know what an ice chest is and what's inside, so it is a good idea to keep food-related items out of sight. If you cannot avoid keeping food out in the open, wrap it and all other odorous items in plastic bags and shove them into a deep crevice well away from camp. Never sleep with food nearby, and burn or bury all food residue.

Poisonous snakes also pose a threat to back-country campers, especially in the Southwest. Although relatively few snakebite victims die, many lose a limb. Again, prevention and awareness are the best protection against snake bites. Wear boots, thick socks, and long pants. Look before you put your hands on a rock or ledge, and carry a walking stick to push tall grasses out of the way. Before climbing into an empty sleeping bag, shake it out to check for any visitors.

Some of the most hazardous wildlife of the back country are insects and poisonous plants, which are far more numerous and familiar than bears. Ticks, which feed by attaching themselves to the skin and feasting on their victim's blood, are extremely common in wooded areas. These creatures can transmit such diseases as Rocky Mountain spotted fever and Lyme disease. Tick bites can be prevented by wearing long sleeves and pants, tucking your pants into your socks, and staying near the middle of trails. The chemical repellent permethrin is an effective tick repellent when applied to clothing.

Poisonous plants are another common hazard. In the United States, the most troublesome plants are poison ivy and poison oak. Both plants are native to the U. S., but poison ivy is more widespread. Poison ivy is frequently found in moist, rainy areas and by river beds. Both of these plants carry urishiol, an extremely irritating oil that causes most people to break out in an itchy, hivelike rash. If you get exposed to urishiol, avoid touching anything—especially your eyes and face—until you can wash thoroughly with soap.

A safe and pleasant experience

When we have the chance to spend a few nights out of doors, we discover in ourselves a kind of self-reliance that can be scarce in today's world of modern conveniences. Camping brings us closer to nature, reminding us that most of our everyday needs are as basic as shelter, warmth, food, and water. However, living in the wilderness is also a reminder of how vulnerable we are to the things our houses protect us from. With good preparation and simple common sense, anyone can enjoy a safe, rewarding camping experience.　•••

For additional information:

Capossela, Jim. *Camp & Trail Cooking Techniques*. Countryman Press, 1994.

Mouland, Michael. *The Complete Idiot's Guide to Hiking, Camping, and the Great Outdoors*. Alpha Books, 1996.

Tilton, Buck and Frank Hubbell. *Medicine for the Backcountry*. ICS Books, 1994.

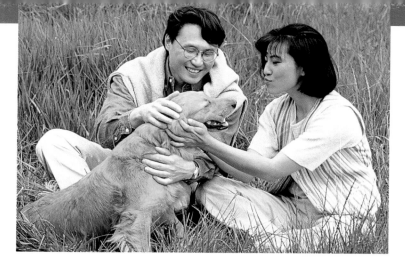

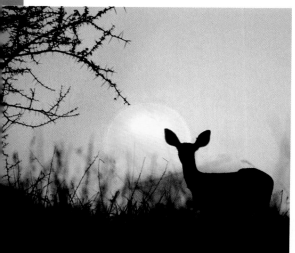

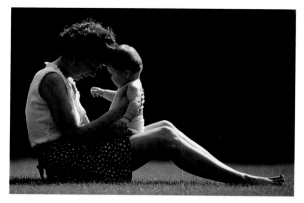

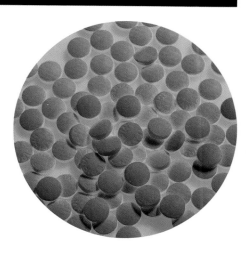

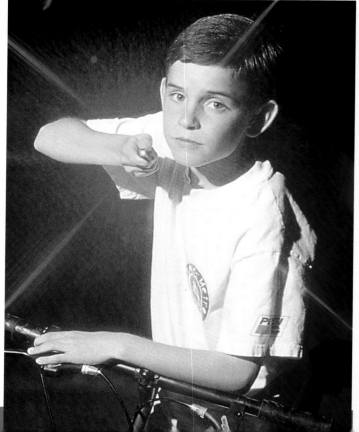

HEALTH UPDATES

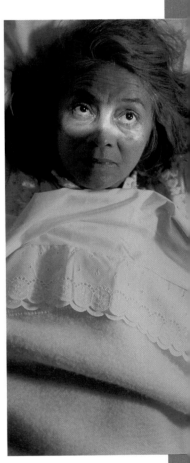

- Vitamin D and hip fractures
- Incontinence control
- Therapy for recurrent depression

A report published in April 1999 by researchers at Brigham and Women's Hospital in Boston concluded that postmenopausal women with low vitamin D levels may be more prone to hip fractures. While a woman is in her 30's, levels of *estrogen*—a hormone produced mainly by the ovaries—begin a gradual decline that accelerates when she reaches her 40's. Hormone levels continue to drop until they become so low that menstruation ceases, a condition that triggers menopause.

The Boston researchers examined 98 postmenopausal women admitted to the hospital for hip replacement.

Of those women, 30 had acute hip fractures and 68 had been admitted for joint replacement. The women provided researchers with information on their lifestyle, childbirth history, dietary calcium intake, and physical activity.

The researchers measured the participants' bone mineral density and tested blood samples to determine the women's levels of vitamin D and their parathyroid hormone levels. (An increase in parathyroid hormone levels occurs when vitamin D levels are low, which in turn promotes bone loss.) The researchers reported that 15 of the women who had hip fractures also had lower levels of vitamin D. Eleven of the women also had elevated parathyroid hormone levels.

The researchers said that daily supplements of vitamin D may prevent such deficiencies, which in turn may reduce the risk of bone fractures and promote fracture repair among postmenopausal women.

Incontinence control. Older people with *incontinence* (involuntary leakage of urine) often suffer from embarrassment, depression, and social isolation. The condition often predisposes them to other health problems. According to a six-year study published in December 1998, patients who are taught skills and strategies for preventing incontinence—called behavioral training—stand a better chance of controlling the disorder than patients who receive drug therapy.

A team of researchers from the University of Alabama at Birmingham, the University of Pittsburgh, the Allegheny General Hospital in Pittsburgh, and St. Vincent's Health Center in Erie, Pennsylvania, examined 197 women who were between the ages of 55 to 92 at the start of the study. All of the women had previously been diagnosed with *urge incontinence*—a leakage of urine associated with either an overactive bladder or reduced bladder capacity—and had at least two episodes of incontinence a week.

The women used a two-week diary to document the pre- and post-treatment incontinence, the amount of urine lost, and the circumstances of

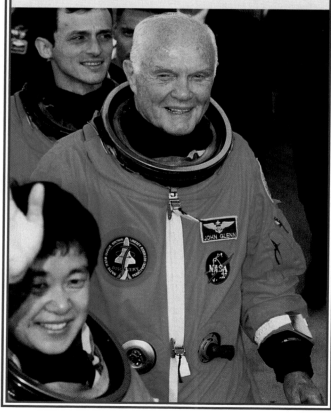

Return to space

On Oct. 29, 1998, John H. Glenn, Jr., the first American to orbit Earth in 1962, became the oldest person to fly in space. Glenn's trip on board the space shuttle Discovery was designed so that scientists could study the effects of space on his body and learn more about the physiology of aging.

each episode. The subjects were divided into groups as having either mild, moderate, or severe incontinence depending on the number of incontinence episodes each week. The researchers then treated the women in each group with either behavior training or oxybutynin chloride, a drug prescribed for the overactive bladder, or gave them a *placebo* (inactive substance).

The women made four clinic visits at two-week intervals during an eight-week period. Before the start of treatment, the frequency of incontinence reported by the women was similar among the three groups. Following the treatment, however, the groups reported significantly different outcomes. Thirty-nine percent of the women who had received a placebo, 69 percent of women who had taken the drug, and 81 percent of the women who had been in the behavioral training group reported improvement in their incontinence.

The level of incontinence improvement perceived by the patient was also greater for those women who had participated in the behavioral training group. Seventy-four percent of those patients reported feeling "much better," compared with 51 percent of those patients who had received drug therapy, and 27 percent of those who received a placebo.

Therapy for recurrent depression.
Researchers at the University of Pittsburgh Medical Center reported in January 1999 that elderly patients diagnosed with recurrent major depression may be able to prevent or delay recurrence of the disorder through treatment with both nortriptyline, a drug for the treatment of depression, and interpersonal psychotherapy (IPT). The researchers found that the treatments worked better in combination than separately. Over the course of the seven-year study, the researchers followed 180 elderly patients. The patients were treated initially with a combination of nortriptyline and psychotherapy.

After 16 weeks of this treatment, the researchers evaluated the patients for symptoms of depression. Those patients who no longer experienced depression were randomly as-

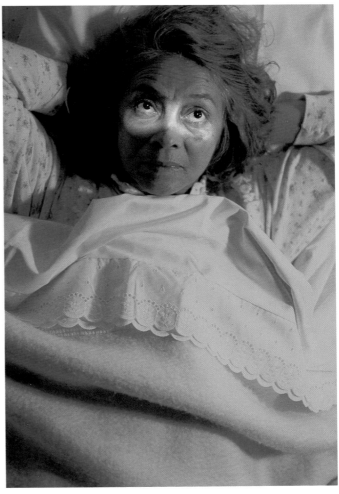

signed to one of four groups. The patients were either treated with nortriptyline; treated with a placebo; treated with monthly IPT and nortriptyline; or treated with monthly IPT and a placebo.

The researchers said that patients who received a combination of drugs and therapy experienced fewer major depressive episodes than patients in the other study groups. Only 20 percent of the patients experienced a recurrence of depression during this three-year phase of the study. In comparison, 43 percent of patients receiving only nortriptyline, 64 percent of patients receiving IPT and a placebo, and 90 percent of patients receiving only a placebo had recurrence of depression.   • Rein Tideiksaar

**Insomnia and
the elderly**
Researchers from Laval University in Quebec, Canada, reported in March 1999 that insomnia in older adults can best be treated with behavioral therapy, with sleep medication, or a combination of drugs and therapy. The researchers compared the treatments in 78 men and women and reported that patients who were educated about better sleep habits were most able to enhance and maintain their quality of sleep.

AIDS

- U.S. AIDS deaths decline
- International AIDS trends
- Cutting AIDS medications
- Opportunistic infections
- New AIDS drugs
- Persistence of HIV
- AZT for babies

Deaths from AIDS (acquired immune deficiency syndrome) in the United States have declined significantly, according to an October 1998 report from the United States National Center for Health Statistics. As a result, the disease dropped from 8th to 14th on the government's list of the leading causes of mortality. AIDS deaths fell by 47 percent in 1997, compared with deaths in 1996.

Researchers credited treatment with combinations of potent drugs, including protease inhibitors that became available in 1995, for the reduction in the number of deaths. These drugs prevent individuals infected with human immunodeficiency virus (HIV—the virus that causes AIDS) from developing full-blown AIDS and reduce the likelihood of those with AIDS dying from so-called opportunistic infections.

In 1997, 16,685 people died of AIDS. Approximately 40,000 individuals became infected with HIV that year, a figure that has remained steady throughout the mid-1990's.

International AIDS trends. In November 1998, the United Nations AIDS Program announced that HIV infections worldwide rose 10 percent in 1997. The number of people infected with HIV soared by 5.8 million, increasing from 27.6 million to 33.4 million worldwide. The great majority

of those infected—95 percent—lived in Africa, Asia, and eastern Europe. Almost half of the new infections were reported in 15 to 24 year olds. Women accounted for 43 percent of people with HIV over age 15.

Cutting AIDS medications. A study published in the *New England Journal of Medicine* in October 1998 indicated that many HIV-positive patients may have to continue taking expensive drug combinations for the rest of their lives. When researchers at the University of California in San Diego attempted to cut back on the number of medications prescribed, the patients' HIV levels rose dramatically.

Typically, people with HIV take a combination of medications totaling 20 to 30 pills each day that include protease inhibitors and drugs called reverse transcriptase inhibitors. The drug combinations cost approximately $15,000 per year. Protease inhibitors often cause side effects such as diarrhea, vomiting, dramatic increases in cholesterol levels, and disfiguring fatty deposits in the upper body. For these reasons, patients had hoped that they would eventually be able to cut down on their use of the drugs. Some researchers believed that, once the drugs reduced blood HIV levels, the levels would remain low even when drug intake was reduced.

However, the San Diego study

AIDS in the United States

The Centers for Disease Control and Prevention in Atlanta, Georgia, reported in November 1998 that the highest rates of U.S. AIDS cases per 100,000 people in 1997 occurred in the northeastern, southeastern, and western states. Most reported AIDS cases (81 percent) were found among residents of large metropolitan areas—those with populations greater than 500,000.

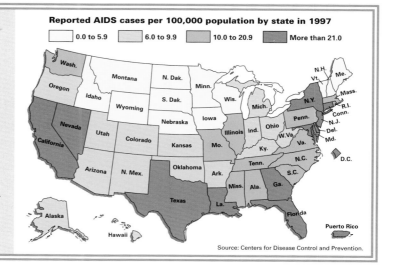

Reported AIDS cases per 100,000 population by state in 1997

0.0 to 5.9   6.0 to 9.9   10.0 to 20.9   More than 21.0

Source: Centers for Disease Control and Prevention.

showed that HIV levels escalate when drug treatment is reduced. Researchers evaluated more than 300 people with HIV who had been taking a triple-drug therapy of indinavir (Crixivan), zidovudine (AZT), and lamivudine (Epivir) for six months. While one-third of the group continued to take all three medications, the others were given either indinavir alone or zidovudine plus lamivudine. Within two months, 23 percent of the patients receiving the reduced drug treatments showed renewed increases of the amount of HIV in their blood.

Opportunistic infections. Two serious HIV-related infections—pneumocystis carinii pneumonia and toxoplasmic encephalitis—can often be prevented by standard triple-drug AIDS therapy. Thus, patients may not require additional treatment with antibiotics. That was the conclusion of a study by Swiss researchers published in the *New England Journal of Medicine* in April 1999.

The researchers evaluated 262 HIV-infected patients whose immune systems had recovered to an acceptable level during treatment with a three-drug AIDS therapy. During the study, the patients continued the three-drug treatment but stopped taking the standard antibiotics prescribed for protection against the two potentially serious opportunistic infections. After 11 months, none of the patients showed any signs of the opportunistic illnesses. The researchers concluded that HIV-infected patients may be able to reduce the number of pills they take each day without further risks to their health.

New AIDS drugs. In September 1998, the U.S. Food and Drug Administration (FDA) approved the first AIDS medication that needs to be taken only once a day. Researchers hoped that the medication—efavirenz (Sustiva)—would provide an alternative for people unable to take the standard regimen of AIDS drugs because of side effects. Although efavirenz is prescribed in combination with other AIDS medications, it will reduce the total number of pills a patient must take each day. Efavirenz

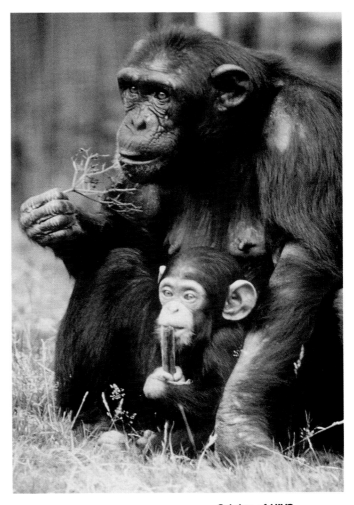

produces side effects similar to those of some other AIDS drugs—dizziness, insomnia, and difficulty concentrating. However, the side effects tend to be mild in most patients and subside over time. Researchers found that efavirenz, when taken with other AIDS medications, dramatically reduces HIV levels in the blood.

Another new AIDS drug, abacavir (Ziagen), won FDA approval in December 1998. The drug, taken twice daily in combination with other medications for HIV-positive patients, suppresses levels of the virus. However, at least 5 percent of patients experienced a potentially life-threatening allergic reaction, including such symptoms as a skin rash, fever, nausea, abdominal pain, and severe fatigue.

Origins of HIV?
A subspecies of chimpanzees in west-central Africa called Pan troglodytes trog-lodytes, *above*, was identified as the carrier of an AIDS-like virus that appears to have evolved into human HIV. Researchers at the University of Alabama in Birmingham reported the finding in January 1999. The scientists analyzed tissue and blood samples from a chimp that died in 1985. The animal tested positive for a simian form of HIV that closely matched HIV-1, the strain that causes 99 percent of human AIDS cases.

Thus, people hypersensitive to the drug would not be able to take it.

Research showed that abacavir was most effective in HIV patients who had not yet taken other AIDS medications. In a study in which patients were prescribed abacavir in addition to AIDS drugs AZT and 3TC, HIV levels declined dramatically in most patients. The virus was no longer detectable in 75 percent of those taking the drug treatment. Abacavir is part of the oldest class of AIDS drugs, called nucleoside analogue reverse transcriptase inhibitors.

In April 1999, the FDA approved the first new protease inhibitor to appear on the market in more than two years. The drug, called amprenavir (Agenerase), may cause some of the same side effects as other protease inhibitors, such as nausea, vomiting, and diarrhea. However, in a 24-week study involving 700 people, it did not raise patients' cholesterol levels, indicating that it would not increase their risk for heart disease as other protease inhibitors do. Researchers hoped that amprenavir would provide an alternative for longer-term HIV patients in whom the virus had *mutated* (changed to another form), making other protease inhibitors useless.

Persistence of HIV. Although medications can reduce amounts of the AIDS virus to levels too low to be measured, HIV may still linger for many years. That was the conclusion of a study at Johns Hopkins University in Baltimore, published in *Nature Medicine* in May 1999. Researchers found that even when HIV-positive patients are treated with multiple AIDS medications, the virus can hide in reservoirs in the body for decades. They analyzed the amounts of hidden HIV in 34 patients and calculated the rate at which HIV deteriorates in the blood. The researchers determined that it could take as long as 60 years for the virus to be eradicated.

Another team of researchers, at the University of Washington in Seattle, reported in *Nature Medicine* in January 1999 a new method for suppressing HIV in patients who may have remnants of the virus hiding in their *lymph nodes,* glands located throughout the body that help filter out harmful substances. This approach is based on the concept that HIV thrives because the body has an inadequate number of immune cells called cytotoxic T lymphocytes (CTL's) to kill the virus.

The researchers injected patients with CTL's that had been derived from each patient's own immune system and *cloned* (duplicated) in the laboratory. These cells carried a tracer molecule that made it possible to monitor their movement in the body. The researchers found that the injected CTL's traveled to the lymph nodes and killed HIV-infected cells. They

S T A T I S T I C S			
AIDS worldwide Region	Total with HIV/AIDS	Infected in 1998	Percentage of adults infected
Sub-Saharan Africa	22.5 million	4 million	8%
North Africa, Middle East	**210,000**	**19,000**	**0.13**
South and Southeast Asia	6.7 million	1.2 million	0.69
East Asia and Pacific	**560,000**	**200,000**	**0.068**
Latin America	1.4 million	160,000	0.57
Caribbean	**330,000**	**45,000**	**1.96**
Eastern Europe and Central Asia	270,000	80,000	0.14
Western Europe	**500,000**	**30,000**	**0.25**
North America	890,000	44,000	0.56
Australia and New Zealand	**12,000**	**600**	**0.1**

The United Nations AIDS Program reported that the number of people in the world infected with human immunodeficiency virus (HIV—the virus that causes AIDS) rose by 10 percent in 1998 over 1997 figures. The agency, headquartered in Geneva, Switzerland, stated that the increase showed a lack of progress in prevention of the disease.

Source: United Nations AIDS Program.

hoped that this approach could become the basis of a treatment to enhance the capacity of CTL's.

AZT for babies. Babies born to women with HIV have a lower risk of becoming infected with the virus if they are treated with the drug AZT within the first two days after birth. Researchers at the New York State Department of Health in Albany reported this finding in November 1998 in the *New England Journal of Medicine*.

Women who are HIV-positive are typically treated with AZT to reduce the chances of passing the virus to their babies. Without this therapy, the babies have a 27 percent chance of becoming infected with HIV. However, some infected women do not receive prenatal care and thus do not take AZT while pregnant.

Researchers analyzed the status of 939 HIV-exposed infants up to 6 months old. They found that when AZT was given to the mothers before birth, the rate of HIV transmission was 6 percent. When mothers took AZT during labor and delivery, the rate was 10 percent. And when the drug was given to babies within the first 48 hours of their lives, the transmission rate was 9 percent. The rate climbed to 18 percent when AZT was given on or after the third day of the baby's life. • Richard Trubo

The Monitoring the Future Study, an annual survey on drug-use trends among 8th-, 10th-, and 12th-graders in the United States, found a slight decrease in the use of illicit drugs in 1998 compared with 1997. The study, conducted by the University of Michigan at Ann Arbor and released in December 1998, also found that the use of alcohol had declined somewhat among students in all three grades.

According to the study, the number of secondary school students using illicit drugs or alcohol on a daily basis was fairly low in 1998. For example, only 3.6 percent of 10th-graders and 5.6 percent of 12th-graders reported using marijuana daily. Similarly, only 1.9 percent of 10th-graders and 3.9 percent of seniors said they drank alcohol every day.

However, alcohol continued to be widely used by teen-agers in 1998. Thirty-three percent of the high school seniors in the study reported that they were drunk at least once in the month before the survey. Moreover, 31.5 percent of the seniors, 24.3 percent of the 10th-graders, and 13.7 percent of the 8th-graders reported consuming five or more drinks in the previous two weeks.

Marijuana also continued to be widely used. Twenty-two percent of 8th-graders and 49 percent of 12th-graders said they had tried the drug at least once. However, only 22.8 percent of the 12th-graders said they had used marijuana in the previous month. Thus, the researchers noted that marijuana appeared to be used infrequently by many students and regularly by just a few.

Educational efforts about the negative effects of illicit drugs seem to be showing results, according to the Monitoring the Future Study. Among 10th-graders, 65.8 percent said they thought there was "great risk" in smoking marijuana regularly; 73.3 percent said there was great risk in regular use of inhalants, such as glues and solvents; and 77.5 percent thought there was great risk in taking crack occasionally.

Heroin users triple. The number of heroin users more than tripled between 1993 and 1997, researchers with the Substance Abuse and Mental Health Services Administration (SAMHSA), part of the U.S. National Institutes of Health (NIH), reported in August 1998. The National Household Survey on Drug Abuse, an annual SAMHSA survey on drug use, attributed the increase mainly to the fact that the majority of new heroin users were sniffing the drug rather than injecting it. The survey also found that many of these new users had tried heroin as early as age 12.

The National Institute on Drug Abuse warned that many young heroin users mistakenly believe that sniffing heroin is less risky and less ad-

Alcohol and Drug Abuse

- Substance abuse declines slightly among students
- Educational efforts
- Heroin users triple
- Treating heroin addiction
- College drinking
- Designated drivers
- Alcohol and drugs in movies
- Coverage for substance abuse

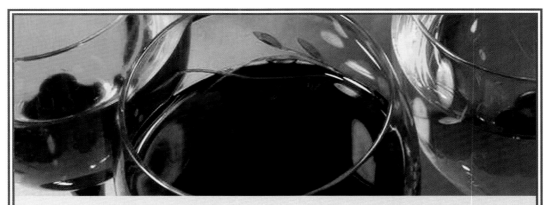

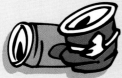

Consequences of alcohol abuse

The effects of alcohol abuse go far beyond health problems. The American Psychiatric Association warns that alcohol can have serious consequences in a number of other areas, including a person's job and family.

Physical consequences

• Liver disease

• Pancreatic disease

• Heart and blood vessel disease

• Stomach and intestinal problems

• Nervous system disorders, such as seizures and intellectual decline

Source: American Psychiatric Association.

• Reproductive system disorders, including effects on fetus

• Cancers, including those of the liver, pancreas, and throat

Psychiatric consequences

• Depression

• Anxiety

• Antisocial personality

Other consequences

• Legal problems, due to such incidents as traffic accidents and violent offenses

• Employment problems, resulting from tardiness, inability to concentrate, or other factors

• Family problems, such as divorce, child abuse, and behavioral problems in children

dictive than injecting the drug. However, the federal institute emphasized that heroin is a highly addictive *opiate* (a drug containing opium) that can change brain chemistry to the point where the pursuit of the drug becomes the abuser's main interest.

Treating heroin addiction. NIH published a report in December 1998 supporting the use of the synthetic opiate methadone to treat heroin addiction. The report presented evidence that methadone maintenance therapy, a common but controversial treatment for heroin addiction, helps decrease drug use and criminal activity among heroin addicts.

Methadone helps addicted individuals stop craving heroin by blocking the initial euphoric high created by the drug. People in methadone maintenance programs are usually given a dose of methadone orally once a day. Although some individuals remain in methadone treatment programs for months or years, the NIH report stressed that the cost to society of these methadone programs is relatively low—averaging about $3,900 per individual per year.

Some physicians criticize methadone maintenance as substituting one drug addiction for another. However, the NIH panel maintained that if methadone is properly prescribed, it does not cause intoxication or sedation and, if coupled with counseling and work, enables addicts to lead productive lives.

Methadone is one example of *pharmacotherapy*—a drug treatment that uses a medication to treat drug addiction. Other pharmacotherapy substances being used in 1999 included naltrexone, a heroin-blocking agent, and levomethadyl acetate hydrochloride (LAAM), a drug similar to, but longer-lasting, than methadone.

College drinking. One in five college students in the United States is a frequent binge drinker, concluded a study by the Harvard School of Public Health in Boston published in September 1998. The Harvard researchers defined binge drinking as having five or more drinks in one sitting.

A drink was defined in the study as a glass of beer or wine or a shot of hard alcohol.

The report stressed that college drinking patterns vary greatly from student to student and school to school. Fraternity and sorority members and athletic team leaders were more likely to be binge drinkers than other students, and they often drank more than double the amount that other binge drinkers drank. These amounts totaled up to 14 or more drinks per week. Half of the college binge drinkers had also binged on alcohol as high school seniors.

Although binge drinking is commonly perceived as the norm in col-

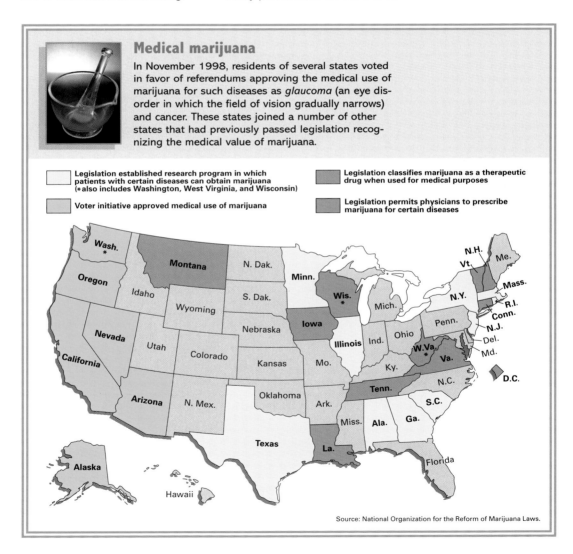

Medical marijuana

In November 1998, residents of several states voted in favor of referendums approving the medical use of marijuana for such diseases as *glaucoma* (an eye disorder in which the field of vision gradually narrows) and cancer. These states joined a number of other states that had previously passed legislation recognizing the medical value of marijuana.

Legislation established research program in which patients with certain diseases can obtain marijuana (∗also includes Washington, West Virginia, and Wisconsin)

Voter initiative approved medical use of marijuana

Legislation classifies marijuana as a therapeutic drug when used for medical purposes

Legislation permits physicians to prescribe marijuana for certain diseases

Source: National Organization for the Reform of Marijuana Laws.

lege, the Harvard study indicated that this perception is not accurate. The study found that when moderate drinkers and nondrinkers were considered, the average amount of alcohol consumed by a college student per week was only 1.5 drinks.

The Harvard researchers encouraged college communities to focus less on the problem of college drinking itself and more on curbing the disruptive behavior of binge drinkers. Because drunken students often cause residence hall problems, damage campus property, and hurt other students, the researchers suggested that addressing such behavior would be more effective than campus-wide crackdowns or bans on alcohol.

Designated drivers. When colleges ban alcohol on campus, many students go off-campus to drink. This often means that students are driving in order to drink, endangering themselves and other individuals. A January 1999 Harvard School of Public Health report described both positive and negative results regarding the use of designated drivers in such circumstances.

On the positive side, the study found that when students served as designated drivers, they either abstained from alcohol or drank very little—1 or 2 drinks per evening. Even students who usually engaged in binge drinking said that they consumed little or no alcohol when they were designated drivers. On the negative side, however, the report found that many of the students who used designated drivers still occasionally rode with alcohol-impaired drivers. Thus, the researchers suggested that educational efforts should stress that students need to designate a driver before they start drinking.

Alcohol and drugs in movies. In April 1999, the White House Office of National Drug Control Policy announced the results of a study that analyzed alcohol and drug use in the most popular American movie videos and music recordings of 1996 and 1997. The study found that the movies were almost four times as likely as the music to depict the use of alcohol or drugs, and that alcohol

was four times more likely to appear in the movies than illicit drugs.

Alcohol appeared in 93 percent of the 200 films in the study, while illicit drugs were seen in 22 percent. Each of these substances was depicted in less than 20 percent of the 1,000 songs in the study.

In more than half the scenes in which alcohol appeared in film, it was associated with wealth, luxury, or sexual activity and had no negative consequences for the user. In 37 percent of the scenes, alcohol was associated with crime or violence. Only 14 percent of the scenes with alcohol depicted an actor refusing to use the substance, and less than 10 percent featured a direct antiuse statement.

The study concluded that the film industry is presenting the misleading message to young people that alcohol use is normal and does not cause problems.

Coverage for substance abuse. In June 1999, President Bill Clinton directed the U.S. Office of Personnel Management to achieve parity for substance abuse for all federal employees. Parity means that health insurance pays for treatment for substance abuse, just as it pays for treating other *chronic* (long-term) disorders, such as asthma and heart disease. Clinton said he hoped this move would serve as an example to private insurance companies, many of which do not provide coverage for substance-abuse treatment.

The National Institute on Alcohol Abuse and Alcoholism estimates that substance abuse costs the United States more than $100 billion per year. Government officials predict that this cost would be substantially reduced if substance-abuse treatment was included in more health insurance benefits.

For example, the National Household Survey on Drug Abuse reported that 73 percent of illegal drug users were employed in 1997. This suggests that if all these individuals had health insurance for substance abuse through their employers, the amount of money that the government spends on treating drug abuse and fighting crime would be greatly reduced.　　　• David C. Lewis

One of the most commonly prescribed medications for long-term control of asthma symptoms contains an ingredient that may actually have a detrimental effect on a patient's condition. The results of a study on racemic albuterol were reported in December 1998 by a team of researchers led by asthma specialist Harold Nelson at the National Jewish Medical and Research Center in Denver, Colorado.

Racemic albuterol is a *bronchodilator,* a drug that relaxes the muscles around the air passages in the lungs. The drug contains equal portions of two related compounds. R albuterol (also called levalbuterol) is the actual bronchodilator. The other compound, S albuterol, was originally believed to be a neutral agent, but several studies in the 1990's suggested that it could exaggerate the sensitivity of air passages, making it more likely for a person to have an asthma attack.

Nelson's group investigated this potential problem in a study of 328 people with moderate to severe asthma. They treated the patients with a certain dosage of either levalbuterol (only the R compound), racemic albuterol (both the R and S compounds), or a *placebo* (an inactive substance). The researchers determined the effectiveness and safety of the drugs with various lung-function tests and the patients' reports of side effects.

The most effective treatment in the study was the largest dose of levalbuterol (1.25 milligrams). However, the smallest dose of levalbuterol (0.63 milligrams) proved to be as effective as the largest dose of racemic albuterol (2.5 milligrams). The researchers concluded, therefore, that the S compound acted against the beneficial effect of the R compound.

All of the people who received medication in the study experienced the common side effects of albuterol drugs, including nervousness, tremors, increased heart rate, increased levels of sugar in the blood, and decreased levels of potassium. The researchers noted, however, that the small dose of levalbuterol resulted in fewer side effects while still effectively controlling the asthma.

Asthma treatment for children. In February 1999, researchers led by asthma specialist James Baker at Kaiser Permanente, a health maintenance organization based in San Diego, California, recommended changes in treatment for infants and young children with asthma. Their study addressed a gap in guidelines for controlling *chronic* (long-term) inflammation of air passages, the primary condition of the disease.

In 1997, the National Asthma Education and Prevention Program—a branch of the National Institutes of Health in Bethesda, Maryland—called for the regular use of anti-inflammato-

Problems with piercings

Researchers at the Helsinki City Center for the Environment in Finland reported in January 1999 that nickel allergies are on the rise. Constant exposure to nickel in inexpensive earring studs and other pierced jewelry can lead to an allergic sensitivity to the metal that can cause skin inflammation.

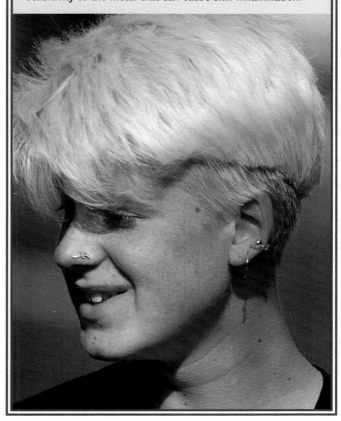

ry agents, such as corticosteroids, early in the treatment of asthma. However, asthma experts did not determine the most effective and safest treatment for young patients.

Most older children and adults inhale anti-inflammatory agents with a device called a metered-dose inhaler, which delivers the medication directly to the lungs. These devices require the person to spray the medication and inhale at the same time—a task that is impossible or difficult for infants and young children.

To help young patients, physicians often prescribe the use of a *spacer,* a small chamber attached to an inhaler that makes the timing of spraying and

inhaling less critical. Other children take corticosteroids with a *nebulizer,* a machine that changes the drug into a mist that can be inhaled through a breathing mask. Unfortunately, not all drugs are easily nebulized, and consequently, children may not receive adequate doses of corticosteroids.

In a 12-week study, Baker's group evaluated the use of an anti-inflammatory drug called budesonide inhalation suspension (BIS), which has properties that make it easy to nebulize. The researchers hoped to determine what dosage level of BIS would be safe and effective for children ages 6 months to 8 years who had moderate, persistent asthma.

The 480 children in the study received certain doses with a nebulizer once or twice day, or they received a placebo. The researchers analyzed the effectiveness of the treatment on the basis of various lung-function tests, daily journals kept by parents, and the number of times children needed to take short-acting medications to control an asthma attack. The researchers determined that taking 0.5 milligrams of BIS once a day was the minimum dosage necessary for controlling chronic inflammation. Determining a minimum dosage is important because a physician's goal is generally to begin treatment with the least amount of medicine as possible.

Baker's team also tested some of the children to determine if BIS affected growth or the regulation of certain hormone levels in the body, known side effects of corticosteroid treatment. At the end of the study, they found no significant changes between the group receiving treatment and the placebo group. The researchers cautioned, however, that their study did not take into account possible long-term effects.

Risks in asthma treatment. In the 1990's, inhaled corticosteroids became the primary line of defense for controlling asthma, but numerous studies had noted the adverse effects of the drugs. In May 1999, respiratory specialist Brian J. Lipworth of the University of Dundee in Scotland reported a review and analysis of 27 studies of corticosteroids that were published since 1996. He noted the

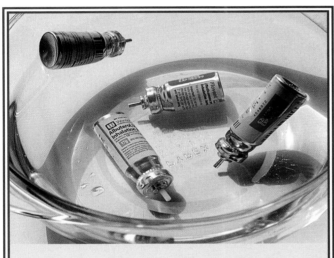

Waiting to inhale—the float test

A simple floating test can help people with asthma determine how much medication is left in the canister of an inhaling device. Family physician Mark A. Rickenbach of Portsmouth University in England reported on the results of tests with 289 inhalers at the September 1998 conference of the World Organization of Family Health Doctors.

- The two canisters floating horizontally below the surface of the water, *center,* are more than 70 percent full.

- The canister floating almost vertically with the valve pointing down, *right,* is between 30 and 70 percent full.

- At about 15 to 30 percent fullness, *left,* the canister floats at about a 30-degree angle with about half of it in the air and the valve end submerged.

- If the valve is at all exposed, then the amount of medication has dropped below 15 percent, a level that is too low for safe use of an inhaler.

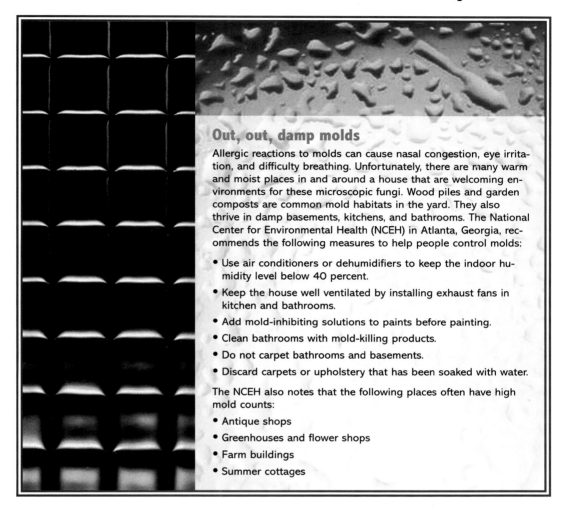

Out, out, damp molds

Allergic reactions to molds can cause nasal congestion, eye irritation, and difficulty breathing. Unfortunately, there are many warm and moist places in and around a house that are welcoming environments for these microscopic fungi. Wood piles and garden composts are common mold habitats in the yard. They also thrive in damp basements, kitchens, and bathrooms. The National Center for Environmental Health (NCEH) in Atlanta, Georgia, recommends the following measures to help people control molds:

- Use air conditioners or dehumidifiers to keep the indoor humidity level below 40 percent.
- Keep the house well ventilated by installing exhaust fans in kitchen and bathrooms.
- Add mold-inhibiting solutions to paints before painting.
- Clean bathrooms with mold-killing products.
- Do not carpet bathrooms and basements.
- Discard carpets or upholstery that has been soaked with water.

The NCEH also notes that the following places often have high mold counts:

- Antique shops
- Greenhouses and flower shops
- Farm buildings
- Summer cottages

consensus of these studies and the need for research in certain areas.

He reported, for example, that studies consistently showed that high doses of inhaled corticosteroids (more than 1.5 milligrams a day) result in significant suppression of the adrenal gland, a condition that can render the body incapable of dealing with emotional and physical stress. One particular corticosteroid called fluticasone porpionate caused adrenal suppression at relatively moderate doses of 0.75 milligrams a day.

Lipworth also cited several studies showing that corticosteroid treatment slowed the rate of growth in children and adolescents. He suggested, however, that the most important outcome to evaluate is long-term growth

and the comparison of a final adult height with the expected height for each individual. Only two studies addressed this final outcome, and both suggested that adults reached their expected height after a delayed growth in adolescence. Lipworth also noted the difficulty of accurately studying this impact of corticosteroids because asthma itself can delay or suppress growth.

The author also reported that long-term, high-dosage treatment with inhaled corticosteroids resulted in a significant loss of bone density and an increased risk for eye disorders, such as glaucoma. Nonetheless, Lipworth concluded that, according to the current research, the benefits of corticosteroids for controlling asthma outweighed the risks of side effects. He stated, however, that the most rational approach to treatment is for doctors to taper inhaled corticosteroid doses to the lowest effective level and to monitor patients carefully for possible adverse effects.

Asthma and adults. An April 1999 report by allergist Charles E. Reed of the Mayo Clinic in Rochester, Minnesota, drew attention to the particular problems of asthma in adults and the risks of irreversible damage to the lungs. Based on a review of research, Reed recommended measures for controlling asthma in middle-age and elderly adults, who are often more

severely impaired by asthma than are children but who are often neglected in asthma research.

Reed's review of several studies showed that people over the age of 50 are more susceptible to *airway remodeling,* the permanent damage to air passages due to uncontrolled, chronic inflammation. Asthma during adulthood, he also noted, is often complicated by other factors, such as respiratory infections and bronchitis, that require careful monitoring. Reed's recommendations included diligent control of inflammation and more research on treatments that prevent irreversible damage to the lungs.   • Dominick A. Minotti

Birth Control

- Emergency contraceptive approved
- Contraceptive failure rates
- Computer-guided birth control

In September 1998, the Preven Emergency Contraceptive Kit became the first prepackaged *emergency contraceptive* (a birth control medication taken after intercourse) approved by the Federal Drug Administration (FDA) for sale in the United States. The kit, manufactured by Gynetics, Incorporated, of Belle Mead, New Jersey, was available by prescription from physicians and other health care professionals.

Birth control pills included in the Preven kit are known as combined emergency contraceptive pills, because they contain both the hormones estrogen and progestin. These are the same two pregnancy-blocking hormones found in many ordinary birth control pills. Estrogen and progestin inhibit *ovulation* (the release of an egg by the ovary) and prevent the *endometrium* (lining of the uterus) from accepting the implantation of a fertilized egg. Unlike RU-486, a drug recommended for approval by an FDA advisory committee in 1996 but still unavailable in the United States as of mid-1999, the Preven pills do not interfere with an established pregnancy.

To be effective, the first dose of the pills must be taken within 72 hours after unprotected sexual intercourse. A second dose must then be taken 12 hours after the first. Studies showed that a woman's risk of pregnancy decreased by an average of 75 percent when the Preven pills were used correctly.

Contraceptive failure rates. Two U.S. studies, published in March and April 1999, reported that approximately 10 percent of American women using *reversible* (nonsurgical) contraceptives experience an unplanned pregnancy within the first 12 months of contraceptive use. The studies, by researchers at Princeton University in Princeton, New Jersey, and the Alan Guttmacher Institute, a reproductive-health research organization based in New York City, were based on data from the National Survey of Family Growth. This survey, of more than 10,000 women, was conducted by the U.S. National Center for Health Statistics between 1991 and 1995.

The researchers reported that long-term birth control methods that did not involve ongoing efforts by the users had very low failure rates after one year. For example, hormonal implants and injectable birth control methods failed in only about 2 to 3 percent of women in the survey. The researchers found that those birth control methods that required more active involvement by users, such as birth control pills and the male condom, had medium-level failure rates. The pill failed in about 8 percent of the surveyed women, while 14 percent of the women reported pregnancies despite the use of the condom. Spermicides, withdrawal, and periodic abstinence showed the highest one-year failure rates—at 26 percent, 24 percent, and 21 percent respectively.

FDA approves emergency contraceptive

The Preven Emergency Contraceptive Kit was approved by the U.S. Food and Drug Administration in September 1998. The kit, manufactured by Gynetics, Incorporated, of Belle Mead, New Jersey, contained birth control pills that could be taken after unprotected intercourse to prevent pregnancy. The Preven kit was available only by prescription. Possible side effects included cramping, breast tenderness, and fluid retention.

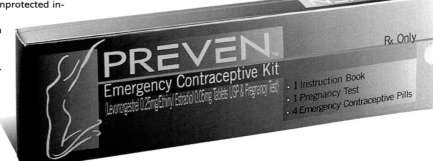

According to the studies, levels of contraceptive failure varied widely depending on the personal characteristics of the user. Women who were poor, younger, unmarried, Hispanic, or African American experienced the highest contraceptive failure rates. The researchers theorized that difficulty in obtaining particular contraceptive methods, inexperience with various methods, and the inconsistent use of contraceptives contribute to many unintended pregnancies.

Computer-guided birth control.
Researchers in 1999 tested the effectiveness of a computer designed to help women chart their menstrual cycles. Women using the Persona computer, manufactured by Unipath Diagnostics Company of Great Britain, insert urine test sticks into the handheld device eight days a month. The computer analyzes hormone levels on the test sticks to determine on which days during a woman's menstrual cycle she can engage in sexual intercourse without becoming pregnant.

According to Unipath, early results of the *clinical trials* (observations of patients) showed the Persona computer to be 93 to 95 percent reliable. Although Persona kits were not yet available in the United States in 1999, the devices were being sold in Great Britain.　　　● Lauren Love

A *mutation* (change) in the gene that encodes *prothrombin,* a protein that is important for blood clot formation, may increase the risk of heart attack. That conclusion was published in January 1999 by researchers at the Laboratory for Experimental Internal Medicine at the University of Amsterdam in the Netherlands.

Prior research had shown that a specific change in the DNA sequence of the gene that encodes prothrombin resulted in increased levels of prothrombin. (DNA—deoxyribonucleic acid—is the molecule that makes up genes.) However, scientists did not know whether individuals carrying the abnormal prothrombin gene were at an increased risk for developing blood clots in their arteries or veins or suffering heart attacks.

The researchers in Amsterdam examined 400 healthy patients and 263 patients who had early development of *atherosclerosis* (fatty deposits in the heart). They reported that 1 percent of the healthy individuals in the study had the abnormal prothrombin gene, while 2.7 percent of those patients in the early stages of atherosclerosis carried the abnormal prothrombin gene.

Furthermore, patients who carried one abnormal and one normal prothrombin gene of the possible two prothrombin genes had an increased risk of heart attack. The researchers said that the risk for those patients

Blood

- Risk of heart attack
- Erythropoietin and transfusions
- TTP cause identified

was four times greater than patients who did not have an abnormal prothrombin gene.

These investigators suggested that people who have the abnormal prothrombin gene also have an increased risk for heart attacks and blood clots.

However, another study contradicted these findings. In a study published in March 1999, researchers at Brigham and Women's Hospital in Boston, led by cardiologist Paul Ridker, reported that of 14,916 men with the defective prothrombin gene, only 833 developed some type of heart ailment. The researchers concluded that there was no proof of an association between patients who carry the abnormal prothrombin gene and the risk of heart attack, stroke, or blood clots.

Erythropoietin and transfusions.

Researchers led by Andreas Laupacis, an epidemiologist at the Ottawa Civic Hospital in Ontario, Canada, in December 1998 reported that using *erythropoietin*, a hormone that increases the amount of red blood cells in the body, decreases the need for blood transfusions from unrelated donors in patients undergoing bone or heart surgery.

The researchers reviewed numerous studies that determined the side effects of giving erythropoietin to patients who had undergone such surgeries. Erythropoietin had already been used successfully to increase red blood cell counts in patients with cancer and those with kidney failure.

The Canadian researchers reported that the studies they examined showed that erythropoietin decreased the need for blood transfusion from unrelated donors in patients and presented no negative side effects. Additional studies taking place in mid-1999 were designed to determine the cost-effectiveness of giving patients erythropoietin versus other treatments to minimize blood transfusion after surgery.

TTP cause identified. A team of international researchers, headed by Miha Furlan of the University Hospital in Bern, Switzerland, reported in November 1998 that they had discovered the cause of inherited forms of thrombotic thrombocytopenic purpura (TTP). TTP is a potentially fatal disease characterized by widespread platelet clots in the small blood vessels. Platelets are the cells responsible for blood clotting. Without such platelets, a person could bleed to death from even a minor cut. Patients with TTP can experience fevers, mental confusion, destruction of red blood cells, decreased platelet counts, and kidney failure.

According to the study, patients with TTP have abnormally large amounts of a protein, called von Willebrand's factor, in their blood.

Safe needle disposal
A safer way to destroy used needles was marketed in 1999 by Bio Medical Disposal in Norcross, Georgia. The battery-powered device, called the SharpX Needle Destruction Unit, *right,* uses an electrical charge to disintegrate a needle in less than 10 seconds. A replaceable drawer collects the debris.

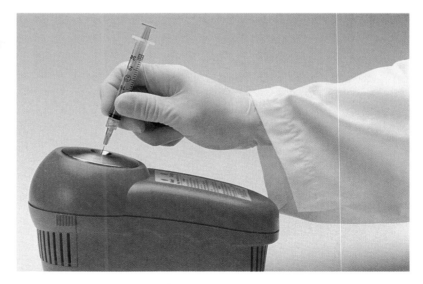

Von Willebrand's factor activates the platelets responsible for the clotting of blood. These proteins can be broken down into smaller pieces by a protein called von Willebrand factor-cleaving protease. (A protease is any one of various enzymes that break down proteins into simpler compounds).

The team of international researchers found that there was a lack of the protease in the majority of patients with an inherited form of TTP. Patients who did not have an inherited form of TTP, however, had an antibody that inhibited the protein that breaks down von Willebrand's factor in their blood.

Furlan's research was supported by a second study also published in November 1998. Researchers led by Han-Mou Tsai at Montefiore Medical Center and Albert Einstein College of Medicine in Bronx, New York City, found that antibodies to the protease were present in patients with TTP. This antibody disappeared when the patients were treated successfully for TTP. However, when TTP recurred in these patients, the antibodies against the protein that breaks down von Willebrand's factor returned. Scientists in 1999 said that identification of the cause of TTP should offer new types of treatments for patients.

• G. David Roodman

Researchers at St. Thomas Hospital and at Whipps Cross Hospital, both in London, England, reported that women who are older, heavier, and have osteoarthritis (OA) in their hands have an increased risk for developing osteoarthritis in the knee. This study was published in the journal *Arthritis & Rheumatism* in January 1999.

OA is the most common form of arthritis. It is a major source of pain and disability in men and women over the age of 45, though it occurs more often in women than in men. OA primarily affects the *cartilage,* a slick, resilient material at the ends of bones that acts as a shock absorber and makes joint motion smooth. In the joints of people with OA, cartilage becomes thin and rough and loses its shock-absorbing properties. Although genetic factors may predispose people to OA, other factors, such as repeated injury to an area, also influence its occurrence.

The researchers studied more than 700 women over 50 years of age. They examined X rays of the women's knees at the beginning of the study and then again four years later. In an average of 3.3 percent of the women each year, the X rays revealed the formation of *osteophytes,* spurs or bony growths that surround joints af-

Bone and Joint Disorders

- Increased risk of osteo-arthritis (OA)
- Heart disease, stroke, and lupus
- A new treatment for rheumatoid arthritis (RA)
- Chemotherapy and arthritis

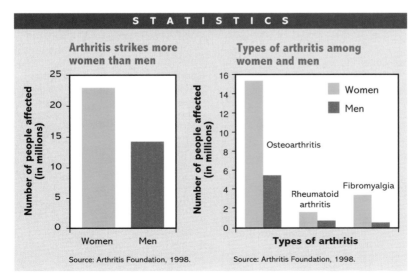

STATISTICS

Arthritis strikes more women than men

Number of people affected (in millions)

Women / Men

Types of arthritis among women and men

Number of people affected (in millions)

Women
Men

Osteoarthritis
Rheumatoid arthritis
Fibromyalgia

Types of arthritis

Source: Arthritis Foundation, 1998.

Source: Arthritis Foundation, 1998.

The Arthritis Foundation reported in 1998 that while both men and women are affected by various forms of arthritis, women tend to be affected more often by the most common and most damaging forms of the disease. Women account for 74 percent of all cases of osteoarthritis, 71 percent of all cases of rheumatoid arthritis, and 89 percent of all fibromyalgia cases.

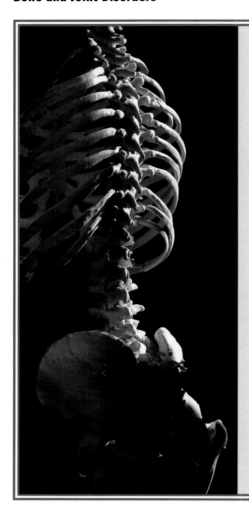

Who is at risk for osteoporosis?

Osteoporosis is a disease that robs bones of calcium and makes them more likely to break. It occurs more commonly in women than in men, primarily in people over the age of 65. According to the National Osteoporosis Foundation, doctors can now predict who is most likely to be in danger of developing the condition.

Primary risk factors

- Previous fractures as an adult, regardless of cause
- Parents or siblings who have had fractures
- Cigarette smoking
- Small, thin body frame

Secondary risk factors

- Race (Caucasians are most at risk)
- Age
- Poor health
- Dementia
- Diet low in calcium
- Eating disorder
- Estrogen deficiency in women
- Testosterone deficiency in men
- Excessive drinking
- Physical inactivity

fected by OA. The women most likely to develop osteophytes were those who were older, heavier, and already had OA of the hands.

A surprising result of the study was the observation that women who had undergone estrogen replacement therapy (ERT) seemed less likely to develop OA. ERT is commonly prescribed for women undergoing *menopause,* a time when the ovaries decrease their production of the female sex hormone estrogen and menstruation stops. ERT reduces symptoms associated with menopause and has been shown to provide protective benefits for the bones and cardiovascular system.

Although OA affects a large number of older people, the investigators concluded that its impact may be lessened by a program of weight reduction and ERT use in women.

Heart disease, stroke, and lupus. Although young women are usually spared from heart disease and stroke, women with an autoimmune disease called systemic lupus erythematosus (SLE or lupus) are at risk of developing these conditions at a young age. A comprehensive survey of hospital records in California, described in the journal *Arthritis & Rheumatism* in February 1999, reported that women with SLE are much more likely to be hospitalized for heart attacks, congestive heart failure, and stroke than women without SLE.

Autoimmune disease is any disorder in which the body treats its own tissues or cells as if they were foreign substances and produces *antibodies* (molecules that normally protect people from disease) to destroy those tissues or cells. In SLE, disturbances in the immune system lead to the production of abnormal antibodies that bind to normal tissue and cause inflammation or disrupt the function of the tissue. Lupus most commonly damages tissue in the skin, joints, kidneys, blood, and nervous system. The disease affects primarily young women in their child-bearing years.

Researcher Michael M. Ward of Stanford University School of Medicine in California reviewed the records of more than 8,700 women over the age of 18 who had been hospitalized in California and who were identified as having SLE. He compared their records with those of hospitalized women who did not have SLE. Ward discovered that women with SLE were hospitalized for heart attacks, heart failure, and strokes 2 to 4 times more often than women without the disease. The risk for heart disease was greater in younger women with lupus than in older women. Since heart attacks are rare in young women because of the beneficial effects of the female sex hormone estrogen, the increased occurrence in women with SLE suggested that the disease may have a powerful effect on blood vessels.

Ward noted that several factors may explain the increased risk for cerebrovascular and cardiovascular disease in women with lupus. These factors include inflammation of the blood vessels, high blood pressure, the effects of medications to treat SLE, abnormalities in blood clotting or in blood *lipids* (fats or fatlike substances) from drugs, and kidney disease. With increasing age, the differences between women with and without lupus may decrease because women without lupus acquire other risk factors for cardiovascular disease.

Ward concluded that, because the study identified a connection between the immune system and cardiovascular and *cerebrovascular* (relating to blood vessels in the brain) disease, patients with SLE should be regularly evaluated for symptoms that suggest heart disease and stroke. Doctors who treat such patients may want to consider prescribing preventive measures, such as medications that lower cholesterol or modify blood clotting.

A new treatment may halt the damage to cartilage and bone caused by rheumatoid arthritis (RA). Researchers reported this finding in the December 1998 issue of *Arthritis & Rheumatism.*

Rheumatoid arthritis is the most common form of inflammatory arthritis. It causes pain, stiffness, and swelling in joints. In people with RA,

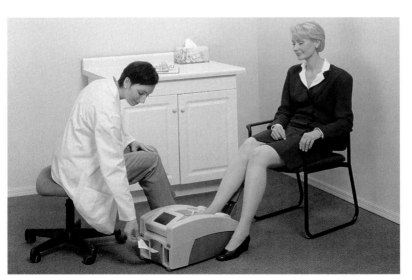

Testing for bone loss
A device introduced in 1999 allows doctors to test a patient's risk for developing fractures due to osteoporosis during routine office visits. An instrument called an ultrasonometer, *left,* uses ultrasound to measure the bone density of the heel. The machine then calculates the patient's *T-score,* a comparison between the density of the patient's bone and that of a young adult who does not have osteoporosis. Patients with low bone mass can then take steps to build stronger bones.

the body's immune system attacks the lining inside a joint and causes inflammation that can damage bones and cartilage. RA usually affects the fingers and wrists, though it can also occur in the feet, knees, ankles, shoulders, and elbows. RA affects approximately 2.1 million Americans, usually beginning between the ages of 20 and 40. It strikes about three times as many women as men.

The new treatment, called interleukin-1 receptor antagonist (IL-1Ra), not only relieves the symptoms of RA but also seems to halt the damage to cartilage and bone that lead to pain and deformity. IL-1Ra is produced by a technique called *recombinant DNA technology* (manipulation of genes).

IL-1Ra, a hormonelike protein, blocks the action of IL-1, a protein that causes inflammation in the joints of people with RA. The researchers found that IL-1Ra binds to the same immune cells as IL-1. As a result, IL-1Ra stops IL-1 from prompting the immune cells to attack healthy joint tissue.

IL-1Ra was tested on more than 400 people between the ages of 18 and 75 who had active and severe arthritis. The patients were treated at 41 centers in 11 European countries. Three groups of patients were given varying doses of IL-1Ra daily by injection. The fourth group received a *placebo* (inactive substance).

After 24 weeks, the group receiving the highest dose of IL-1Ra experienced marked reduction in pain and swelling. In addition, X rays showed that this group had 41 percent less damage to their joints than the group treated with a placebo. The groups receiving lower doses of IL-1Ra improved as well.

Since visible damage in joint X rays predicts the extent of future cartilage and bone destruction, the investigators were optimistic that IL-1Ra could modify the long-term course of the disease. However, they noted that future research will be needed to determine the best way to use IL-1RA both alone and in combination with other therapies.

Chemotherapy and arthritis. High-dose *chemotherapy* (drug therapy often used to treat cancer) may provide a new way of treating people with serious autoimmune diseases. Researchers at Johns Hopkins University School of Medicine in Baltimore and at Hahnemann University in Philadelphia, Pennsylvania, reported their findings in the December 1998 issue of *Annals of Internal Medicine*.

The investigators administered high doses of a drug called cyclophosphamide (sold as Cytoxan) to eight patients who had a variety of autoimmune diseases, including RA and SLE. (The patients' illnesses had previously proven resistant to other treatments for autoimmune diseases.) Cytoxan is

New drugs for rheumatoid arthritis (RA)

The U.S. Food and Drug Administration approved several new drugs in 1998 and 1999 for the treatment of RA, a form of inflammatory arthritis that causes pain, stiffness, and swelling in joints.

RA can destroy cartilage and bone and lead to crippling and deformity. Doctors have generally treated RA with nonsteroidal anti-inflammatory drugs (NSAID's), such as aspirin and ibuprofen.

Type of drug	Generic and (brand) names	Cost per month	The way it works
Disease-modifying antirheumatic drug (DMARD)	Leflunomide (Arava)	$200 to $300	Slows the progression of RA by blocking a protein that causes the immune system to attack the joints. In studies performed thus far, Arava seems not to significantly affect the immune system's ability to fight infections.
Biologic response modifier	Etanercept (Enbrel)	$1000	Self-injected by patients twice a week. Slows the progression of RA by attacking a protein called tumor-necrosis factor that causes joint inflammation and tissue damage.
COX-2 inhibitors	Celecoxib (Celebrex) Rofecoxib (Vioxx)	$100 to $200	Limit pain and swelling by inhibiting hormones that cause them. Unlike older NSAID's, COX-2 inhibitors do not block the enzyme COX-1, which protects the stomach lining.

a powerful drug commonly used to treat cancer, because of its ability to cause damage to DNA and kill cells. The drug had been used to treat autoimmune diseases, but usually only at relatively low dosages to reduce the likelihood of serious side effects such as the suppression of *bone marrow,* the source of red and white blood cells in the body. In the 1998 study, the investigators gave the eight patients Cytoxan in doses sufficient to destroy bone marrow cells.

The investigators reasoned that Cytoxan, given at high doses, could kill the white blood cells that cause autoimmune disease, while sparing the precursor or stem cells that allow the bone marrow to return after a period of suppression. Thus, the blood cells that eventually return lack the abnormal factors that cause autoimmunity. The patients were given drugs to help speed recovery of the bone marrow, after Cytoxan treatment.

Four of the patients experienced complete remission of their disease, and two others had partial remission for approximately two years. The therapy appeared to cause few side effects. Future studies, however, need to determine the long-term safety of this dose therapy and the chance that the autoimmune diseases will recur.

• David S. Pisetsky

See also DRUGS.

The following books on health and medicine topics were written for the general reader. All were published in 1998 and 1999.

Aging. *RealAge: Are You as Young as You Can Be?* by Michael F. Roizen with Elizabeth Anne Stephenson. Internist and anesthesiologist Roizen and science writer Stephenson discuss lifestyle choices that can extend life. They review such issues as diet, exercise, stress reduction, and driving safety. (Cliff Street Books, 1999. 335 pp. $25.)

Alternative medicine. *Radical Healing: Integrating the World's Great Therapeutic Traditions to Create a New Transformative Medicine* by Rudolph M. Ballentine. Ballentine, director of the Center for Holistic Medicine, draws on more than 30 years of practice as a physician and psychiatrist. He discusses alternative therapies including herbs, homeopathy, and Eastern traditions of medicine. (Harmony Books, 1999. 612 pp. $27.50.)

Anesthesia. *Patient's Guide to Anesthesia: Making the Right Choices* by A. J. Hill. Anesthesiologist Hill dispels common myths about surgery and anesthesia. He describes what one may see, hear, and feel during surgery, making the process less mysterious and frightening. (Kensington Books, 1999. 270 pp. $13.)

Cancer. *Healing Lessons* by Sidney J. Winawer with Nick Taylor. Winawer, a specialist in cancer of the digestive system, recounts his wife's struggle with stomach cancer that spread to her liver. Straddling the worlds of both physician and patient, he describes his wife's treatments—based on both traditional and alternative therapies—and the effects of her disease on his work and on their marriage. (Little Brown, 1998. 273 pp. $24.95.)

One Renegade Cell: How Cancer Begins by Robert A. Weinberg. Weinberg, the director of a cancer research lab and a professor of biology at the Massachusetts Institute of Technology, explains the forces driving malignant growth. He draws on discoveries of the late 1900's and new insights that are beginning to change how cancers are diagnosed and treated. (Basic Books, 1998. 170 pp. $18.90.)

Chronic illness. *Surviving Your Spouse's Chronic Illness* by Chris McGonigle. McGonigle, whose husband was diagnosed with multiple sclerosis at the age of 32, recounts her feelings over 15 years of his illness. She examines such issues as communication, sex, anger, money, parenting, and spirituality. (Henry Holt, 1999. 238 pp. $13.95.)

Drugs. *The American Pharmaceutical Association Practical Guide to Natural*

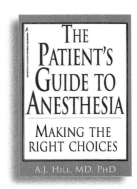

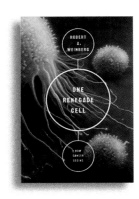

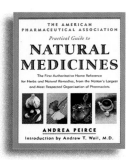

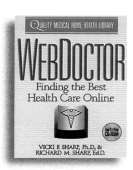

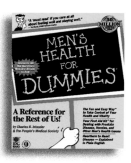

Medicines edited by Andrea Peirce. Medical editor Peirce provides scientific evidence of the safety and effectiveness of more than 300 natural substances. For each substance, she lists the source, scientific and common names, side effects, and uses. (Morrow, 1998. 728 pp. $35.)

Magic Molecules: How Drugs Work by Susan Aldridge. A professional science writer and fellow of the Royal Society of Medicine, Aldridge describes the action of drugs in treating pain, heart problems, cancer, infections, and mental disorders. She also includes herbs and food supplements. (Cambridge University Press, 1998. 269 pp. $24.95.)

Eye care. *The Eye Book* by Gary H. Cassel, Michael D. Bilig, and Harry G. Randall. Three eye-care specialists detail how the eye works, what can go wrong, how to recognize emergencies, and how best to cope with low vision. They also discuss eyeglasses, contact lenses, and the effects of disease and medications on sight. (Johns Hopkins University Press, 1998. 367 pp. $18.95.)

Family health. *The Doctor's Book of Home Remedies for Preventing Disease* by Hugh O'Neill and the editors of *Prevention* magazine. The authors consulted hundreds of experts and explored current research to find home remedies for over 130 common health problems. They include help for allergies, fatigue, bursitis/tendonitis, jet lag, back and knee pain, and menopause symptoms. (Rodale Press, 1999. 637 pp. $29.95.)

Family Health for Dummies by Charles B. Inlander, Karla Morales, and the People's Medical Society. The authors outline preventive measures for good health. Special sections cover children, teens, parents, managing medical conditions, making the most of medical visits, and stretching the medical dollar. (IDG Books, 1998. 385 pp. $19.99.)

Surviving Modern Medicine by Peter Clarke and Susan H. Evans. Clarke, a University of Southern California (USC) professor of preventive medicine and communications, and Evans, a research scientist at the USC Institute for Health Promotion and Dis-

ease Prevention, provide advice on getting a doctor's attention, making good medical decisions, seeking support from family and friends, and maintaining lifelong health. (Rutgers University Press, 1998. 308 pp. $17.)

Health care online. *Web Doctor* by Richard M. Sharp and Vicki F. Sharp. The authors list Web sites that contain relevant and timely health care information. They have chosen sites that are effectively organized in stable locations, are updated regularly, and acclaimed by other reviewers as valuable, reliable, and authoritative. The publication includes a CD-ROM with links compatible with Internet Explorer and Netscape Navigator. (St. Martin's Griffin, 1998. 557 pp. $29.95.)

Hypertension. *Essential Guide to Hypertension* by the American Medical Association. The authors discuss how the body controls blood pressure, how hypertension hurts the body, and how the condition—which affects 1 out of 4 adults in the United States—is diagnosed and treated. They also explain how hypertension is related to other diseases, explore current research in the field, and answer common questions. (Pocket Books, 1998. 228 pp. $14.)

Menopause. *Menopause and the Mind: The Complete Guide to Coping with Memory Loss, Foggy Thinking, Verbal Slips and Other Cognitive Effects of Perimenopause and Menopause* by Claire L. Warga. Warga, a neuropsychologist and researcher, provides scientific explanations for the mental symptoms experienced by many women as estrogen levels decrease. She includes a self-screening test and guides for treating symptoms including diet, hormone replacement, and memory improvement methods. (Free Press, 1999. 388 pp. $24.)

Men's health. *Men's Health for Dummies* by Charles B. Inlander and the People's Medical Society. Inlander recommends that men take charge of their health by making careful choices about personal health maintenance and insurance. He also discusses strategies for losing weight and reducing stress and for specific problems such as pain, hair loss, insomnia, depression, chronic illnesses, and sexual health. (IDG Books Worldwide, 1999. 380 pp. $19.99.)

Mental health. *Straight Talk About Psychiatric Medications for Kids* by Timothy E. Wilens. Wilens surveys the mental, emotional, and behavioral conditions in children that are treated with medications. He explains conditions and symptoms, treatment options, how to use medicines and their short- and long-term effects. (Guilford, 1999. 279 pp. $14.95.)

Your Mental Health by Allen Francis and Michael B. First. Francis and

First, the chairman and editor, respectively, of DSM-IV, the standard psychiatric reference, present 20 screening questions for a variety of mental illnesses and systematically address the diagnoses indicated by the answers. They describe the conditions and offer advice. (Scribner, 1998. 445 pp. $27.50.)

Sleep. *Power Sleep* by James B. Maas and others. The authors list the symptoms of sleep deficiency and provide tips and strategies for getting the sleep needed for mental and physical well-being. (HarperPerennial, 1999. 222 pp. $13.)

• Margaret E. Moore

Pharmaceutical researchers reported in July 1999 that they used a vaccine made from a common protein to prevent a brain condition similar to Alzheimer's disease in laboratory mice. The report was the first evidence that vaccination may help prevent this degenerative brain disorder.

Alzheimer's disease, which affects about 4 million people in the United States—most of them elderly—causes a progressive loss of memory and, eventually, a complete loss of mental function. The disease is characterized by the degeneration and death of brain cells. As the brain cells die, they form *amyloid plaques,* tangled masses

of cells and proteins. Scientists do not fully understand how or why these plaques develop. There is no effective treatment or cure for Alzheimer's disease.

Researchers at Elan Pharmaceuticals in South San Francisco, California, said they developed a vaccine that prevented the growth of amyloid plaques in mice that had been genetically altered to develop the human disorder. The researchers reported that the vaccine also halted the growth of plaques in mice with advanced plaque conditions.

The vaccine was made from a protein called beta-amyloid, the same

Brain and Nervous System

• Experimental vaccine for Alzheimer's disease
• Controlling Huntington's disease
• Growing new brain cells
• Blood cells from the brain
• How memory works

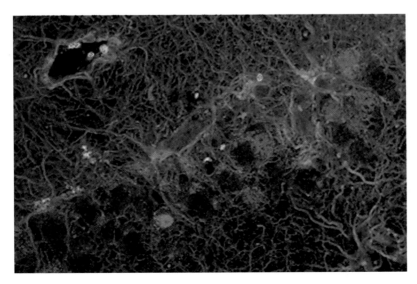

New cells in adult brain
In November 1998, scientists reported that they used chemical dyes to prove that the human brain can grow new nerve cells (green cells, *left*) in adulthood—overturning a long-held belief to the contrary. The scientists, at the Salk Institute for Biological Studies in La Jolla, California, and Sahlgrenska University Hospital in Sweden, said the finding offered hope to patients with degenerative brain disorders.

The slow decline of Alzheimer's disease

Individuals with Alzheimer's disease, an incurable brain disorder characterized by a progressive loss of mental skills, show a slow decline in the ability to perform daily activities. The disease may last 10 years or more, during which time patients become increasingly disabled in one activity after another. As a result of their declining abilities, Alzheimer's patients often need nursing-home care between 6 and 12 years after the onset of the disease.

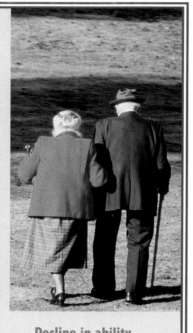

Activity	Decline in ability (years after onset of disease)
Shopping	1-5
Managing finances	1-5
Bathing	4-7
Bladder/bowel control	5-8
Feeding self	8-11

Source: Philip D. Sloane, University of North Carolina at Chapel Hill School of Medicine.

venting amyloid plaques would stop the loss of mental function in Alzheimer's patients. Some researchers believe that plaques may be a side effect of Alzheimer's disease rather than a cause.

Elan officials said they hoped to obtain approval from the U.S. Food and Drug Administration to begin preliminary human tests of the vaccine by the end of 1999. They planned to test the vaccine on patients who show early signs of Alzheimer's disease.

Controlling Huntington's disease. Scientists delayed the onset and slowed the progression of a mouse version of Huntington's disease, a hereditary human disorder in which brain cells are destroyed, according to a May 1999 report. The research, led by neurosurgeon Victor O. Ona of Harvard Medical School in Boston, brought the degenerative disease under control in mice by blocking an *enzyme* (a protein that speeds up chemical reactions) called caspase-1. The scientists hoped that additional research into this enzyme would lead to new treatments for Huntington's disease and other degenerative brain disorders.

Caspase-1 is one of the major enzymes involved in *apoptosis* (programmed cell death). Apoptosis is a genetically programmed process that causes the breakdown of the cell nucleus and cell wall.

All normal cells in the human body carry this self-destruction plan in their genes, to be activated when needed. For example, apoptosis is responsible for killing cells when they become cancerous. However, apoptosis can harm the body when it happens to normal, healthy cells—as in Huntington's disease.

Huntington's disease occurs because of a *mutation* (change) in a gene that codes for the production of a protein called huntingtin. The scientists noted that mice with this mutated gene developed a neurological disease similar to the human disorder, with seizures, tremors of the legs, and difficulty in walking. Associated with these abnormalities was a degeneration of *neurons* (nerve cells) in a part of the brain called the striatum.

protein present in amyloid plaques. The researchers said they were not sure why the vaccine prevented the development of the plaques. However, they speculated that vaccination with the protein may prompt immune-system cells in the blood to produce *antibodies* (substances that attack proteins foreign to the body). The antibodies, in turn, may induce immune-system cells in the brain— which normally fail to respond to amyloid plaques—to destroy the harmful protein.

Other Alzheimer's researchers, though encouraged by these findings, cautioned that more research would be needed to determine if such a vaccine would work in humans. They also said they were not sure if pre-

The scientists bred these mice with a strain of mice that carried a defect in the gene that codes for the production of caspase-1. The offspring of these two mouse strains had the mutated huntingtin gene, which would tend to cause the degenerative disorder. But they also had the mutated caspase-1 gene, which blocked apoptosis. Although the mice eventually developed tremors and seizures, the onset of these symptoms was greatly delayed and the life span of the mice was increased compared with mice with normal caspase-1.

For the final step of the experiment, the scientists used mice with the mutated huntingtin gene and normal caspase-1 gene. The researchers injected the mice with a drug made up of *peptides* (small pieces of proteins). The drug inhibited the action of caspase-1. Although these mice developed neurological disease, the symptoms were milder than in those mice that had not received the drug. In addition, the treated mice had a 25 percent greater life span than the untreated animals.

These results indicated that it is possible to decrease the death of neurons by inhibiting the actions of key enzymes necessary for apoptosis. However, the scientists noted that more research work needed to be done to ensure that altering apoptosis would not harm the human body.

Growing new brain cells. Several laboratories in 1998 and 1999 reported that, contrary to long-held beliefs, new cells can form in the adult brain. These findings offered hope to millions of people who have lost brain tissue due to strokes, trauma, or degenerative diseases.

One example of such research was reported in March 1999 by a team of biologists led by Su-Chun Zhang and Ian D. Duncan of the University of Wisconsin at Madison. These researchers demonstrated that cells taken from the mature brains of rats have the capacity to form new cells that produce *myelin,* the fatty insulation around nerve fibers. Myelin is destroyed in such diseases as multiple sclerosis, a disorder that can cause paralysis and vision loss.

Zhang and Duncan extracted brain cells called neural stem cells from a part of the adult rat brain called the subependymal region. These cells have the capacity to develop into any of the different types of brain cells. The scientists then grew the stem cells in a laboratory culture solution to obtain pure populations of the cells. Finally, the researchers transplanted the cells into the brains of other adult rats.

The scientists reported that the transplanted neural stem cells produced normal sheaths of myelin in the rat brains. Zhang and Duncan said that if similar results could be

Beethoven builds brains
Many years of playing a musical instrument causes the *cerebellum,* the part of the brain that controls balance and muscle coordination, to grow in size. This finding, reported in November 1998 by scientists at Beth Israel Deaconess Medical Center in Boston, suggested that the precise finger movements needed to play an instrument spur new nerve growth in the brains of musicians.

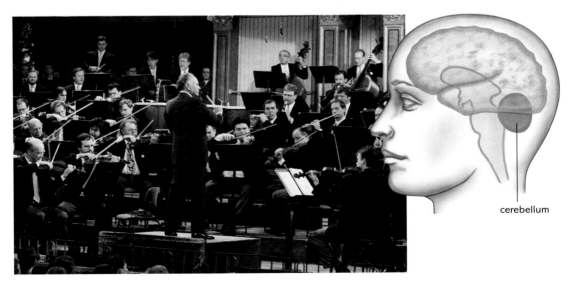

cerebellum

obtained with neural stem cells in human brains, it would be possible to repair some of the damage caused by myelin-destroying disorders.

Blood cells from the brain. Scientists reported in January 1999 that neural stem cells have the ability to develop into blood cells when transplanted into mice whose own blood-forming tissue has been destroyed. This research highlighted the potential of using neural stem cells in treatments for blood disorders and other medical conditions, in addition to neurological disorders.

A research team led by neurobiologist Angelo Vescovi of the National Neurological Institute in Italy transplanted neural stem cells from the brains of mice into the bodies of other mice. The mice that received the neural stem cells had previously undergone radiation to eliminate most of their *bone marrow,* the tissue where blood cells are formed. Following the transplantation, the animals redeveloped normal blood cells and bone marrow.

This experiment showed for the first time that the adult brain contains cells with the capacity to form cells unrelated to the brain. However, scientists said they still needed to learn what makes a neural stem cell become one cell type or another. Once this knowledge is obtained, new treatments could become available for a variety of disorders, according to researchers. These disorders include *severe combined immunodeficiency,* an illness characterized by the lack of certain infection-fighting cells, and *aplastic anemia,* a condition in which the body does not produce enough red blood cells.

How memory works. New clues into the mystery of how memory works were reported in January 1999 by a team of researchers led by psychologist Robert A. Jensen of Southern Illinois University at Carbondale. Jensen's group found that electrical stimulation of the vagus nerve, which extends from the *medulla* (brain stem) to organs in the abdomen, improved the memory of several individuals. The researchers said this finding might lead to new treatments for peo-

ple with brain disorders that result in memory loss.

The vagus nerve regulates the body's *vegetative functions*—the unconscious functions that control internal organs such as the heart, stomach, and intestines. For example, electrical impulses carried by the vagus nerve tell the brain that the stomach is full and that the heart needs to beat faster during exertion.

To determine if there is a connection between the vagus nerve and memory, the scientists studied 10 individuals with uncontrollable epilepsy, a brain disorder characterized by seizures. Because the seizures of these patients could not be managed with medication, they were treated with a form of therapy called vagal nerve stimulation. In this treatment, an implanted device delivers rapid electrical shocks to the vagus nerve to control seizures. (Scientists do not know how stimulation of the vagus nerve is able to control seizures.)

Jensen and his colleagues performed experiments in which they asked their subjects to read a series of paragraphs. After waiting a short time, the researchers asked the patients to recall 42 words from the paragraphs. The scientists then repeated the test, but in this instance they stimulated the vagus nerve of each individual immediately after he or she read the paragraphs.

The scientists noted that if the rate of vagus nerve stimulation was less than that required to control epileptic seizures, the patients' ability to remember words increased by 36 percent compared with when the nerve was not stimulated. The scientists also found that when the vagus nerve was stimulated at a rate necessary to control the seizures, the patients lost their improved memory.

The researchers did not know the reason for the dramatic increase in memory resulting from stimulation of the vagus nerve. Nonetheless, Jensen said the technique might serve as a useful tool to speed the recovery of patients with memory loss caused by stroke or trauma. He also said the technique might be able to improve the memory of patients with Alzheimer's disease. • Gary Birnbaum

See also MENTAL HEALTH.

A study released in February 1999 found evidence that supports the long-held belief that eating lots of fresh and processed tomatoes can lower the risk of some kinds of cancer. The study, led by researchers at Harvard Medical School in Cambridge, Massachusetts, used 72 studies that had examined the link between various cancers and the consumption of tomatoes and tomato-based products like spaghetti sauce and ketchup.

Some of the studies also examined the blood levels of lycopene, a compound principally found in tomatoes that protects cells from substances that have been linked to cancer. In all, 57 of the 72 studies linked tomato consumption with a reduced risk of cancer. The data were most compelling for cancers of the prostate gland, lung, and stomach.

The results of the Harvard study were supported by a study released in April 1999 which found that lycopene lowers the risk of prostate cancer. Researchers at the Karmanos Cancer Institute in Detroit, Michigan, studied 33 men who were due to have a cancerous prostate gland removed. Each day for three weeks the researchers gave 21 men 30 milligrams of pure tomato extract that contained lycopene. The remaining 12 men received no such treatment.

Men who took the tomato extract had smaller tumors than those who did not take the extract and the tumors in the treated group showed fewer signs of aggressive growth. Men treated with lycopene were about half as likely as men in the other group to have cancer that had spread to the edge of the prostate gland or beyond.

Debate on chemotherapy. Four major studies published in April 1999 showed that high-dose chemotherapy followed by a bone-marrow transplant, a grueling procedure held out as a hope to many women with advanced breast cancer, does not prolong survival. But the medical group that announced the findings cautioned that it was still too soon to pass final judgment on the procedure.

Many patients and doctors had hoped that the studies would finally determine whether it was worthwhile for women to undergo the drastic and costly treatment, which involves extremely high doses of chemotherapy. But the findings may instead fuel the long-standing disagreement between the procedure's advocates and its detractors and do little to help women decide whether to undertake the treatment.

The idea behind the treatment is to try to wipe out the cancer with high doses of chemotherapy. But those drugs also destroy the bone marrow, which produces the stem cells that generate the cells of the blood and

Cancer

- Tomatoes linked to reduced cancer rate
- Debate on high-dose chemotherapy
- Liver cancer rates on the rise
- Breast cancer and fat
- Reducing colon cancer rates
- Preventive mastectomies
- Cancer rates decline in the United States

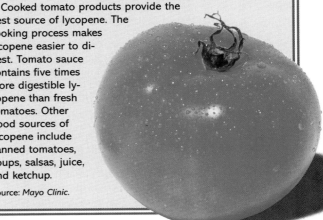

The low-down on lycopene

Research suggests that there is more to love about tomatoes than their fresh taste and versatility. Researchers believe lycopene, the substance that gives tomatoes their red color, is a potent antioxidant. Antioxidants are thought to neutralize *free radicals*, harmful substances in the body that may contribute to cancer and cardiovascular disease.

Researchers in 1998 and 1999 published several studies on the health effects of lycopene. One study of more than 1,300 European men suggested that individuals who consumed high quantities of lycopene-rich foods had about half the risk of heart attack as other men. Another study of 4,800 men found that those individuals who ate 10 servings a week of cooked tomato products had the lowest risk of prostate cancer. Their risk was one-third that of men who ate less than two servings a week. Other studies suggested that lycopene may help reduce the risk of other cancers, including breast, colon, and rectal cancer.

Cooked tomato products provide the best source of lycopene. The cooking process makes lycopene easier to digest. Tomato sauce contains five times more digestible lycopene than fresh tomatoes. Other good sources of lycopene include canned tomatoes, soups, salsas, juice, and ketchup.

Source: *Mayo Clinic.*

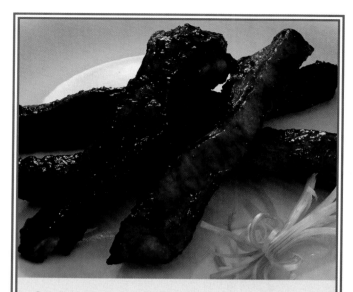

Overcooked meat and cancer risk

In November 1998, a team of researchers led by Wei Zheng of the University of South Carolina reported in the *Journal of the National Cancer Institute* that breast cancer is four times more common among women who eat beef and bacon cooked very well done than among women who eat rare or medium meat. Cooking meat has long been known to produce cancer-causing chemical compounds called heterocyclic amines (HCA's). In April 1999, *Science News* reported that J. Ian Gray of Michigan State University in East Lansing had discovered a novel solution for inhibiting HCA's: adding fruit to meat. Gray and his research team found that substituting ground tart cherries for 11.5 percent of the meat in hamburger suppressed HCA formation.

immune system. After high-dose chemotherapy, a patient will die unless the marrow is restored by a transfusion of bone marrow or stem cells harvested from a donor or from the patient's own body before treatment.

The studies, published by the American Society of Clinical Oncology, involved more than 2,000 patients treated at many different medical centers. The studies included breast cancer patients who had a poor prognosis because cancer had invaded 10 or more lymph nodes in the underarm or had spread to organs or bones, a condition known as metastic disease.

Four of the studies found no difference in survival between patients who had high-dose chemotherapy

with transplants, and those who had lower-dose chemotherapy. A fifth study did find a benefit in patients with cancerous lymph nodes, suggesting that the treatment might help some women.

The National Cancer Institute said the studies had not shown that high-dose therapy was better than standard treatment, but noted that some of the findings might change as the patients were studied longer.

Liver cancer rates on the rise.
Hepatocellular carcinoma, the most common form of liver cancer, is on the rise in the United States, and the increase is expected to continue until hepatitis B and C are brought under better control. These conclusions were reached by a study published in a March 1999 issue of *The New England Journal of Medicine.*

Researchers at the Veterans Affairs Medical Center in Albuquerque, New Mexico, found that the incidence of the cancer rose 71 percent from the mid-1970's to the mid-1990's. The researchers found that hospitalization and death rates for all types of liver cancer were rising at a similar pace.

Liver cancer struck an estimated 14,500 Americans in 1999, according to the American Cancer Society. Most of these people will get hepatocellular carcinoma.

Hepatocellular carcinoma is almost always fatal. Only 5 percent of sufferers are alive five years after the disease is diagnosed, because the tumors are usually found only after the cancer has spread.

The cancer is often caused by chronic hepatitis B and hepatitis C, viral diseases that lead to liver scarring, or cirrhosis, which in turn can result in liver cancer. Hepatitis can also cause other changes in liver cells that make them cancerous.

Breast cancer and fat. A 14-year study of nearly 89,000 women found no evidence that a high-fat diet promotes breast cancer or that a low-fat diet protects against it. Researchers from Harvard University published these findings in a March 1999 issue of *The Journal of the American Medical Association.*

Health experts were quick to note,

however, that a low-fat diet is still good for the heart and other aspects of health. They said the study indicated a need to look more carefully at how diet may affect the risk of breast cancer.

Doctors had long theorized that eating large amounts of fat increases the risk of breast cancer. They had based their thinking on animal studies, international comparisons, and studies of women who developed breast cancer and women who did not. Other experts had suggested that the crucial factor is the type of fat consumed rather than the amount, or that contaminants stored in fat promote breast cancer.

The Harvard study tracked 88,795 women in the continuing Nurses' Health Study. The women, ages 30 to 55, completed detailed questionnaires about their eating habits every four years from 1980 to 1994. Diets of the women without breast cancer were compared with those of 2,956 women whose breast cancer was discovered during the study.

Breast cancer was found to be no more common among women who ate large amounts of fat, or among those who ate a high proportion of animal fat, *polyunsaturated fat* (vegetable fat) or *transunsaturated fat* (partially hydrogenated oils, like those used in margarine).

Nor was breast cancer any less common in women who got a high proportion of their fats from fish oil or who got less than 20 percent of their total calories from fat.

Reducing colon cancer rates. A simple screening test for blood in the bowel can reduce by up to a third the death rate from colon cancer, the second leading cause of cancer death in the United States. The finding, published in a March 1999 issue of the *Journal of the National Cancer Institute*, promoted a campaign to encourage people over age 50 to take the test, because they account for most of the country's 56,000 colon cancer deaths each year.

Minnesota researchers monitoring the health of 46,000 volunteers since 1976 found that those who took the fecal occult blood test each year had 33 percent fewer deaths from colon cancer than people who did not take the test. Those tested every other year, the study found, had a 21 percent reduced rate.

Preventive mastectomies. Removing both breasts while they are still healthy reduces the risk of getting breast cancer by 90 percent, according to a study published in January 1999. Health care experts regarded the findings as the most reliable information to date on the long-term effectiveness of the operation.

Surgeons had been performing the procedure, bilateral prophylactic mas-

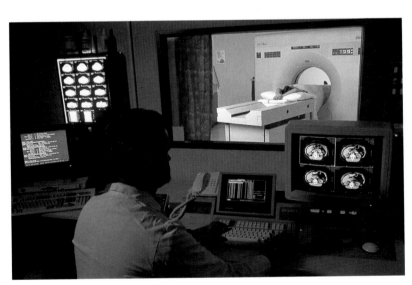

CT scans effective in detecting lung cancer
Computed tomography (CT) scans are effective in detecting early-stage lung cancer in people at high risk for the disease, according to a study published in February 1999. Researchers at the Early Lung Cancer Action Program in New York studied 1,000 smokers or former smokers age 60 or older. CT scans detected 19 out of 24 early stage cancers. Chest X-rays found only three.

tectomy, on women since the 1960's, assuming it would reduce a woman's cancer risk. But they did not know whether it really did, or by how much, since there is no guarantee that all the problem tissue had been removed.

Mastectomy can remove only 90 percent to 95 percent of breast tissue, and many researchers feared that the tissue left behind might harbor rogue cells that could one day turn malignant.

Researchers at the Mayo Clinic in Rochester, Minnesota, studied the effects of the surgery on 639 women who had their breasts removed between 1960 to 1993. The women were considered at high risk because of a strong family history of breast cancer or a personal history of breast lumps needing biopsies.

Among the women studied, the researchers concluded that at least 20 and as many as 40 women would have died if they had not had their breasts removed. Only two of the women died.

Health experts pointed out that high-risk women can try to protect themselves by having regular mammograms and breast examinations in hopes of detecting the disease early enough to cure it with surgery, chemotherapy, and radiation. The only other way such women can protect themselves against breast cancer is by taking the drug tamoxifen, which in a large study in 1998 was shown to reduce the risk of the disease by about 45 percent.

Cancer rates decline in the U.S.

Fewer Americans are stricken with cancer every year, largely because of the decline in smoking, the American Cancer Society reported in April 1999. And though men have a higher incidence of cancer than women, in 1998 the rate of new cancer cases was dropping eight times faster for men than for women.

Over all, cancer incidence has dropped 2.2 percent a year since 1992, according to the organization's annual report on cancer, which analyzed cancer trends through 1996, the latest data available. Declines in lung cancer among men who quit smoking in the 1970's and 1980's helped fuel the overall declines in cancer cases and deaths. But health officials warned that a high smoking rate among teen-agers and the popularity of cigars could reverse the trend.

Cigarette smoking by high school students rose 32 percent during the 1990's, the report said. And cigar smoking—which a study published in an April 1999 issue of the Journal of the National Cancer Institute concluded to be as cancer-causing as cigarettes—has reversed a 20-year-decline, rising 50 percent since 1995.
• Laura Bushie

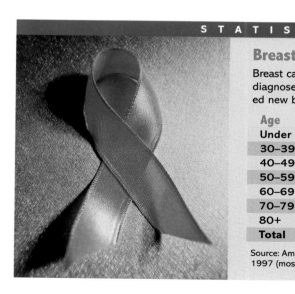

S T A T I S T I C S

Breast cancer rates

Breast cancer accounts for one out of every three cancers diagnosed in the United States. Following are the estimated new breast cancer cases per year in women by age.

Age	Estimate	Percent of total
Under 30	600	0.6
30–39	8,600	4.8
40–49	32,600	18.1
50–59	33,000	18.3
60–69	36,600	20.3
70–79	43,500	24.2
80+	25,300	14.0
Total	180,200	100.0%

Source: American Cancer Society, Surveillance Research, 1997 (most recent available).

In November 1998, researchers at Stanford University in California announced that they had uncovered the first known difference in the way the brain functions in children with attention-deficit/hyperactivity disorder (ADHD). The researchers expressed hope that their discovery would lead to an effective diagnostic test for the disorder.

ADHD is characterized by poor attention and concentration skills and low impulse control. In 1999, as many as 6 percent of school-age youngsters in the United States had the condition.

The Stanford investigators used a method known as functional magnetic resonance imaging to study the blood flow in the brains of 16 boys ages 8 to 13 while they participated in simple mental tests. Ten of the boys had been diagnosed with ADHD and six had not.

The researchers found that a structure in the brain called the basal ganglia was less active in youngsters with ADHD. They also reported that methylphenidate (sold as Ritalin)—the drug most commonly prescribed for ADHD—intensified brain activity in the basal ganglia in children with ADHD but decreased the activity in the other youngsters.

The study confirmed earlier theories that ADHD is associated with a particular deficit in the functioning of the brain, instead of being a personality problem or the outcome of poor parenting. The Stanford researchers cautioned, however, that 200 or more children will need to be studied with the imaging technique to confirm that the method can be used in the diagnosis of ADHD.

The availability of a diagnostic tool could prevent the use of Ritalin in children without the disorder. In the late 1990's, critics expressed concern that Ritalin was overprescribed and that it was taken by many youngsters who do not actually have ADHD.

Effects of lead. Researchers at Queensland University of Technology in Brisbane, Australia, reported in the *Journal of the American Medical Association* in December 1998 that the effects of children's exposure to lead early in life are only partially reversible. Earlier research had shown that children exposed to high lead levels experience delayed mental development, reflected in poor performance on tests measuring intellectual performance. But until the Australian study, it was unclear whether these negative effects were reversed when the levels of lead in the youngsters' blood declined.

In the study, researchers collected blood samples for 11 to 13 years from 375 children who had been ex-

New pennies—new risk
Doctors at Duke University Medical Center in Durham, North Carolina, reported in January 1999 that pennies may pose a danger to children who swallow them. Pennies minted after 1982, *below left,* contain 98 percent zinc, unlike older pennies, which had only 5 percent zinc. Zinc corrodes rapidly in stomach acid, *below right,* and can cause ulcers. While most pennies pass quickly through a child's system, the doctors recommended that parents who suspect their child has swallowed a penny consult a doctor if it is not excreted within a day.

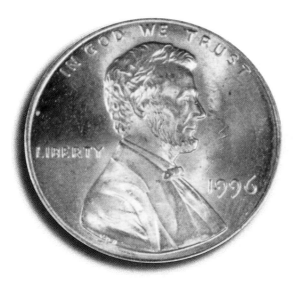

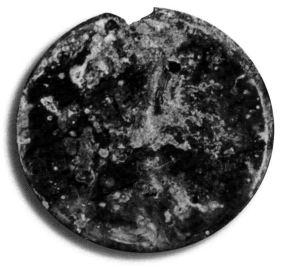

Is your computer child friendly?

Children sitting at computer equipment set up for adults are at risk of developing repetitive-strain injury, a condition that affects 20 million adults in the United States. Researchers at Cornell University in Ithaca, New York, observed children at computer workstations and found that 4 in 10 were at risk of serious injury. The American Occupational Therapy Association recommends some simple steps that parents can take to make the family computer safer to use for the whole family.

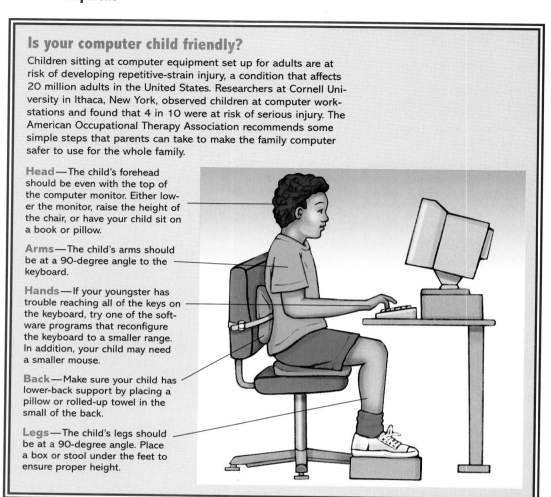

Head—The child's forehead should be even with the top of the computer monitor. Either lower the monitor, raise the height of the chair, or have your child sit on a book or pillow.

Arms—The child's arms should be at a 90-degree angle to the keyboard.

Hands—If your youngster has trouble reaching all of the keys on the keyboard, try one of the software programs that reconfigure the keyboard to a smaller range. In addition, your child may need a smaller mouse.

Back—Make sure your child has lower-back support by placing a pillow or rolled-up towel in the small of the back.

Legs—The child's legs should be at a 90-degree angle. Place a box or stool under the feet to ensure proper height.

posed to lead from a *smelter* (refinery that melts ore to get metal) near their homes. The children were also regularly tested to assess their developmental status and cognitive abilities.

The researchers found that many of the children whose blood lead levels were high at two years of age continued to have high blood lead levels at ages 11 to 13. They noted that even in children whose blood lead concentrations decreased, those who had had higher lead exposure showed little improvement in their mental ability with age. The researchers concluded that because the effects of lead may be irreversible, adults should concentrate on reducing children's exposure to environmental lead at a very early age.

Babies and language. Psychologists at New York University in New York City and at Amherst College in Massachusetts concluded that even in the first months of life, infants are instinctively learning the ways in which language is structured. Their findings were reported in the January 1999 issue of *Science*.

The researchers devised an artificial language of three-word "sentences" that had specific structures (such as "li na li" and "li na na"). They played a two-minute recording of one of these sentence patterns for 45 7-month-old babies. Then they played recordings of a mixture of sentence patterns. The infants paid attention longer (by about nine seconds) to the unfamiliar sentence structures than they did to those they had previously heard. Ninety-four percent of the babies apparently recognized the particular structure to which they had first been exposed.

Earlier studies had found that infants are able to recognize differences between words of varying syllable lengths. The new study concluded that babies could also recognize simple sentence patterns and rules, even when they do not yet understand what the words mean.

Learning environment. In a report published in the journal *Child Development* in October 1998, researchers at California State University at Northridge and at Fullerton studied the effect that mental stimulation at home can have on a child's motivation to learn. They found that when home environments provided learning activities and opportunities, youngsters had a greater desire to excel in school.

The researchers examined the home environments of 100 8-year-old youngsters. They noted such factors as whether the family encouraged children to develop hobbies and to take lessons to support their talents. They evaluated whether the children went to the library at least once a month, visited museums, and took trips on planes, trains, or buses.

The researchers also studied the children's use of home computers and access to musical instruments. In addition, they evaluated how often each child's family discussed political and social issues, how often they attended plays or concerts, and how often the family watched television. The psychologists then evaluated the child's motivation to achieve academically at ages 9, 10, and 13.

The investigators reported that children from homes with strong learning environments were more self-motivated to academic achievement than children from homes with fewer opportunities for mental stimulation. The benefits of a stimulating environment were evident from childhood through early adolescence.

Early intervention. A study at the University of Washington in Seattle found that negative adolescent behavior such as crime, drug abuse, and sexual activity can be reduced by boosting the self-esteem and academic interest of youngsters earlier in life. This type of intervention is more effective than programs aimed at children who have already reached their teen-age years. The researchers published their findings in the *Archives of Pediatrics and Adolescent Medicine* in March 1999.

The study was conducted in elementary schools (grades one through six) in high-crime areas of Seattle. The researchers evaluated about 600 students until they were 18 years old.

Resistant head lice
Some of the chemical products available to eliminate head lice may no longer be as effective as they were in the past. Researchers at Harvard University in Cambridge, Massachusetts, reported preliminary findings in 1998 that head lice in the United States may be developing a resistance to the chemicals in some of the products. As many as 6 million to 12 million people worldwide are infected by lice each year.

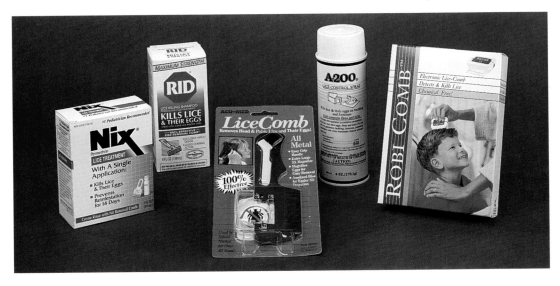

The researchers gave the students' parents and teachers guidance on how to develop interest in academics among the children and how to reinforce positive behaviors. The youngsters themselves were taught how to relate socially to others in ways that would positively affect their behavior.

The researchers found that the students who completed the program had fewer problems—such as violent, delinquent acts, heavy drinking, and pregnancy—by age 18 than those students who did not participate in the program. For example, 11 percent fewer program participants reported engaging in violent behavior than students who were not in the program. Heavy drinking was reported by 10 percent fewer students in the program. Program participants also demonstrated a greater commitment to schoolwork, with lower dropout rates, greater academic achievement, and fewer behavior problems at school.

A separate analysis of the research conducted by the Washington State Institute for Public Policy found that communities could save money by establishing similar programs. The program's costs were more than offset by the savings associated with fewer felonies being committed by adolescents.

Working moms. Psychologists have long wondered whether young children whose mothers work outside the home are at greater risk of behavioral and academic problems later in life. A large, long-term study at the University of Connecticut in Storrs concluded that children of working mothers suffer no lasting psychological damage. The research was published in the journal *Developmental Psychology* in March 1999.

The researchers evaluated about 6,000 children whose mothers worked during the first three years of their lives. They evaluated the youngsters for as long as 12 years, specifically in terms of the effects of their mothers' employment on behavioral problems, academic success, self-esteem, and language development. No significant differences were found among children of working mothers, when compared with children of stay-at-home moms. The researchers reported that certain issues, including the bond between mother and child and the quality of the day-care experience, are critical to the well-being of children of working mothers.

Quality child care. When youngsters are cared for in quality day-care settings, they tend to demonstrate greater confidence in their relationships with other children and are more cooperative in their interactions with adults. At the same time, however, the dominant influence in a child's life remains his or her family, despite the time they spend being cared for by others. These conclusions were presented in January 1999 at the American Association for the Advancement of Science meeting in Anaheim, California.

Previous research had suggested that children who spent long periods in child care were less cooperative and more aggressive than children cared for at home by their mothers. Educational psychologists at the University of Wisconsin in Madison presented a study of child care involving 1,300 families and investigators at 14 universities. The investigators observed the children during the first three years of their lives. They found that in settings where caregivers were sensitive, warm, responsive, and capable of creating positive experiences, children developed good social and linguistic skills.

The researchers pointed out that day care services need to improve in the United States. They also stressed the need for basic standards of care for children.

In related research presented at the same conference, a federally funded study concluded that fewer than 10 percent of children under 3 years of age receive excellent care; 53 percent of the available care is fair; and about 30 percent is good.

The researchers found that the highest quality day care is usually offered in smaller settings (fewer than three children per adult for very young children). Excellent child care is also characterized by a stimulating and safe environment and caregivers who are educated and experienced.

• Richard Trubo

Dental amalgam, a mixture of silver and mercury used in millions of tooth fillings each year, does not lead to Alzheimer's disease, a study concluded in February 1999. Stanley R. Saxe, a specialist in geriatric dentistry at the University of Kentucky at Lexington, headed the study. Mercury is one of several metals found in increased amounts in the brains of Alzheimer's patients. Alzheimer's disease, which affects millions of older Americans, causes increasing loss of memory and other mental abilities.

Researchers checked mercury levels in various parts of the brain in 68 people with Alzheimer's disease and 33 control subjects without the disease. They also collected information about each individual's exposure to dental amalgam and other sources of mercury. They found no evidence that dental amalgam contributed in any important way to levels of mercury found in the brain, or that mercury is a contributing factor in the development of Alzheimer's disease.

Oral piercing. The American Dental Association (ADA) announced in December 1998 that it had classified oral piercing as a public health hazard, and it urged that the practice be stopped. The ADA said oral piercing has become more common with the growing popularity of body piercing. It involves using a needle to make a hole in the tongue, lips, cheeks, or other areas of the mouth. Jewelry is then inserted into the hole. Piercing is usually done with no anesthetic.

People who undergo oral piercing face a number of dental health risks, the ADA said. Infection sometimes occurs because bacteria in the mouth can enter tissues through the needle hole, which may take four to six weeks to heal. An infection can lead to pain and swelling that interferes with breathing. Other risks include fractured teeth from accidentally biting oral jewelry, hypersensitivity to metals used in the jewelry, and choking after accidentally swallowing oral jewelry.

Passive smoking and gum disease. Nonsmokers who inhale cigarette smoke in places where cigarette smoking is allowed may have an increased risk of developing gum disease, scientists at the University of Buffalo School of Dentistry reported in March 1999. Researchers believe that tobacco smoke has an irritating effect on the gums which contributes to gum infection.

Previous studies have shown that cigarette smokers themselves are at greater risk of developing gum disease. Gum disease is the leading cause of tooth loss in adults. It leads to inflammation and destruction of gums and other tissues that hold teeth firmly in the jaw.

In the study, headed by Sara G.

- Dental amalgam
- Oral piercing
- Passive smoking and gum disease
- Tooth loss from cigars and pipes

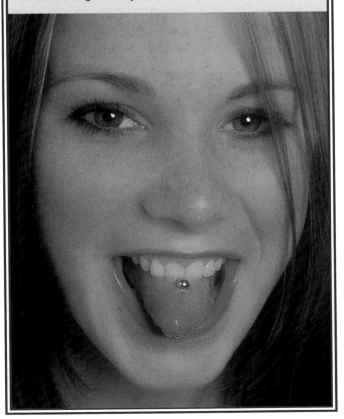

Dentists take stand against piercing

The American Dental Association (ADA) condemned oral piercing as a public health hazard in December 1998. During an annual meeting, the ADA passed a resolution opposing the practice, citing risks for infection, tooth damage, and breathing difficulty.

Diabetes

Cigar damage risks

Cigar smokers have tooth loss rates similar to those of cigarette smokers, the Boston University School of Dental Medicine reported in January 1999. Researchers found that cigar smoking increases the risk for tooth and jawbone loss.

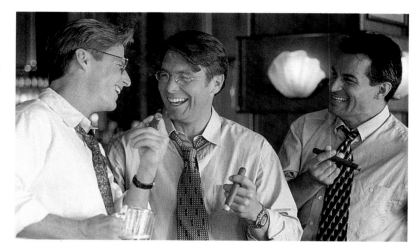

Grossi, an oral biologist, researchers analyzed medical records of 13,798 men and women who participated in a nationwide health survey conducted from 1988 to 1994. They found that nonsmokers who were routinely exposed to cigarette smoke at home had up to a 70 percent greater risk of developing gum disease than people with no smokers in the home. Researchers took into account family income and other factors that might affect dental health.

Tooth loss from cigars and pipes.

In January 1999, researchers at the Boston University School of Dental Medicine announced the results of

the first study showing that cigar and pipe smokers face a greater risk of tooth loss than nonsmokers. The researchers said the findings were important due to cigar smoking's growing popularity. Many people mistakenly believe cigars and pipes are safer than cigarettes, said Elizabeth A. Krall, a specialist in dental public health who headed the study.

Krall's group monitored 690 cigar smokers, pipe smokers, cigarette smokers, and nonsmokers over a 23-year period. The cigar and pipe smokers had tooth loss rates similar to those of cigarette smokers. Cigar smokers also had an elevated rate of jaw bone loss.   • Michael Woods

---

Diabetes

- Tight blood sugar control reduces complications
- Quality-of-life issues
- New medication
- Rezulin restrictions
- Youthful obesity raises risk
- Laser test

In September 1998, a large British study provided strong evidence that when medications are used to achieve tight blood-sugar control in patients with Type II diabetes, the risk of serious long-term complications, such as eye and kidney damage, can be reduced. The findings, by researchers at Oxford University and other British institutions, stressed the importance of treating Type II diabetes aggressively.

Some physicians had previously avoided intensive therapy for Type II diabetes, because the medications for this disease can cause problems, such as weight gain.

Type II diabetes is the most common form of diabetes. It occurs when

the body does not effectively use the hormone insulin, produced by the pancreas, to regulate *glucose* (blood sugar) levels. The disease may lead to blindness, kidney failure, or blood-vessel disorders.

In the British research, called the United Kingdom Prospective Diabetes Study, investigators studied more than 3,800 patients with Type II diabetes. Approximately half of the patients were given intensive drug treatment, such as insulin or sulfonylurea drugs, to keep their *fasting glucose levels* (the blood sugar levels before breakfast) below 108 milligrams per deciliter. The other half of the group controlled their glucose levels mainly through diet, and were given drugs only if their glucose levels exceeded 270 milligrams per deciliter.

The researchers found that after 10 years of treatment, those patients receiving the intensive drug therapy had a 25 percent lower risk of serious eye and kidney damage than the patients who regulated their glucose levels with the less aggressive, conventional method. Despite this benefit, the researchers discovered no significant difference between the two groups in the incidence of major blood-vessel diseases, such as heart disease and stroke.

Quality-of-life issues. A November 1998 report showed that when Type II diabetics have their blood sugar effectively managed with medication, they experience improvements in their quality of life and job productivity. The study, conducted by researchers at Harvard University in Cambridge, Massachusetts, was the first to demonstrate that moderate improvements in glucose levels produce greater physical and emotional well-being, less days missed from work, fewer canceled activities, and fewer visits to the doctor.

In the study, 569 people with Type II diabetes received either diabetes medication plus dietary management, or dietary management and a *placebo* (inactive substance). The medication used in the study was glipizide, a drug that helps the body produce more insulin. During the study, the patients also filled out questionnaires providing information about their psychological and physical well-being.

After 12 weeks of treatment, those patients in the drug-plus-diet group experienced better control of their glucose levels than the diet-plus-placebo patients. The group taking medication also reported an improved quality of life in every area evaluated by the questionnaire. For example, the patients treated only with diet were almost five times as likely to miss a day of work due to their disease, compared with the patients taking glipizide.

New medication. In May 1999, the United States Food and Drug Administration (FDA) approved the use of a new oral medication called Avandia,

or rosiglitazone, for the treatment of Type II diabetes. Tests of the drug on patients showed that Avandia, manufactured by SmithKline Beecham PLC of England, reduced glucose levels an average of 76 milligrams per deciliter in diabetes patients without causing serious side effects.

Avandia is a member of a class of diabetes drugs called thiazolidine-diones, which help the body efficiently use the insulin it makes. A diabetes medication that went on the market in March 1997 called Rezulin, or troglitazone, also belongs to this class of drugs. Rezulin, manufactured by Warner-Lambert Company of Morris Plains, New Jersey, has been

Earlier diabetes testing
People should get their blood tested for Type II diabetes beginning at age 25, 20 years earlier than previously recommended, according to a November 1998 report by the U.S. Centers for Disease Control and Prevention. The report said that earlier diagnosis would help prevent such diabetes complications as blindness and kidney failure.

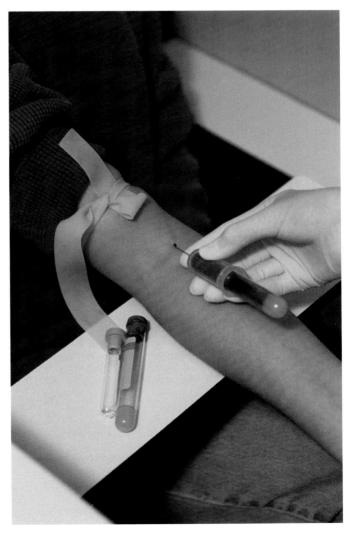

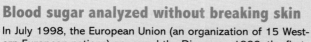

Blood sugar analyzed without breaking skin

In July 1998, the European Union (an organization of 15 Western European nations) approved the Diasensor 1000, the first device designed to analyze *glucose* (blood sugar) levels without breaking the skin. To use the device, made by Biocontrol Technology, Incorporated, of Pittsburgh, Pennsylvania, a person rests his or her forearm in the groove and presses a button. Infrared light then passes through the skin into the blood and is reflected back to a sensor. Software inside the Diasensor 1000 analyzes the level of reflected light to calculate a glucose level, which is displayed on the screen. In 1999, the U.S. Food and Drug Administration was considering Biocontrol's application to market a similar device in the United States.

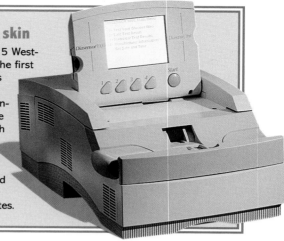

linked to serious liver problems. The FDA said its studies revealed no evidence of liver problems with Avandia.

Rezulin restrictions. The FDA cautioned physicians in June 1999 to avoid prescribing Rezulin as an initial treatment for Type II diabetes. The agency said the drug should be used only after other diabetes medications have been tried but failed to effectively manage glucose levels.

An FDA advisory panel had recommended that restrictions be placed on Rezulin in March 1999, after at least 28 deaths caused by liver failure were attributed to the drug. FDA *epidemiologist* (expert on the spread of disease) David Graham said Rezulin may have caused as many as 400 cases of liver failure.

Youthful obesity raises risk. Men who are overweight at age 25 are more than three times as likely to develop diabetes later in life than are their peers whose weight is normal. That conclusion was announced in May 1999 by researchers at the Johns Hopkins Medical Institutions in Baltimore.

Obesity in middle age has long been known to be a risk factor for the development of Type II diabetes. However, the Johns Hopkins research highlighted the importance of maintaining proper weight at younger ages for preventing the disease.

The researchers studied 916 former medical students over a period of about 30 years. None of the men had diabetes while in medical school, though some were overweight. The researchers found that those men who were overweight at age 25 had a much higher incidence of diabetes after age 50 than the other men. Furthermore, the study showed that the men who became overweight at age 35 or 45 also increased their risk of becoming diabetic in their 50's.

The researchers said their results indicated the importance of targeting diabetes-prevention efforts at young adults as well as middle-aged people.

Laser test. Self-testing of glucose levels can now be performed without pricking a finger with a razor-sharp lancet. In December 1998, the FDA approved a portable, battery-operated laser device that diabetics can use at home to evaluate their blood several times a day.

The patient places his or her finger into a slot on the device, called the Lasette, and presses a button. A beam of light is emitted, penetrating a tiny bit of skin and releasing a drop of blood for testing.

The Lasette, manufactured by Cell Robotics International, Inc., of Albuquerque, New Mexico, was expected to benefit patients who do not test their blood sugar as often as recommended because of the pain caused by lancets. Patients reported that using the Lasette, available only by prescription, was easy and painless.

• Richard Trubo

In December 1998, the United States Food and Drug Administration (FDA) approved the first of a new class of arthritis drugs, called COX-2 inhibitors, which relieve pain and inflammation, while reducing the risk of side effects associated with pain relievers, such as stomach pain and *peptic ulcers* (sores in the digestive system). G. D. Searle & Company in Skokie, Illinois, began marketing the new drug, Celebrex, in January 1999. Merck & Co., Inc. of Whitehouse Station, New York, received FDA approval in May for their COX-2 inhibitor, Vioxx.

Two of the most common forms of arthritis are *osteoarthritis,* the wearing out of joints, and *rheumatoid arthritis,* inflammation mostly in smaller joints and the deterioration of the tissues surrounding them. Most people with these conditions take several daily doses of nonsteroidal anti-inflammatory drugs (NSAID's), such as ibuprofen. NSAID's inhibit the action of an immune-system chemical called cyclooxygenase-2 (COX-2), which causes inflammation. They also inhibit the action of a different form of the chemical called COX-1, which protects the lining of the stomach and small intestines. NSAID's, therefore, make people with arthritis vulnerable to problems in the digestive system.

Celebrex and Vioxx, however, were designed to inhibit only the action of COX-2, allowing the stomach to remain protected. The FDA approved Celebrex for osteoarthritis and rheumatoid arthritis and approved Vioxx for osteoarthritis, as well as severe pain and menstrual cramps.

New drug for Crohn's disease. In August 1998, the FDA approved a new drug designed to treat the symptoms of Crohn's disease, a painful, often debilitating, and incurable intestinal disease. Crohn's disease results in *chronic* (long-term) inflammation of the large or small intestine, a condition that can lead to bleeding ulcers, abdominal cramps, diarrhea, and *fistulas* (abnormal growths) that connect the intestines to the surface of the skin.

The new drug, infliximab, is a laboratory-designed protein similar to a naturally occurring immune system protein. Infliximab fights another protein that causes inflammation. Clinical trials found that the drug eliminated symptoms in 48 percent of the patients after four weeks of treatment.

The FDA approved infliximab for patients with moderate to severe cases of Crohn's disease who did not respond well to other medications. Centocor Inc. in Malvern, Pennsylvania, began selling the drug under the name Remicade.

The ulcer bug and indigestion. Two studies published in December 1998 showed opposite results in the search for a link between indigestion

- Gentler pain reliever
- New drug for Crohn's disease
- The ulcer bug and indigestion
- Ulcer bug in the water supply?
- Listeria outbreak

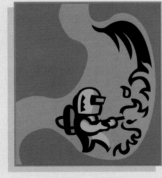

When heartburn endures

Heartburn is the common name for the condition that occurs when stomach acids flow backward into the *esophagus,* the tube connecting the stomach to the mouth. These acids can cause a burning sensation in the chest and a bad taste in the mouth. If a person experiences *chronic* (long-term) heartburn, the condition is known as gastroesophageal reflux disease (GERD). GERD can sometimes damage the wall of the esophagus or narrow the passage, making it difficult or painful to swallow. GERD may also cause chronic chest pain and coughing.

Although a physician may prescribe medication for GERD, treatment often depends on changes in everyday habits. Doctors may suggest the following measures to eliminate or reduce symptoms:

- Quit smoking.
- Avoid alcoholic beverages.
- Avoid beverages with caffeine.
- Avoid highly acidic foods, such as oranges and tomatoes.
- Avoid foods with chocolate, spearmint, and peppermint.
- Do not eat large meals. Eat smaller meals more often if necessary.
- Do not eat anything for three to four hours before going to bed.
- Do not sleep on your side.

Source: American Academy of Family Physicians.

and *Helicobacter pylori* (*H. pylori*), the bacterium that causes the majority of peptic ulcers. *Gastroenterologists* (digestive system specialists) hoped that if *H. pylori* were a culprit in non-ulcerous forms of indigestion, then antibiotics could be used to treat symptoms of indigestion, such as gas, nausea, and stomach pain.

Gastroenterologist Kenneth McColl of the University of Glasgow in Scotland led a study of people infected with *H. pylori* who had chronic indigestion but no ulcers. The patients received either a two-week treatment of antibiotics or a *placebo* (inactive substance). A year later, the doctors could not detect the bacteria in 85 percent of the patients treated with antibiotics, and 21 percent of those patients no longer experienced indigestion. The bacteria was undetectable in 12 percent of the patients who received the placebo, and only 7 percent of those patients reported no symptoms of indigestion. The researchers concluded that *H. pylori* may have caused indigestion.

Another study, however, revealed no clear link between *H. pylori* and indigestion. A team of researchers led by gastroenterologist Andre Blum at Universitaire Vaudois in Lausanne, Switzerland, found in a similar study that indigestion was reduced or eliminated in 21 percent of people who received placebos and 27 percent of those given antibiotics. The researchers concluded that *H. pylori* is not a leading factor in causing indigestion.

Ulcer bug in the water supply?

The source of *H. pylori* is a long-standing mystery for scientists. In April 1999, microbiologist Donald Reid and his colleagues at Robert Gordon University in Aberdeen, Scotland, theorized that the bacteria breed in the slimy film that coats the inside of water pipes.

This film, or biofilm, is a colony of microorganisms that live in all water distribution systems. The Scottish scientists grew biofilm in pipes in a laboratory and injected the biofilm with *H. pylori* to determine if it was a hospitable environment for the bacteria. The researchers then flushed the pipes with nonchlorinated water to see if the bacteria could be washed away. After 192 hours of flushing, the bacteria survived.

The researchers concluded that water pipes may be a major source of *H. pylori*. They noted that their study demonstrated the risks of nonchlorinated water supplies and speculated that even chlorinated water may not kill all the *H. pylori* in biofilm.

***Listeria* outbreak.** From December 1998 to February 1999, a rash of food recalls marked a resurgence of the deadly bacterium *Listeria monocytogenes*. There were only a few reports of *Listeria* contamination in the United States between 1993 and 1998. But in the 1998-1999 outbreaks, U.S. officials found the bacteria in meat products in 22 states.

The bacterium usually causes only short-term problems in the digestive systems of healthy adults, but it can be deadly for children, the elderly, and people with weakened immune systems. Normally carried in animal intestines, *Listeria* can contaminate raw meat, dairy products, raw vegetables, and precooked meats. Unlike many other bacteria, *Listeria* can grow in refrigerators and freezers.

The first reports of *Listeria* contamination came in August 1998, when people fell ill after eating hot dogs and deli meats from Bil Mar Foods of Zeeland, Michigan, a subsidiary of the Chicago-based Sara Lee Corporation. Four months later, Sara Lee voluntarily recalled about 15 million pounds of meat from supermarkets and shut down the Michigan plant.

According to the U.S. Centers for Disease Control in Atlanta, Georgia, *Listeria* contamination resulted in 100 cases of illness and 21 deaths, including 6 miscarriages or stillbirths. By March 1999, the U.S. Department of Agriculture (USDA) had announced recalls from nine different companies.

To decrease the chance of *Listeria* infection, public health officials advised consumers to cook all meats, including deli meats, thoroughly, wash all raw fruits and vegetables, and wash hands and utensils after handling raw meat. They also warned that microwave ovens usually do not kill bacteria and that all leftovers should be thoroughly reheated.

• Lorna Luebbers

After many years during which no unique arthritis drugs were developed, four new drugs to treat arthritis received U.S. Food and Drug Administration (FDA) approval in less than nine months in 1998 and 1999. Two of these medications, celecoxib and rofecoxib, were the first in a new class of drugs called "super aspirins," designed to treat pain and inflammation without the side effects of aspirin and related drugs like ibuprofen and naproxen. The FDA approved celecoxib (marketed as Celebrex) in December 1998, and approved rofecoxib (marketed as Vioxx) in May 1999.

Like aspirin and ibuprofen, the new medications are nonsteroidal anti-inflammatory drugs (NSAID's). However, they are a new type of NSAID known as COX-2 inhibitors. Earlier NSAID's work by inhibiting COX-1 and COX-2, enzymes associated with inflammation and the sensation of pain. However, COX-1 also plays a role in protecting the lining of the stomach. Because NSAID's block COX-1, they can cause stomach irritation and ulcers in some patients. COX-2 inhibitors, however, do not affect COX-1, which enables celecoxib and rofecoxib to provide relief of pain and inflammation with a smaller risk of gastrointestinal complications.

Both celecoxib and rofecoxib were approved for the treatment of *osteoarthritis,* a degenerative joint disease that causes the cartilage between bones to break down. In addition, celecoxib was approved for the treatment of *rheumatoid arthritis,* a disease in which inflamed tissue and other factors in a joint erode the bone and cartilage. Rofecoxib was also approved for treating acute general pain and acute menstrual pain.

Like other NSAID's, these drugs are not to be taken by patients who are allergic to aspirin or another NSAID. In addition, celecoxib must not be taken by patients who are allergic to sulfas, which are included, for example, in products that are commonly used in the treatment of urinary tract infections.

In late 1998, the FDA had approved leflunomide and etanercept to treat rheumatoid arthritis. In September 1998, the FDA approved leflunomide (marketed as Arava) for the treatment of rheumatoid arthritis. In addition to reducing arthritic symptoms, leflunomide was the first orally-administered drug shown to slow the worsening of this disorder. The drug blocks the production of immune cells that cause joint inflammation.

The most dangerous side effect of leflunomide is that it may cause birth defects if used by pregnant women. The drug remains in the body for a long time, so women who take the drug and later wish to become pregnant must make certain that the drug has been completely eliminated from their systems.

A potential wonder drug

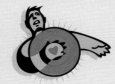

In April 1999, researchers announced that a still experimental cancer-fighting compound may also be effective against heart attacks and strokes. In 1997, researchers, led by Judah Folkman of Harvard Medical School and Children's Hospital in Boston, first reported that two experimental drugs, angiostatin and endostatin, eliminated cancerous tumors in mice. These drugs block the growth of new blood vessels, cutting off the blood supply that certain tumors need in order to survive.

In 1999, researchers in Folkman's lab revealed that endostatin can also prevent the build-up of *plaque* (deposits of cholesterol, white blood cells, and muscle cells) in the arteries. Theoretically, endostatin should inhibit the formation of plaque deposits by choking off the blood supply that cells in the plaque need to survive. In a study to verify this effect, endostatin reduced the rate of plaque build-up in laboratory mice by as much as 85 percent. Endostatin was set to begin testing in human cancer trials in mid-1999.

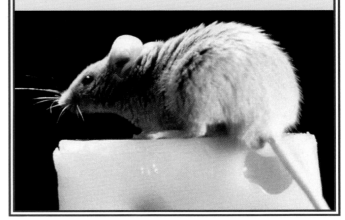

In November 1998, the FDA approved etanercept (marketed as Enbrel), a genetically engineered drug that acts by inhibiting a naturally occurring protein known as tumor necrosis factor (TNF). TNF plays an important role in causing the inflammatory symptoms of rheumatoid arthritis. The drug, which is administered by injection, can produce quick and dramatic results. It does not cure rheumatoid arthritis, but it is recommended for patients with moderate to severe symptoms who have not responded well to other drugs.

Because TNF plays a role in the body's defenses against infection, the FDA warned, etanercept can make a patient more vulnerable to infection or cause an existing infection to worsen. Therefore, patients with an active infection must not start treatment with etanercept. Patients who develop an infection while being treated with the drug must be monitored closely, and the drug should be discontinued if the infection worsens.

Drug for severe Crohn's disease. The FDA on August 24, 1998, approved the first new drug for the treatment of Crohn's disease in more than 30 years. Infliximab (marketed as Remicade) is given intravenously to treat moderate to severe Crohn's disease in patients who have not responded well to conventional therapy.

Crohn's disease is a disorder of the immune system that causes the body to attack and destroy its own digestive system. Some Crohn's patients develop open, draining fistulas, a painful complication in which deep wounds in the bowel wall perforate the surface of the skin. Infliximab is the first drug approved to treat fistulizing Crohn's disease.

Infliximab is a monoclonal antibody, a specialized type of artificial protein designed to attack a specific substance in the body. Specifically, it attacks a substance known as tumor necrosis factor alpha (TNF-alpha), a protein that causes inflammation, thereby providing a unique and important means to manage Crohn's disease. Infliximab was also being studied as a treatment for patients with other inflammatory conditions, such as rheumatoid arthritis, psoriasis, and asthma.

The return of thalidomide. In July 1998, the FDA approved thalidomide—with significant restrictions—in patients with leprosy who develop painful skin nodules and other severe symptoms. The drug was marketed as Thalomid. Few medications have had as dramatic an impact on drug development and regulation as thalidomide, a drug that, in the late 1950's and early 1960's, was marketed in Canada and Europe as a sedative and morning-sickness treatment. Only after thalidomide was marketed did researchers learn that the drug could cause birth defects.

Doctors recommend new Lyme disease vaccine

In December 1998, the United States Food and Drug Administration (FDA) approved LYMErix, the first vaccine against Lyme disease. Lyme disease is a bacterial infection spread by ticks that live in wooded or grassy areas. The ticks are carried on the bodies of white-tailed deer and certain other wild animals. The disease infects approximately 16,000 people in the U.S. each year. The disease commonly causes a ring-shaped rash and flulike symptoms, and severe cases can lead to more severe illnesses.
A series of three shots over a one-year period is needed to produce maximum protection. The FDA approved the vaccine for people age 15 to 70. Individuals living in the Northeast and the northern Midwest, where Lyme disease is most common, are most at risk. LYMErix was not recommended for children, pregnant women, or the elderly. Testing on these groups was to be completed in 1999.

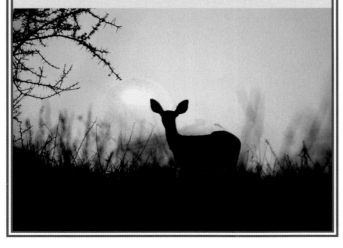

By the time warnings about this danger were issued, more than 10,000 babies with serious deformities had been born to women who took the drug while pregnant. This tragedy caused thalidomide to be removed from the market. Except for a few limited research initiatives, little attention was given to this infamous drug for the next three decades. By the 1990's, however, researchers had developed a renewed interest in thalidomide and, in particular, in its use to treat leprosy.

Leprosy is a chronic infectious disease that primarily affects the skin, the mucous membranes (especially those in the nose), and the peripheral nervous system, which includes nerves that connect the spinal cord to the muscles. Patients with untreated or neglected infections may develop crippling deformities of the hands and feet. Studies suggest that thalidomide may also be useful in treating many other disorders, including AIDS wasting syndrome, rheumatoid arthritis, lupus erythematosus, Crohn's disease, and even malignant brain tumors. Studies of the drug in patients with these disorders were ongoing in 1998 and 1999.

Even a single dose of thalidomide taken during pregnancy can cause severe birth defects, and the drug must not be used by pregnant women or by women who wish to become pregnant. It was approved for marketing only under a restricted distribution program called the System for Thalidomide Education and Prescribing Safety (STEPS). Under this program, only prescribers and pharmacists registered with the program are permitted to prescribe and dispense the drug. In addition, patients must sign a special consent form and comply with the requirements of the STEPS program in order to receive the medication.

Obesity drug has a new approach.

In April 1999, the FDA approved orlistat (marketed as Xenical) for the management of obesity when used in conjunction with a reduced-calorie diet. While previous antiobesity drugs work by suppressing the patient's appetite, orlistat takes a different approach. Orlistat interferes with en-

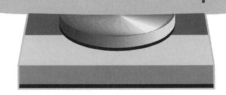

Error: Illegal Internet pharmacy

On March 3, 1999, members of the United States House of Representatives Commerce Committee expressed concern about the growing trend of purchasing prescription drugs over the Internet. Online pharmacies boomed especially after the sensation caused by the March 1998 debut of the anti-impotence drug Viagra. By early 1999, the U.S. Food and Drug Administration (FDA) had identified more than 30 Web sites selling Viagra (or counterfeits of the drug) to people whether or not they had a valid prescription.

Many such sites either offered prescriptions without a physical exam or sold prescription drugs to anyone who wanted them. In a March 22, 1999, meeting, the National Association of Boards of Pharmacy supported a plan to educate the public about the potential dangers of buying prescription drugs from unregulated sources and to verify the licensing of pharmacies doing business on the Internet.

zymes that break down dietary fat into smaller components, which permits the fat to be absorbed by the body. As a result, orlistat cuts the absorption of dietary fat by about 30 percent. In one year, most patients in clinical trials experienced weight loss ranging from 5 to 10 percent of their initial body weight.

However, orlistat also reduces the absorption of fat-soluble vitamins (vitamins A, D, E, and K) and beta-carotene. Patients taking the drug are also advised to take a multivitamin product containing fat-soluble vitamins. Orlistat is taken three times a day with each main meal containing fat. The most common side effects associated with Orlistat include intestinal cramping, oily spotting, gas, and diarrhea. The frequency of these events increases with the amount of fat consumed.

New narcolepsy drug. In December 1998, the FDA approved the use of modafinil (marketed as Provigil) for the treatment of narcolepsy. Described as a "wakefulness-promoting agent," it was the first new drug marketed for this disorder in more than 40 years. Narcolepsy is a chronic neurological sleep disorder of unknown origin that affects an estimated 125,000 Americans. The most common and disabling symptoms of narcolepsy are uncontrollable daytime sleepiness and persistent drowsiness.

Some of modafinil's side effects, which include nervousness or anxiety, increased blood pressure and heart rate, and insomnia, are similar to those of amphetamines and methylphenidate (sold as Ritalin). However, the new drug may be better tolerated by some patients, with fewer side effects and addictive qualities. These problems frequently cause patients to stop taking the other drugs.

Modafinil may interfere with the action of some contraceptive drugs. Physicians therefore advise women using such drugs to adopt alternative or additional birth control methods while taking the drug and for one month afterward.   • Daniel A. Hussar

Ear and Hearing

• Hearing tests for newborns
• Ear shape
• Hearing aid use
• The perils of headphones

The American Academy of Pediatrics recommended in February 1999 that all newborns be evaluated for hearing loss before they are discharged from the hospital. By performing this test shortly after birth—or at most before 3 months of age—the academy believes that doctors can diagnose and treat hearing impairments at a time when problems with language development can still be minimized.

Significant hearing loss is one of the most common major abnormalities present at birth, occurring in about 3 of every 1,000 infants. Usually, these hearing difficulties are not detected until a youngster is an average of 14 months old, when he or she may already be having trouble developing normal speech. If hearing problems are detected much earlier, however, babies can often be fitted with hearing aids that can help reduce any lag in the development of language skills.

Physicians use a number of tests to screen infants for hearing loss. In a technique called *evoked otoacoustic emissions,* tiny microphones detect and measure sound waves in the *cochlea* (inner ear) in response to clicks or tones. Another method, called *auditory brainstem response,* measures brain waves that occur in reaction to clicks or other sounds. These tests are noninvasive (usually done while a baby is asleep), take less than five minutes to conduct, and cost only $7 to $26 per child.

Ear shape. Researchers at the University of Nijmegen in the Netherlands reported in September 1998 that the unique shape of a person's ears appears to play a key role in the way he or she processes sounds. The scientists were testing the assumption that as sounds are reflected in the *pinnae* (the outer ear and its unique ridges and folds), the brain learns over time to interpret the sounds and the direction from which they are coming. To test their theory, researchers fitted plastic molds that altered the shape of the outer ear on people in a study group. They found that people wearing the devices initially lost their ability to judge the height from which a particular sound was emanating. Over several weeks, however, they regained that ability.

Hearing aid use. Although the use of hearing aids increases with age, the devices may still be underused. That was the finding reported by researchers at the University of Wisconsin Medical School in the *Journal of the American Geriatrics Society* (JAGS) in September 1998. The researchers examined the medical histories and evaluated the hearing of 1,629 adults, ages 48 to 92 years. They found that only 14.6 percent of the men and women with a hearing loss used a hearing aid. The investigators concluded that physicians need to improve hearing screening and intervention programs for older adults.

In a separate study published in the same issue of JAGS, researchers at the Center for Aging Study in Padova, Italy, investigated the prevalence of hearing impairment in older Italians. In a questionnaire, nearly 2,400 people ages 65 and older reported whether they believed they had hearing problems. Then researchers tested their hearing. They discovered that many people who did not think they had hearing problems did, in fact, show signs of hearing loss. About 8 percent of the men and 7 percent of the women surveyed said they had trouble hearing at home. And 11 percent of men and 9 percent of women reported difficulty hearing in social situations. However, tests showed that 19 percent of men and women had hearing problems.

The perils of headphones. Researchers at the National Acoustic Laboratories in Sydney, Australia, reported in December 1998 that personal stereo systems are associated with impaired hearing. The scientists evaluated a number of lifestyle risk factors and administered a hearing test to 1,724 people ages 10 to 59. According to the researchers, users of personal stereo devices consistently had poorer hearing than nonusers. This hearing loss was even greater in individuals who also were exposed to workplace noise.   • Richard Trubo

---

How well does your baby hear?

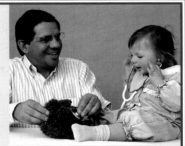

Many parents do not recognize a hearing problem in their baby until the child reaches almost 2 years of age. Yet experts say that if a child's hearing loss is diagnosed early, many problems with speech and language development can be minimized. According to the National Institute on Deafness and Other Communication Disorders, the following behaviors are signs of normal hearing development.

Birth to 3 months
- Startled by loud sounds.
- Is awakened by voices or sounds.
- Recognizes and is soothed by parent's voice.

3 to 6 months
- Turns toward a sound.
- Repeats sounds such as "ooh" and "aah."
- Enjoys toys that make sounds.

6 to 10 months
- Responds to own name and common words such as "bye-bye."
- Babbles, even when alone.
- Responds to requests such as "come here."

10 to 15 months
- Imitates simple words or sounds.
- Points to familiar objects when asked to do so.
- May use single words.

15 to 18 months
- Knows 10 to 20 words.
- Speaks in 2-3 word sentences.
- Follows simple directions such as "Bring me your shoe."

18 to 24 months
- Understands yes/no questions.
- May sing or hum spontaneously.
- Enjoys being read to.

In May 1999, the United States Federal Appeals Court for the District of Columbia ruled that air pollution standards established in 1997 by the U.S. Environmental Protection Agency (EPA) could not be enforced. The new regulations were designed to control smog-causing ozone and microscopic particles of soot by placing stricter limits on the amount of pollutants from automobile and truck tailpipes, factories, and other sources. (Ozone is a gas produced by a chemical reaction between sunlight and airborne pollutants.)

The 1990 amendment to the Clean Air Act of 1970 had charged the EPA with reviewing and updating air pollution regulations periodically. Opponents of the 1997 standards charged that the new measures would cost U.S. industries more than $10 billion to implement by a 2010 deadline. The court decision, however, rested on more technical arguments.

By a two-to-one vote, the judges ruled that the EPA had overstepped its authority by setting ozone standards without a clearly defined criterion for determining what levels of ozone pose a health risk. The court also ruled that the EPA had arbitrarily set standards for small airborne particles. The EPA planned to appeal the ruling, but some observers believed that new legislation would be necessary for the EPA to revise air pollution standards.

Environmental Health

- Air pollution standards struck down
- Bad air in rinks
- Risks in plastics?
- Pesticide risk
- Radon dangers
- Coal poisoning

Bad air in rinks. Some ice-resur-facing machines used in indoor ice-skating rinks emit dangerous levels of pollution, according to a December 1998 report by researchers at the Harvard School of Public Health in Boston. The exhaust from resurfacing machines can result in the accumula-tion of the toxic gas nitrogen dioxide. Exposure to this gas can lead to res-piratory problems such as coughing, tightness in the chest, and shortness of breath.

The Harvard team studied 19 rinks over three years and found that rinks with propane-powered machines had average nitrogen dioxide concentra-tions of 206 parts per billion. Rinks with gasoline-powered machines av-eraged 132 parts per billion, while the level for those with electric ma-chines was only 37 parts per billion. Previous research had associated in-creased levels of respiratory disease with *chronic* (long-term) exposure to nitrogen dioxide at concentrations of 100 parts per billion.

Risks in plastics? A 30-year-old concern over the possible toxicity of a chemical that is added to plastics re-emerged in 1999, focusing partic-ularly on plastic intravenous (IV) bags and tubing used in the hospitals. The so-called plasticizers, a group of chemicals known as phthalate esters, are added to rigid polyvinyl chloride (PVC) to make it more flexible. The medical industry in the United States uses an estimated 400 million IV bags containing plasticizers annually.

Because phthalates do not chemi-cally bond to PVC, small quantities of the chemical can leach out into fluids in IV bags. Some studies with animals have shown that plasticizers can cause liver tumors, kidney problems, and decreased fertility. Other studies, however, have shown that the amount of plasticizers a person absorbs is proportionally smaller than the levels believed to be harmful in animals.

In April, EPA researchers reported on the common plasticizer called di(2-ethylhexyl)phthalate (DEHP). The scientists administered DEHP and a related chemical to female rats and then studied their male offspring. The team found that the males pro-duced abnormally low levels of the male hormone testosterone and had a variety of abnormalities, including missing testicles, feminized breasts, and unusually small *epididymides,* the structures that store sperm. Because of the severe results, the researchers said they would conduct further stud-ies with doses closer to those that humans may take in.

Also in April, the National Institute of Environmental Health Sciences in Bethesda, Maryland, announced that it would convene a panel to examine the health effects of the chemicals. And the largest manufacturer of IV bags, Baxter International, Inc. of Deerfield, Illinois, announced that it would phase out PVC bags.

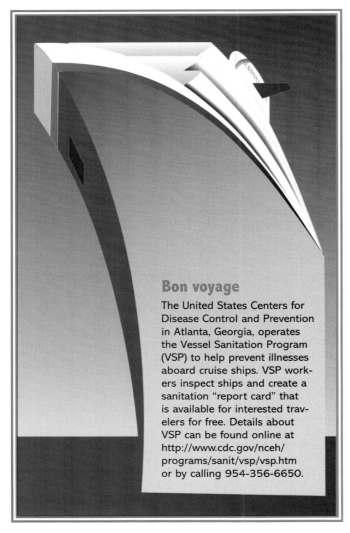

Bon voyage

The United States Centers for Disease Control and Prevention in Atlanta, Georgia, operates the Vessel Sanitation Program (VSP) to help prevent illnesses aboard cruise ships. VSP work-ers inspect ships and create a sanitation "report card" that is available for interested trav-elers for free. Details about VSP can be found online at http://www.cdc.gov/nceh/ programs/sanit/vsp/vsp.htm or by calling 954-356-6650.

Pesticide risk. Exposure to the pesticide dieldrin, a chemical thought to mimic the effects of estrogen, doubles the risk of breast cancer, scientists reported in December 1998. The study conducted at the Center for Preventive Medicine in Glostrup, Denmark, was the largest investigation yet of the possible link between pesticides and breast cancer.

Dieldrin was used on such crops as corn and cotton beginning in the 1950's. Although it was banned in most countries in the 1970's, dieldrin residues remain in the soil.

In the Danish study, the researchers took blood samples from 7,712 women in 1976 to check for levels of various pesticides. In 1996, they retested the blood of 240 women who had developed breast cancer and 477 women who had not. The scientist found that dieldrin was the only pesticide that appeared to increase the risk of breast cancer.

Radon dangers? Radon in homes may not be as dangerous as researchers had previously believed, according to a January 1999 report by scientists at Columbia University in New York City. Radon, a radioactive gas that is found in nearly all soil and rock, can enter a house through basement floors and walls.

Because high concentrations of radon released in mining operations are a known cancer threat, scientists had also assumed that the lower concentrations found in houses are also a hazard. To investigate this possible risk, the Columbia scientists exposed 250,000 mouse cells to radon radiation at the levels typical of homes. They found no unusual incidence of *mutations* (genetic changes) that would be the first step toward the development of cancer. The findings supported a University of Pittsburgh study from March 1998 that failed to find any correlation between average lung cancer levels in U.S. counties and radon levels in 500,000 houses.

Coal poisoning. Millions of Chinese are being poisoned by toxic metals released from burning coal, scientists at the U.S. Geological Survey and the Institute of Geochemistry in Guiyang, China, reported in February 1999.

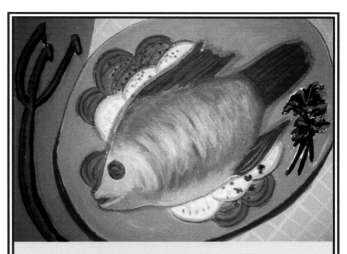

Hooking a safe one

Some fish caught in lakes and streams can harbor harmful chemical pollutants. The U.S. Environmental Protection Agency (EPA) offers the following suggestions for helping you to know when it is safe to eat your catch.

- Check with a local EPA office for pollution warnings.
- Eat younger fish—generally the smaller, less impressive catch—which contain lower levels of chemicals.
- Eat bluegill, perch, stream trout, and other fish that feed mostly on insects. These fish carry fewer contaminants.
- Avoid fatty fish, such as lake trout, and bottom-feeding fish, such as carp and catfish, which tend to have higher concentrations of chemicals.
- You can lower the risks of ingesting chemicals if you discard the head, guts, kidneys, liver, and fat before cooking.

The researchers surveyed various studies to show the health impact on the estimated 70 percent of China's 1.2 billion people who use coal in their homes for cooking and heating.

The researchers found that much of the coal in China is contaminated with lead, arsenic, fluorine, and other metals, which are released in smoke and baked into the food or inhaled. In Guizhou province, authorities identified thousands of cases of arsenic poisoning from coal use. In Guizhou and the surrounding areas, scientists estimated that there were 10 million cases of fluorine poisoning, often resulting in soft or misshapen bones. The researchers called for solutions to reduce coal consumption or to make it safer.   • Thomas H. Maugh II

Exercise and Fitness

- Exercise reduces the risk of stroke
- Exercise guidelines revised
- Flexibility increases strength
- Aging gracefully

A study published in October 1998 in the American Heart Association journal *Stroke* found that men who engaged in regular, moderate exercise during middle age reduced their risk of stroke as they reached retirement age. Paradoxically, however, the study also found that men who were very active seemed to benefit less. The study was led by I-Min Lee of the Harvard School of Public Health and Ralph S. Paffenbarger, Jr., of Stanford University in Stanford, California.

The investigators surveyed 11,120 male Harvard alumni whose average age was 58. The same men had responded to a 1997 survey of physical activity levels. The researchers found that men who burned 2,000 to 3,000 calories per week reduced their risk of stroke by 46 percent, compared with those who engaged in little or no physical activity. However, even small amounts of exercise showed significant benefits. People who burned 1,000 to 2,000 calories a week (roughly equivalent to 30 minutes of walking 5 times a week) cut their risk by 24 percent.

Among the men who burned more than 3,000 calories per week, however, the risk of stroke decreased by only 22 percent. Those who burned more than 4,000 calories per week reduced their risk by only 18 percent.

The researchers commented that further investigation was needed to determine why the benefits seemed to taper off as exercise levels reached higher intensities. They also said that the results should not discourage people who exercise vigorously. Nor do the results indicate that these people should cut back on their exercise routines. Exercise has been proven to help reduce risk factors common to heart attacks and strokes, including body fat and cholesterol levels.

Exercise guidelines revised. New guidelines published in November 1998 by the American College of Sports Medicine (ACSM) may be easier for the average person to follow. The new guidelines represented a significant shift from the first ACSM guidelines, which were issued in 1978. The older guidelines recommended 15 to 60 minutes of *aerobic exercise* (exercise that increases the body's use of oxygen) three to five days per week at an intensity of at least 50 percent of a person's maximum heart rate. Health advocates hoped that the new guidelines would encourage more people to exercise regularly.

The revised recommendations were based on a review of 262 studies on health and exercise. Much of this pool of research showed that three 10-minute exercise sessions per day may be as beneficial as one 30-minute

Fitness with a kick

Tae-Bo, *right,* a workout regimen combining elements of boxing, martial arts, and aerobic exercise, became popular in 1998 and 1999. Although Tae-Bo was a copyrighted system of routines, fitness buffs across the country flocked to local classes, where instructors led routines that were similar to Tae-Bo in many respects, but which were not officially licensed by Tae-Bo's originator.

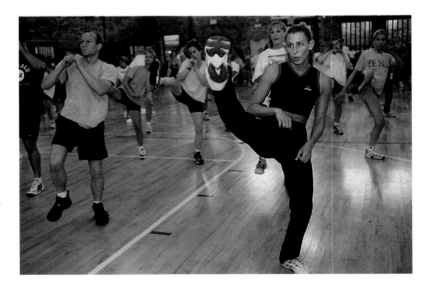

Fitness in 200 minutes a week

Fitness experts advise that 200 minutes of exercise per week is the minimum amount necessary for the average person to gain lasting cardiovascular benefit. But for many people, setting aside that amount of time can be difficult. In an effort to inspire more Americans to exercise, many fitness advisers in 1998 and 1999 encouraged people to be creative in making time for fitness.

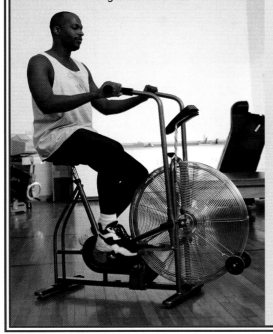

The following tips can be used to fit 200 minutes of weekly exercise into a hectic lifestyle. The tips incorporate new guidelines published in November 1998 by the American College of Sports Medicine.

- **Break it down:** Working out for 200 minutes is about the same as exercising 30 minutes each day. Or 40 minutes five times a week. Or an hour every other day.

  Don't have 30 minutes to spare? Do three 10-minute mini-workouts per day instead. Any aerobic activity (including walking) you can do for at least 10 minutes counts toward your goal of 200, so look for ways to get in a quick 10.

- **Keep moving:** Incorporate activity into your daily life. Bike instead of drive. Work up a little sweat cleaning. Park in the back of the lot and walk. Use the stairs instead of the elevator.

  Have 10 minutes before the start of your TV show? March in place. Try a little dancing. Rake leaves for 10 minutes before taking a break.

- **Variety is key:** Spend some of those 200 minutes doing strength training and flexibility exercises. Lift hand weights. Stretch after a brisk walk. (Building lean muscle mass will help your body burn calories even when you are not exercising. And stretching regularly after exercise may increase the results you get from strength training.)

- **Add it up:** Keep track of your time and reward yourself for reaching (or exceeding) 200 minutes.

Source: Mayo Clinic

daily session. The new guidelines also called for stretching 2 to 3 times per week to maintain flexibility and improve the range of joint motion. Finally, the ACSM reiterated its recommendation, first made in 1991, that fitness programs incorporate strength training. Weightlifting and calisthenics enhance overall strength, muscular endurance, and increase lean body weight, which helps the body burn fat. The ACSM recommended one set of 8 to 12 repetitions for each of the major muscle groups 2 to 3 days a week. Older and more frail individuals should lift lighter weights for more repetitions.

Although the 1978 recommendations were still considered valid, especially for people interested in higher fitness levels or competition, the 1998 guidelines acknowledged that many people do not have the time or inclination to exercise so intensely. The ACSM hoped that people would find the shorter exercise periods easier to incorporate into their daily activities. Even such minor modifications in a person's daily routine as taking the stairs instead of an elevator can make a difference in health.

Flexibility increases strength. Researchers in Massachusetts published a study in January 1999 that showed that weightlifting programs that incorporated stretching not only increase a person's flexibility, but increase strength as well. The study was conducted by Wayne Westcott, director

Exercise and Fitness

You're never too old
A number of studies in 1998 and 1999 indicated that older people benefit significantly from physical activity. Inactivity, the data suggest, is responsible for most of the physical decline that occurs in old age. Even moderate daily exercise has been shown to help older people improve their coordination, balance, and strength—which helps them remain independent in their daily lives and even improves emotional and psychological well-being.

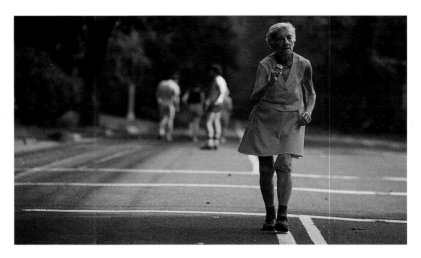

of fitness research at the South Shore YMCA in Braintree, Massachusetts.

For the study, 53 people were enrolled in a 10-week strength-training program. The participants were divided into three groups, each of which completed the same weight-training circuit using 13 standard weightlifting machines. One group performed no flexibility exercises; the second group did stretching exercises after completing the circuit; and the third group stretched between each workout station.

While all the participants grew stronger and more flexible after 10 weeks, the group that stretched after completing the circuit showed the most gains—in strength as well as flexibility. Participants in this group increased their strength by an average of 54 percent, compared with 37 percent in the group that stretched between machines and 29 percent in the group that did no stretching exercises. However, the group showing the best improvement may also have benefited from the one-on-one stretching instruction they received. The other groups had an instructor present only for their first time through the circuit.

Aging gracefully. A number of health studies have shown that exercise can help slow the aging process. Investigators offered substantial evidence that exercise can help older adults maintain their health in a report published in the June 1998 is-

sue of the journal *Medicine & Science in Sports & Exercise.*

Aging is a complex process that involves many variables, including *aerobic capacity* (ability to effectively process oxygen), heart rate, cardiovascular disease risk, loss of muscle mass, and posture. The authors of the study concluded that regular physical activity benefits each of these factors and contributes to the general physical and psychological well-being that defines healthy aging.

Exercise helps increase the body's aerobic capacity, and the ability to pump oxygen through the system depends on how efficiently the heart beats. In adults over age 25, the pumping ability of the heart generally decreases by about 5 to 15 percent per decade. But older adults who engage in endurance exercise benefit from better oxygen uptake and more flexible arteries, both of which contribute to increased flow of oxygen to the body and brain.

In order to boost the body's aerobic capacity, experts recommend rhythmic and aerobic forms of exercise that employ the large muscles, such as walking, running, cycling, and swimming. Lifting weights can also slow the progressive loss of muscle mass that begins after age 30. In older adults, weight training helps reduce the risk of developing such age-related diseases as osteoporosis, helps improve balance and motor skills, and contributes to better health and well-being.   • Renée Despres

- Nightlights linked to nearsightedness
- LASIK safe for myopia
- Guarding against eye injuries
- Paintball eye injuries
- Disposable bifocal contacts

Children who sleep in a lighted bedroom before the age of 2 may have a higher risk of developing *myopia* (nearsightedness) when they become older, researchers at the University of Pennsylvania Medical Center in Philadelphia reported in May 1999. The findings suggested that a nightly period of complete darkness may be necessary for the normal development of the eye, according to the researchers.

People with myopia have eyeballs that are longer than normal. Because of this, images come into focus in front of the *retina,* the light-sensitive tissue at the back of the eye.

The researchers compared the sleeping conditions of 479 young children, asking their parents if the children slept in a dark or lit room. They found that 34 percent of the children who slept in a bedroom lit by a dim nightlight during the first two years of their lives later developed myopia. This figure rose to 55 percent for those children who slept with a bedroom lamp turned on. By contrast, only 10 percent of the children who slept in a dark bedroom before age 2 later became myopic.

A number of eye specialists disputed the link between bedroom lights and myopia. These experts said the Pennsylvania researchers had failed to account for other factors, such as heredity, that may have caused the children to develop myopia.

LASIK safe for myopia. A popular laser technique for correcting myopia rarely results in complications, researchers at Emory University in Atlanta, Georgia, reported in January 1999. The technique, called laser in-situ keratomileusis (LASIK), was widely used in 1999 to correct or reduce moderate to high levels of nearsightedness. Although the United States Food and Drug Administration had not specifically approved LASIK, the agency permitted the procedure to be performed because it used the same type of laser device approved for photorefractive keratectomy, another procedure for treating myopia.

A surgeon performing LASIK first cuts a tiny flap in the outer layer of the cornea. The cornea, the transparent coat of the eye, works with the lens to focus images. The surgeon then uses a computer-controlled laser device called an excimer laser to remove a thin layer of tissue from the exposed part of the cornea. Removing the tissue flattens the cornea, so that objects focus closer to or on the retina. Finally, the flap is replaced and heals without sutures.

The Emory study examined the effect of LASIK on 1,062 eyes of 574 nearsighted patients. The researchers found that surgical complications, such as overcutting or undercutting the cornea flap, occurred in about 5 percent of cases. However, these

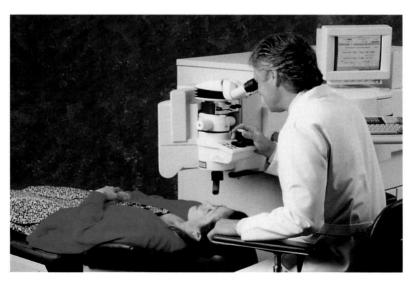

Laser treats hyperopia
A surgeon uses an instrument called an excimer laser to correct a patient's vision. The excimer laser, used since 1995 to treat *myopia* (nearsightedness), was approved by the U.S. Food and Drug Administration in November 1998 to correct *hyperopia* (farsightedness). To improve the focus of a farsighted eye, the surgeon directs the laser to cut a circular trough around the *cornea* (transparent coat of the eye).

complications rarely left patients with a significant loss of vision. The study revealed that complications were more likely in patients who had undergone previous eye surgery.

Guarding against eye injuries. Schools and youth athletic leagues should require all children participating in athletic programs to use protective eye wear, according to an April 1999 recommendation by the American Academy of Ophthalmology (AAO). The AAO, based in San Francisco, is the largest professional organization of ophthalmologists, who study the structure, function, and diseases of the eye.

The AAO maintained that the mandatory eye protection was needed because of a large number of serious eye injuries in youth sports. The organization noted that each year more than 100,000 sports-related eye injuries—one-third of them involving children—result in a trip to the doctor. According to the AAO, 90 percent of these eye injuries could be prevented by shatterproof eye wear.

The AAO advocated eye protection made from polycarbonate plastic. This material is as clear as the lenses in everyday eyeglasses but 20 times stronger. The organization expressed its hope that people who begin wearing eye protection in youth sports will continue to do so as adults.

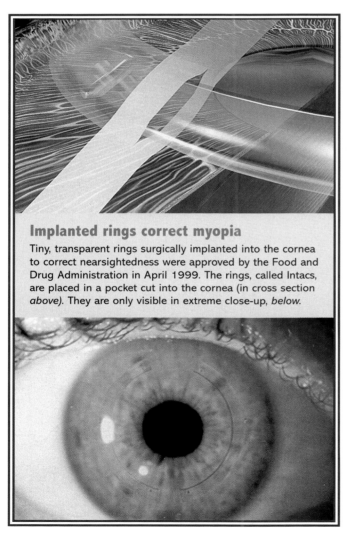

Implanted rings correct myopia

Tiny, transparent rings surgically implanted into the cornea to correct nearsightedness were approved by the Food and Drug Administration in April 1999. The rings, called Intacs, are placed in a pocket cut into the cornea (in cross section *above*). They are only visible in extreme close-up, *below*.

Paintball eye injuries. Ophthalmologists reported in March 1999 that severe eye injuries from paintball pellets continue to occur despite efforts to make participants use protective eye shields. Paintball is a combat-simulation game in which players fire projectiles of gelatin-coated paint at each other. The projectiles, fired from carbon-dioxide powered guns, can move as fast as 400 feet (122 meters) per second.

The team of ophthalmologists, led by Allen B. Thach of Walter Reed Army Medical Center in Washington, D.C., described 13 patients treated for paintball-related eye injuries. The injuries included severe bleeding inside the eye, detached retinas, and ruptures of the eyeball. Eleven of the injured people were not wearing eye protection when they were hit by the paint pellets, and as a result, eight of them were blinded.

The researchers noted that most paintball organizations require players to wear protective eyeglasses, and some clubs even require full facial protection covering the cheeks, ears, and eyes. However, the researchers said that injuries occur when players ignore the rules, or when paintball pellets, tree branches, or other objects dislodge the eye protection.

The ophthalmologists urged paintball players to always wear full facial shields. They said such shields provide the best protection for the face and are unlikely to be knocked off during play.

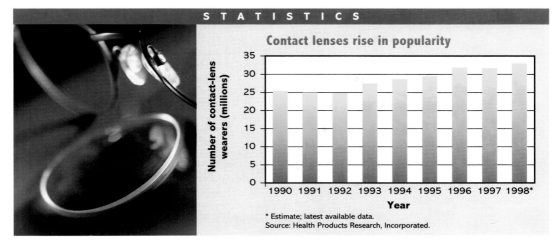

Contact lenses rise in popularity

Number of contact-lens wearers (millions)

Year

* Estimate; latest available data.
Source: Health Products Research, Incorporated.

Disposable bifocal contacts. The first disposable bifocal contact lens went on the market throughout the United States in April 1999, offering 89 million people with *presbyopia* (lens hardening) a new option for improving their eyesight. The Acuvue Bifocal Contact Lenses are manufactured by Johnson & Johnson Vision Products, Inc., of Jacksonville, Florida.

Presbyopia usually begins to occur around the age of 40, as the eyeball starts to lose the elasticity needed to change focus from near to far. People find themselves unable to read or focus on other close-up objects. The condition often occurs in people who are already nearsighted, so they need bifocal spectacles that correct for both visual problems.

The Acuvue lenses consist of five concentric rings made from a cellophane-thin plastic material that allows wearers to focus back and forth between distant and near objects. Although the FDA had approved the Acuvue bifocals in 1997, they had only been available in a small number of cities until 1999.

Johnson & Johnson said tests showed that Acuvue lenses corrected vision in 70 percent of the patients who tried them. This compared favorably with older types of bifocal contacts, which worked well in only 25 percent of patients. • **Michael Woods**

The number of people wearing contact lenses in the United States rose from 25.5 million in 1990 to about 33 million in 1998. In 1999, contact-lens manufacturers planned to introduce new types of lenses to continue this trend. For example, Ciba Vision Corporation of Duluth, Georgia, and Bausch & Lomb, Incorporated, of Rochester, New York, were each testing a contact lens that could be worn continuously for 30 days.

Scientists in Canada and the United States published research in April 1999 challenging earlier work that suggested a genetic basis for male homosexuality. Neuroscientists George Rice, George Ebers, and Carol Anderson at the University of Western Ontario in London, and geneticist Neil Risch at the Stanford Medical School in Palo Alto, California, attempted to replicate a highly publicized 1993 study at the National Cancer Institute in Bethesda, Maryland.

In that study, molecular biologist Dean Hamer and his colleagues analyzed DNA (deoxyribonucleic acid), the molecule genes are made of, from 40 pairs of gay brothers. Hamer's group focused on DNA from the X chromosome, one of the two sex chromosomes in humans. The 23 pairs of human chromosomes in the nucleus of each cell contain the cell's DNA. A female has two X chromosomes. A male has one X and one Y. He inherits the X chromosome from his mother. Hamer's team focused on the X chromosome because they found that many subjects had gay relatives on their mother's side of the family—a phenomenon suggesting that homosexuality may be linked to genes inherited from one's mother.

Analysis of X-chromosome DNA revealed *markers* (segments of DNA) that appeared more often in both gay brothers in a family than would be expected by chance. The markers

Genetic Medicine

• Genetic link to homosexuality?
• Genes and the heart
• Rates of harmful mutations

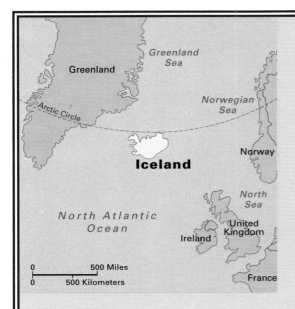

combined with a national health database, will make the search for genes associated with diseases considerably easier than it is in populations that are not as similar genetically and that do not have detailed genealogies.

One of the most controversial aspects of the law is that it grants only one company the right to establish the database and to use the research results to develop new commercial products such as genetic tests and new drugs. The company, deCODE Genetics, headquartered in Reykjavik, the capital, will have exclusive rights for 12 years. The company's chief executive officer, geneticist Kari Stefansson, says that such a long-term guarantee is necessary to protect deCODE's investment in the project.

Opposition to the new law arose from several quarters. Some of the country's leading scientists think that deCODE's ability to control the data-base and the research results will stifle research elsewhere in Iceland. Other Icelandic scientists and physicians are equally concerned about the privacy of genetic information in such a database. They fear that employers and insurance companies will use that information to discriminate against people who have genes associated with certain diseases.

Scientists from the United States and Europe expressed similar concerns. Despite those concerns, polls showed that a sizable majority of Iceland's citizens support the new law.

• Joseph D. McInerney

Iceland's genetic database

On Dec. 16, 1998, the Althing, Iceland's parliament, passed landmark legislation paving the way for establishment of the first nationwide genetic database. The controversial new law established a central database for the health records of all Icelanders, about 275,000 people.

Iceland is geographically—and, consequently, genetically—isolated. In addition, the Icelanders have maintained extensive family histories dating back many generations. Those facts,

---

were in a region of the X chromosome called Xq28. Hamer's group, therefore, contended that this region might contain a gene that contributes to the development of homosexuality.

Ebers and Rice's team set out to test Hamer's findings. They studied 52 pairs of gay brothers from Canada, measuring the extent to which they shared four DNA markers in the Xq28 region of the X chromosome. Their results showed that the brothers shared the DNA markers no more frequently than one would expect by chance. This research, therefore, did not support Hamer's findings.

Hamer contended that the new research was not an appropriate test of his work because the scientists did not choose subjects who had gay rel-

atives in their mothers' families. Ebers and Rice's group dismissed Hamer's objection, stating that they found no patterns of maternal transmission among their prospective subjects.

Additional research may or may not resolve this disagreement, which illustrates the difficulty of investigating genetic contributions to complex traits, especially behavioral traits. Most scientists agree that all complex traits result from a combination of genetic and environmental influences, and it is difficult to determine the relative impact of each component. Ebers and Rice noted that further research was needed because their study did not examine whether a genetic link to homosexuality exists somewhere else in human genes.

Genes and the heart. Early in the 1900's, geneticist William Bateson offered an enduring bit of scientific wisdom—"treasure your exceptions." In other words, scientists can tell a good deal about normal processes in nature by examining phenomena that are out of the ordinary. Such was the case in February 1999, when scientists from the United States and Japan identified a gene that plays a critical role in the development of the heart.

Cardiologist and developmental biologist Deepak Srivastava and his colleagues at the University of Texas Southwestern Medical Center in Dallas collaborated with cardiologist Rumiko Matsuoka from Tokyo Women's Medical University to investigate DiGeorge syndrome (DGS), one of the leading causes of *congenital* (present at birth) heart defects. In babies born with DGS, the major vessels that carry blood from the heart to the lungs and the rest of the body do not connect properly to the chambers of the heart. Other problems, such as facial abnormalities, are also associated with the syndrome.

Research done in the 1980's demonstrated that about 90 percent of people with DGS are missing a portion of DNA in chromosome 22, a region known as 22q11. This deletion involves as many as 20 million pairs of chemical subunits in DNA called bases. Each gene is a particular sequence of base pairs. If a portion of DNA in a chromosome is missing, or deleted, any gene that would normally reside there would likely be missing as well. A segment with 20 million base pairs could contain numerous genes, but all of those genes may not be relevant to DGS symptoms.

To narrow their search for genes related to DGS, Srivastava's group began looking at a relatively well-understood gene that codes for the production of a protein called DHAND. In mice, this protein helps regulate embryonic development of the heart. Mice that lack the gene for DHAND show abnormal development of the heart—abnormalities that are very much like those present in humans who have DGS.

An investigation of the genes activated by DHAND led them to one particular gene called UFD1. In healthy mice embryos, UFD1 was *expressed* (turned on) in structures that eventually became part of the heart and facial structures. The scientists also noted that UFD1 was *down-regulated* (not very active) in the heart cells of embryonic mice that lacked the DHAND protein. The research team confirmed the gene's link to DGS in a study of 182 people who had a 22q11 deletion. All of them lacked the human UFD1 gene.

Many biologists acknowledged the importance of the new findings for understanding the cause of DGS, but they called for further research to determine if other genes contribute to the symptoms of the disorder. Nonetheless, Srivastava's team revealed an important component in the normal stages of development of the heart and some facial structures. They also demonstrated the importance of animal models in studying humans systems.

Rates of harmful mutations. In January 1999, scientists provided the most accurate measure to date of the rate of harmful *mutations* (changes in genetic material) in humans. In the process, they also contributed support for a long-standing hypothesis about the evolution of sexual reproduction. Evolutionary biologists Adam Eyre-Walker from the University of Sussex in England and Peter D. Keightley from the University of Edinburgh in Scotland used the extensive collection of DNA sequences in electronic databases to study human mutations.

Certain mutations have favored the survival of some organisms during the history of life on Earth. Other mutations are harmful, compromising the survival of the organisms that carry them. These genetic advantages and disadvantages are the basis for evolution by natural selection.

Eyre-Walker and Keightley began their investigation of human mutation rates by comparing the DNA of humans and chimpanzees, the closest living relatives of humans. When they found a difference in DNA sequence, they looked at the same genetic region in gorilla DNA. If the gorilla DNA was identical to the chimpanzee

DNA, they labeled the change in human DNA a mutation.

They estimated that the human genetic mutation rate was 4.2 mutations per person per generation (every 25 years). Further analysis revealed that about 1.6 mutations per person per generation are harmful. The analysis was based on the assumption that humans have about 60,000 genes.

Eyre-Walker and Keightley noted that the rate of harmful mutations for humans is relatively high and that harmful mutations tend to stay in the human population in higher proportions than they do in other species. Biologists who study evolutionary genetics know that it is easy for mutations to become well established in small populations—and the human population has been fairly small during most of its evolutionary history.

A harmful mutation can be eliminated from a population only when the individual that carries it fails to produce offspring. However, if the individual with the harmful mutation does reproduce offspring that survive, the mutation can spread. An accumulation of such mutations eventually makes it more difficult for the group as a whole to survive. If humans have such a high mutation rate and large accumulation of harmful mutations, why did the species survive?

Part of the reason for human survival might have to do with sexual reproduction. When a sperm fertilizes an egg, new combinations of genes arise. A harmful gene from one parent can get lost in the shuffle of genetic recombination, or several harmful mutations can be brought together in a single offspring—making the offspring unlikely to survive. These results, the researchers noted, might explain the evolution of sexual reproduction. In organisms that produce *asexually* (without sex), such genetic recombination does not occur.

Eyre-Walker stated that sexual reproduction is probably only part of the explanation for our ability to overcome a high mutation rate. He added that the impact of some mutations was very small and that humans "had several important adaptive substitutions, like higher intelligence."

The continued presence of inherited diseases demonstrates that sexual reproduction does not eliminate all harmful genes. Also, better medical care has allowed people with some harmful genetic mutations to live long enough to reproduce. Harmful mutations, therefore, remain in the population, and could eventually accumulate in the population more quickly than they are removed by natural selection. The authors noted that an increased accumulation of mutations in the future could be damaging to human health.

• Joseph D. McInerney

- More data on estrogen and cancer
- Low estrogen and bone loss in men
- Getting a bad wrap?

The issue of whether estrogen replacement therapy increases a woman's chance of developing breast cancer has been extensively studied in the 1990's. However, clinical trials have yielded mixed results. In June 1999, investigators at the Mayo Clinic Cancer Center in Rochester, Minnesota, and Northwestern University Medical School in Chicago published yet another study on the topic. This study, a large, well-designed clinical trial, offered persuasive evidence to support the argument that estrogen replacement and breast cancer were probably not associated.

Many middle-aged women elect to receive hormone replacement therapy to minimize the effects of declining estrogen levels, which occurs naturally as the result of *menopause* (the end of the menstrual cycle that normally occurs between the ages of 45 and 55). Estrogen replacement is known to lower a woman's significant risk of developing heart disease and *osteoporosis* (a disease in which bones become weak and brittle) after menopause. However, studies showing that the treatment may be linked to a slightly higher risk of breast cancer have caused concern among women and their physicians.

The Mayo study followed 37,105 women ages 55 to 69, about 40 percent of whom had taken hormone replacement therapy. Of the entire group, 1,520 women developed breast cancer, and the women who had not taken hormone replacement therapy showed no increased incidence of the disease. However, the researchers did find an increased risk of other types of cancer. Fortunately, the cancers that did arise were generally types that responded better to treatment and were less likely to spread than breast cancer. Although these results were encouraging, most experts agreed that the link between estrogen replacement and breast cancer had not yet been ruled out.

Low estrogen in men. Medical researchers have long known about the link between osteoporosis and falling levels of the hormone estrogen in postmenopausal women. But findings presented at a meeting of the American Society for Bone and Mineral Research and the International Bone and Mineral Society in November 1998 showed that estrogen levels in men also decline with age, and that this was associated with a decrease in bone mass. Although men also produce estrogen, women produce much higher levels of this hormone.

Estrogen slows down the bone loss that occurs naturally with age. In women, osteoporosis is linked to the sharp drop in estrogen after menopause. However, osteoporosis in men has been traditionally associated with low levels of the male sex hormone testosterone, a rare condition called hypogonadism.

In one study, researchers followed 382 elderly white men for eight years, tracking changes in bone density, estrogen levels, and signs of hypogonadism. The data indicated that the men who had the highest estrogen levels had the highest bone density. The study found no significant connection with hypogonadism.

In another study, German researchers studied 300 men with osteoporosis for five years. They measured bone density, as well as estrogen and testosterone levels, and found that 40 percent of the men had low estrogen, while only 20 percent had low testosterone. The researchers did not see a pronounced effect of testosterone on the men's bone mineral density.

More than 10 million Americans have osteoporosis, and at least 1.5 million are men. However, the disease is often not diagnosed in men, so the actual number of men with the disease could be much higher.

Getting a bad wrap? Plastic wrap is one of the most popular food-storage materials available, but research in the 1990's fueled a debate about the safety of some kinds of plastic wrap. Some food-storage wraps are made with di-(2-ethylhexyl)adipate, or DEHA, a substance that adds clinginess to the wrap, enabling it to seal foods more effectively. However, some data suggest that DEHA is an *endocrine disrupter* (substance imitates or interferes with the action of

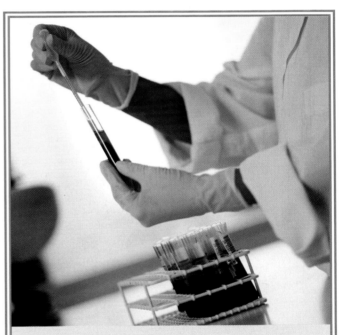

Blood test helps battle prostate cancer

According to three research papers published in the June 16, 1999, issue of the *Journal of the National Cancer Institute,* an observed decline in prostate cancer deaths in recent years may be due in part to the introduction of a blood test to detect the disease. The test for prostate specific antigen (PSA) was approved by the Food and Drug Administration in 1986. By 1999 it was widely used, frequently detecting potential signs of prostate cancer before symptoms are present. This has more men receiving treatment while the disease is still in its earliest stages. However, researchers believed that PSA testing alone did not account for the entire decline.

certain hormones). Some research has suggested that endocrine disrupters can cause breast cancer, birth defects, and other health problems.

DEHA is found in at least one brand of household plastic wrap, as well as the wrap used by many grocery stores to wrap meat and cheese. Research published in June 1998 indicated that certain foods (especially food with a high fat content, like meat and cheese) can absorb plasticizers on contact. In the study, researchers analyzed 19 brands and varieties of cheese, 7 of which were wrapped in plastic wrap that contained DEHA. All seven pieces of cheese were found to contain high levels of DEHA. Although researchers acknowledged that there was no conclusive evidence that the levels of DEHA found in the cheese were harmful, it said that there was cause for concern. The DEHA levels were significantly above the maximum safe limit set by health safety regulators in the European Union (an organization of 15 Western European nations). In the 1980's, British manufacturers replaced DEHA with a safer plasticizer.

American regulatory agencies, however, were not overly concerned about the results of such studies. Both the U.S. Food and Drug Administration (FDA) and the Environmental Protection Agency maintained that there was not enough evidence to demonstrate that DEHA causes hormone disruption. According to the American Plastics Council, an advocacy group for the plastics industry, at the levels documented by the researchers, a 150-pound (68-kilogram) adult would need to consume 1,000 pounds (450 kilograms) of plastic-wrapped cheese every day in order to produce health risks. Despite this position, the Natural Resource Defense Council, an environmental-affairs group based in San Francisco, countered that several studies done since 1996, the year of the FDA's last statement on the topic, have shown that DEHA is almost certainly an endocrine disrupter with potential adverse effects on health. Experts on both sides of the debate agreed that more research was needed to resolve the issue.

Individuals can reduce their exposure to DEHA by limiting the amount of contact between foods and cling wrap. The simplest solution is to rewrap cold cuts or cheese packaged in plastic wrap at home, after scraping off a thin layer where the wrap touched the food. In addition, they should purchase meats and cheeses that have not been prepackaged and have them wrapped in paper or plastic bags. If storing food in a bowl covered with plastic, don't let the plastic touch the food. Finally, plastic wrap should never be permitted to touch food while it is cooking in a microwave oven.　　• Renée Despres

Health Care Issues

• Medicare reform
• Managed care controversy
• SCHIP program successful
• Health care and elections
• Food poisoning
• Editor dismissed

Efforts to revamp the federal Medicare program were at the top of the health care agenda in 1999. The Medicare program covers the cost of many health care services for Americans over the age of 65. Both United States President Bill Clinton and the U.S. Congress supported basic—though very different—reforms.

In 1997, both Congress and the president had called for a National Bipartisan Commission on the Future of Medicare. The commission began meeting in 1998 and continued to meet until early 1999. The 17-member committee was cochaired by Senator John Breaux (D., Louisiana) and Representative Bill Thomas (R., California).

The panel tried to address many complex issues, including whether Medicare should be changed from a government program to one in which its beneficiaries used public money to buy private insurance, and whether Medicare should be expanded to include coverage of prescription drugs in settings other than hospital inpatient care. Medicare traditionally pays for such drugs when they are provided to hospital *inpatients* (patients who spend the night in the hospital, as opposed to going home after treatment).

The commission focused on what Breaux called a defined contribution approach to changing Medicare. Under his plan, each beneficiary would receive a fixed sum of money with which to buy insurance, which could be provided by managed care plans or by the traditional government program. However, the commission expected that traditional Medicare would cost more than the sum provided, thus forcing beneficiaries to pay the difference if they wanted to stay in the original Medicare program.

Although both Democratic and Republican committee members supported the plan, it failed to gain the 11 votes that were necessary to send it to Congress as a recommendation. The panel voted 10 to 7 in favor of the defined contribution proposal. The commission disbanded in March 1999 without making a recommendation to Congress. Breaux, however, vowed to continue to push for his idea in Congress in 1999.

On June 29, President Clinton unveiled his own proposal for Medicare reform, the centerpiece of which was a new prescription drug benefit. Under his proposal, each Medicare beneficiary, beginning in 2002, would have the option of paying $24 a month in drug benefit premiums. Medicare would then pay half the cost of outpatient prescription drugs, up to an annual total limit of $2,000.

The premiums would gradually increase to $44 a month by 2008, and the annual total spending limit would rise to $5,000. Under the president's proposal, the federal government would pay the premiums for individuals with annual incomes up to $11,000 and couples with annual incomes up to $17,000.

Democratic legislators praised the proposal while Republicans criticized it, saying it was too expensive. Republican legislators also said that the plan should be limited to the 15.5 million Medicare beneficiaries who did not already have extra private health insurance that covered prescription drugs, rather than all 39 million beneficiaries.

President Clinton's plan also called for Medicare to pay the total cost of certain preventive health services, part of which beneficiaries have traditionally had to pay. He further asked that beneficiaries pay for 20 percent of laboratory tests and a larger share of the cost of visits to physicians and hospital clinics.

Although there was broad support for an expanded pharmaceutical benefit, many health care professionals expressed doubts that the president's plan would be approved by Congress.

The future of Medicare, which is facing a huge increase in costs as the *Baby Boomer generation* (a large group of people born in the United States from 1946 to 1964) retire and become eligible for benefits beginning around 2011, got some welcome news in March 1999. Trustees of the Medicare Hospital Trust Fund,

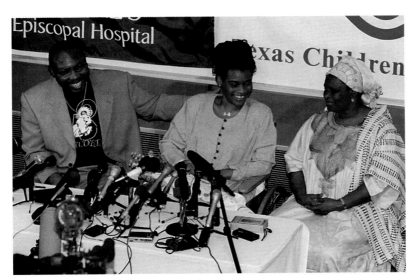

Birth of octuplets

Nkem Chukwu, *center,* her husband Louis Udobi, *left,* and her mother Janet Chukwu, *right,* face the press in December 1998 after Chukwu gave birth to the first known surviving set of octuplets. On December 20, Chukwu gave birth to the last of eight infants. The first child was born on December 8. The smallest infant died on December 27.

which makes Medicare payments to hospitals, reported that the fund would remain solvent until 2015.

Managed care controversy. In July 1998, the House of Representatives approved the Patient Protection Act, which was designed to increase protections for patients who belong to managed care plans such as health maintenance organizations (HMO's).

The bill, which was supported primarily by Republicans, included such measures as allowing women access to *obstetricians* (physicians who specialize in childbirth) and *gynecologists* (physicians who specialize in women's health) without referrals. Democrats proposed an alternative plan that would have allowed patients to collect punitive damages from managed care providers that denied them appropriate care.

The Senate considered similar legislation, but failed to pass any managed care legislation by the end of 1998. However, President Clinton had vowed to veto either bill, saying neither did much to protect patients from unacceptable managed care practices.

In 1998, 100.5 million Americans belonged to HMO's or similar forms of managed care plans. Despite such growth, there continued to be some resistance to these plans, usually based on the belief that managed care did not allow patients enough access to care they needed or sufficient choice of physician, and that they interfered with the freedom of health care providers to adequately serve patients.

When Congress convened in January 1999, Speaker of the House Dennis Hastert (R., Illinois) promised that representatives would vote on managed care patient protection sometime during the 1999 session. Although several bills were submitted early in the year, no action had been taken by late June 1999.

Medicare and managed care collided unexpectedly in late 1998, when officials with managed care plans, who had complained that Medicare was not paying them enough, decided to stop offering coverage to the program's beneficiaries in some markets, leaving the patients scrambling for other coverage.

The situation was troubling to the Clinton administration and Congress. Both had hoped that an increased enrollment of Medicare beneficiaries in managed care would save the program money.

However, when the plans asked for payment increases, Nancy-Ann DeParle, administrator of the Health Care Financing Administration, which oversees Medicare, refused. By mid-October 1998, more than 500,000 Medicare beneficiaries had lost coverage because of managed care plan pullouts.

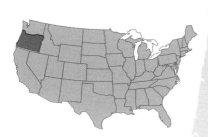

Assisted suicide law in Oregon

A report published in February 1999 by the Oregon Health Division revealed that 15 terminally ill people had used that state's physician-assisted suicide law in 1998. The report, which was issued one year after Oregon became the first state to permit physicians to prescribe lethal drugs for terminally ill patients, showed no signs of abuse on the part of patients. State officials also reported that no one who used the law to end their lives had suffered during the procedure, as some opponents had feared.

Kevorkian guilty. A Michigan judge in April 1999 sentenced Jack Kevorkian to 10 to 25 years in prison for his role in the 1998 physician-assisted suicide of a Michigan man. Kevorkian, a retired pathologist, was the nation's most visible proponent of physician-assisted suicide. A jury in March 1999 convicted Kevorkian of second-degree murder in connection with the death of 52-year-old Thomas Youk. Since 1990, Kevorkian had claimed to have participated in the suicides of at least 130 terminally ill people.

In September 1998, Kevorkian injected Youk, who suffered from amyotrophic lateral sclerosis, or Lou Gehrig's disease, with a lethal dose of chemicals at Youk's request. Kevorkian videotaped the assisted suicide and sent the videotape to the CBS news program "60 Minutes," which aired portions of the video.

Health care and Y2K. Health care officials were among those people concerned about a computer glitch known as the Year 2000 (Y2K) problem. Many older computer components and programs could read only the last two digits of a year. As a result, they could not tell the difference between the year 2000 and 1900 and might malfunction beginning Jan. 1, 2000. Experts said those computers could include some machines that are critical to patient care.

However, a survey released in March 1999 by the American Hospital Association (AHA) in Washington, D.C., showed that most hospitals in the United States expected to be Y2K compliant by Jan. 1, 2000. The AHA surveyed 2,000 hospitals across the country about their Y2K preparedness for information systems such as billing, medical equipment, and day-to-day operations.

Of those hospitals, 98 percent reported that their information systems were ready or would be ready in time; 96 percent reported that their medical devices were ready or would be in time; and 96 percent reported that their building computers were ready or would be ready by 2000.

In each case, less than 1 percent of those hospitals surveyed expected noncompliance. Almost all hospitals

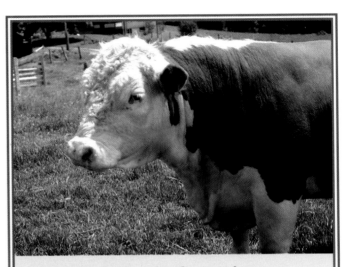

Mad cow disease death rates increase

The rate of death from the human form of "mad cow disease"—called Creutzfeldt-Jakob disease—more than doubled in the fourth quarter of 1998. That finding was published in a January 1999 edition of the British medical journal *Lancet*. Nine people in Great Britain died of the disease in the last three months of 1998, according to the report. Mad cow disease is a brain infection in cattle that causes odd behavior, difficulty in walking, and eventual death. Beef made from infected cows may lead to the human form of the disease. In June 1999, a study published in the *Journal of the American Medical Association* concluded that chances of the disease spreading to the United States are minimal. Researchers said the disease has never been shown to exist in the United States and that there are adequate regulations to prevent such an occurrence.

were preparing emergency plans in the event the computers failed.

However, some hospital officials in mid-1999 were concerned that hospital patients might be at risk if providers of blood, pharmaceuticals, and other critical materials were not Y2K compliant. The AHA urged hospitals not to stockpile or hoard supplies, but rather to keep a normal inventory and develop back-up plans with their key suppliers.

Health insurance problems. A study published in December 1998 by the Employee Benefit Research Institute, a Washington, D.C.-based organization that follows employee benefit issues, revealed that in 1997, 43 million people, or about 18 percent of the U.S. population under age 65, lacked health insurance coverage. The report, which used data compiled by the U.S. Census Bureau, also showed that 36 percent of Hispanics were uninsured, as were 14 percent of whites and 23 percent of African Americans.

SCHIP program successful. The National Governors' Association announced in March 1999 that 828,000 children nationwide had obtained insurance coverage in 1998 through a federal insurance program.

Congress passed the State Children's Health Insurance Program (SCHIP) in 1997 in an attempt to aid the estimated 10 million U.S. children who did not have health care coverage. Under SCHIP, the federal government provides grants to states to enroll uninsured children in private insurance or in Medicaid, a state-run program that covers some health care costs for certain low-income individuals. State officials hoped that by the early 2000's, some 2.5 million children would benefit from SCHIP.

Health care and elections. Several health care related issues were put to a vote in state elections in November 1998. Voters in Michigan rejected an initiative to make physician-assisted suicide legal. Voters in Alaska, Arizona, Nevada, Oregon, and Washington state approved the use of mari-

juana as a medical therapy under certain circumstances.

In spite of those votes, the federal government stood by its position that marijuana use is illegal under federal law. Federal officials said that anyone who used it, even in states where medical use was legal, risked federal arrest and prosecution.

Food poisoning. In December 1998, the Sara Lee Corporation ordered the recall of approximately 15 million pounds of hot dogs, turkey, and other prepared meats that had been processed at a Bil Mar Foods plant in Zeeland, Michigan. Bil Mar Foods is a division of Sara Lee.

Officials feared that the foods contained the bacterium *Listeria monocytogenes*. The bacterium usually causes only short-term problems in the digestive systems of healthy adults, but it can be deadly for the elderly, pregnant women, newborns, and people with weakened immune systems.

Editor dismissed. In January 1999, the American Medical Association (AMA) fired George D. Lundberg, editor of the *Journal of the American Medical Association*, after 17 years. The AMA accused him of trying to influence the impeachment trial of President Clinton, then underway in Congress, by publishing an article about a 1991 study on the definition of sex. • Emily Friedman

Heart and Blood Vessels

- Heart attacks more deadly among women
- Monitoring fainting episodes
- Leeches to treat heart attack
- Laser therapy for heart pain

In people under 50 years of age, heart attacks are far less common in women than in men, but when they do occur, women are more than twice as likely to die. These findings were reported by researchers at the Yale University School of Medicine in a July 1999 issue of the *New England Journal of Medicine*.

Researchers had long known that over all, women with heart attacks fare worse than men, but the large difference in the younger age groups was not known before the Yale study. The difference between women and men who have heart attacks diminishes with age, as men's risk goes up, but women's risk of death stays higher than men's until the age of 75.

The reasons for the difference are not fully understood, and scientists say that the study's findings, based on a study of the hospital records of 155,565 women and 229,313 men who had heart attacks and were treated at 1,658 hospitals, mean that younger women who suffer heart attacks are a high-risk group needing special study and attention.

In the same issue of the journal. a study by researchers at St. Luke's-Roosevelt Medical Center in New York City , involving 3,662 women and 8,480 men with heart problems, also found that over all, women with heart attacks were more likely than men to die. They were more likely to have weakened heart muscle, dangerously low blood pressure, and electrocardiograms that initially made it difficult to tell whether they were having a heart attack.

In addition, women's heart attacks tended to have different causes than men's: in men, blocked arteries were more likely to bring on heart attacks, whereas women had clearer arteries. But the women still had heart attacks, which researchers said were probably caused by large blood clots and spasms in arteries.

Heart disease is the leading cause of death in the United States. According to the American Heart Association, 9,000 women age 29 to 44 had heart attacks in 1997, compared with 32,000 men. The association did not have death rates, but in the Yale study, 6.1 percent of women unger age 50 died from their heart attacks, compared with 2.9 percent of the men.

Monitoring fainting episodes.
In January 1999, investigators from the University of Western Ontario in London, Ontario, Canada, reported on a new implantable heart monitor to help physicians diagnose *syncope* (severe fainting episodes caused by disorders of the heart rhythm). The device, known as the Reveal Insertable Loop Recorder, is a tiny electrocardiogram recorder that is surgically implanted under the skin. The advantage of an implanted device is that it is available at the push of a button to record the information needed to make an accurate diagnosis. Once an event is recorded and a diagnosis is made, the device can easily be removed.

Fainting is a common complaint and most fainting episodes are usually not harmful. Patients with syncope, however, suddenly and unexpectedly lose consciousness due to reduced blood flow to the brain. This can lead to serious injury or death. A reliable diagnosis of syncope requires a physician to confirm irregular heart activity during a fainting spell. Without a diagnosed cause, it is difficult to treat the patient and prevent further episodes.

Traditional techniques to evaluate such patients fail to determine the cause of syncope in up to 50 percent

of the patients. More aggressive testing in the hospital still leaves 25 percent of patients without a diagnosis. Other portable recording devices, which are worn externally, have been used by patients with syncope in the past. But these devices were often of limited value in brief episodes because they could not be activated in time.

Reveal, which was already in use in the United States in 1999, is an electrocardiogram recorder weighing just 0.6 ounces (17 grams). The device is activated using a remote control, which can be used by the patient or caregiver in the event of an episode of syncope. Pressing a button on the

Mechanical heart therapy
Implanted mechanical pumps called left ventricular assist devices (LVAD's), *inset,* help patients with heart failure survive the wait for a heart transplant. In November 1998, a clinical study revealed that LVAD's, which are powered by external battery packs, *below,* may also help diseased heart tissue recover some of its lost function, perhaps eliminating the need for a transplant.

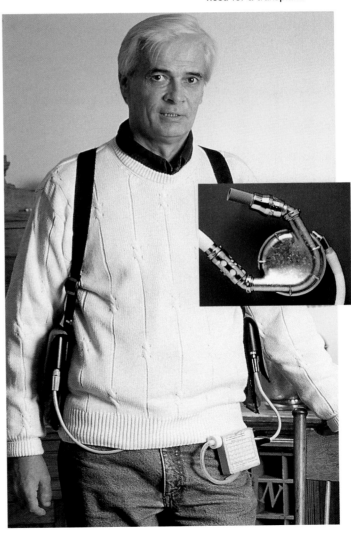

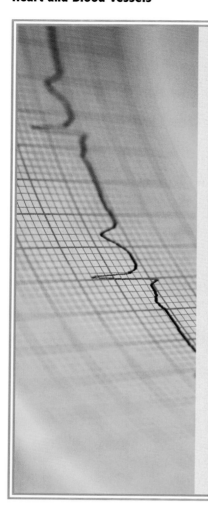

Top 10 heart research advances

In December 1998, the American Heart Association (AHA) published its annual list of the year's top 10 research advances in heart disease and stroke. The list, introduced in 1996, recognizes achievements in basic and clinical research that may have the greatest impact in improving the prevention and treatment of cardiovascular disease. The top 10 advances of 1998 were:

- Genetic therapy can create "natural" bypasses around obstructions in the blood vessels of the heart.
- New "super aspirins" (celecoxib and rofecoxib) do a superior job in fighting heart attack and stroke.
- In addition to preventing blood clots, aspirin may reduce inflammation in blood vessels near a clot, a condition that may increase the risk of a heart attack.
- The development of nonsurgical imaging technology helps detect the early stages of heart disease.
- Damaged heart tissue may recover some of its function with the help of an implanted left ventricular assist device.
- People who smoke fewer than 10 cigarettes daily have a 30 percent higher risk of death than non-smokers.
- Low-fat diet and exercise can significantly reduce harmful blood cholesterol levels, especially in high-risk patients.
- Community education campaigns result in more people with symptoms of a heart attack coming to the emergency room.
- The AHA in 1998 changed the way it computes age-adjusted death rates from heart attack and stroke, which should result in more accurate statistics.
- The Nobel Prize-winning discovery of nitric oxide's action in the bloodstream has present and future implications for treating cardiovascular disease and stroke.

activator turns on the device and records the patient's heartbeat. After the episode, a physician can transfer the information to a standard electrocardiograph to examine the heart rhythm.

The investigators implanted the Reveal unit in 85 patients with undiagnosed syncope for up to 18 months. After implantation, symptoms recurred in 58 patients. Arrhythmia was detected in 21 of these patients. Almost all the cases were readily treatable by implanting a heart pacemaker. The only complication was that three patients developed an infection of the surgical incision. There were no deaths or injuries related to recurrent syncope. The investigators concluded that the Reveal device was a safe and

effective way to diagnose the cause of syncope.

Leeches to treat heart attacks.
A group of cardiologists called the Organization to Assess Strategies for Ischemic Syndromes (OASIS) reported in February 1999 that a new drug derived from leech saliva is an effective treatment for heart-attack patients. The drug is a synthetic version of a *polypeptide* (molecule that forms part of a protein) found in the saliva of the medicinal leech, *Hirudo medicinalis*.

Heart attacks are caused by blood clots in the *coronary arteries* (arteries that supply blood to the heart muscle). Clots often form when a buildup of fatty deposits in the arteries reduces or blocks the flow of blood to the heart. One of the traditional methods for treating a developing heart attack is to administer *anticoagulant* (anticlotting) drugs, such as aspirin and heparin, which dissolve clots or prevent their formation. However, 5 to 10 percent of patients who receive anticoagulant therapy still have a heart attack.

Leeches feed by biting a victim and drinking its blood. The polypeptide, known as hirudin, prevents the blood from clotting while the leech feeds. Although hirudin's anticoagulant properties have been recognized for decades, the development of a hirudin-based anticoagulant drug became possible only after genetic-engineering techniques enabled researchers to manufacture an artificial version of the substance in sufficiently large quantities.

The OASIS team compared the effectiveness of the new drug, known as recombinant hirudin (r-hirudin), with heparin in 10,141 patients admitted to a hospital with symptoms of an impending heart attack. The patients were randomly treated with aspirin and either heparin or r-hirudin for 72 hours. After seven days, researchers found that 213 people in the heparin group had either died of cardiovascular causes or suffered a heart attack. In the r-hirudin group, 182 people died or had a heart attack.

Fifty-nine patients in the r-hirudin group had to end their treatment early, within the first 72 hours of treatment, due to major bleeding complications caused by the drug's powerful blood-thinning capabilities. In comparison, heparin caused only 34 cases of major bleeding. Almost all of these episodes were due to bleeding in the lining of the stomach. The incidence rate of stroke or other complications between the groups was similar.

The investigators concluded that r-hirudin was superior to heparin in preventing heart attacks in patients with heart-attack symptoms. Although bleeding complications were more common with r-hirudin, the overall rate of these complications was low enough for the drug to be considered generally safe.

Laser therapy for heart pain. At the annual meeting of the American College of Cardiology in March 1999, cardiologist Steven Oesterle of Massachusetts General Hospital in Boston reported on the effectiveness of a surgical procedure for *angina* (chest pain caused when the heart muscle is starved of oxygen-rich blood). The technique employed a laser guided by a fiberoptic catheter. People with coronary-artery disease often suffer from angina, and many of them do not respond to traditional drug treatment or are unable to withstand surgery.

Traditional methods of treating angina include administering drugs

Laser procedure offers angina relief

Angina is chest pain caused when the heart muscle is starved of oxygen-rich blood. In 1999, a new variation of a laser surgical technique was reported to offer patients superior benefits over traditional surgery or drug therapy. A laser beam, delivered via a fiberoptic cable, is used to cut several tiny "channels" into the heart muscle. Creation of multiple channels appears to promote blood flow through the affected region of the heart.

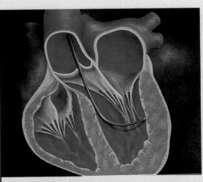

A catheter, introduced through an arm or leg artery, is threaded into the heart and positioned against the wall of the left ventricle. This method eliminates the need to open the chest to expose the heart, as is done in conventional surgery.

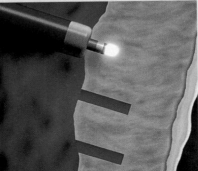

A fiberoptic cable inside the catheter delivers a laser beam to the surgery site. The beam vaporizes the tissue, "drilling" 15 to 30 channels in the heart wall, permitting blood to penetrate. New blood vessels form as the cuts heal, improving blood flow.

that lower cholesterol or that widen the coronary arteries. Surgical options include *angioplasty* (inflating a tiny balloon inside the affected artery to widen the vessel) or creating a bypass around the blockage using blood vessels from elsewhere in the patient's body. However, some angina patients are unresponsive to drugs or unsuitable for surgery for various reasons. Laser treatment may provide relief to many of these patients.

Many animal species do not have coronary arteries to supply blood to the heart muscle. Instead, the heart muscle is filled with tiny channels that permit the blood to penetrate the muscle tissue. Scientists reasoned that producing similar channels in the human heart might enable more blood to penetrate the muscle, preventing angina.

In the mid-1990's, surgeons experimented with this technique during coronary bypass surgery. They used a laser to drill tiny channels into the outer wall of the heart in areas where artery bypass was not feasible. Encouraging results from these trials led to a trial that compared surgical laser treatment in angina patients with traditional drug therapy. But the one-year survival rate was better in the drug-treatment group (96 percent) than in the laser group (89 percent), and 5 percent of patients in the laser group died due to surgical complications. Although the surviving surgical

patients reported reduced angina, they showed only slightly better increases in exercise endurance than the drug-treatment group. The investigators concluded that the risks associated with laser surgery did not outweigh the slight benefit over drug therapy.

Oesterle inserted a fiberoptic catheter into an arm or leg artery and ran it into a chamber of the heart to a point near the blockage site. This enabled the laser beam, running through the fiber, to cut channels into the heart muscle from the inside out.

Oesterle used the new procedure on 221 patients with severe angina who were unsuitable for angioplasty or bypass surgery. Half received aggressive drug therapy and half had laser surgery. After three months, 46 percent of the surgical patients experienced significantly less pain, compared with 6 percent of the drug therapy patients. In addition, the laser-treated group showed a 25-percent increase in their ability to exercise, compared with only 5 percent in the drug-treated group.

After six months, the initial results were maintained and no adverse effects of the laser treatment were found. Oesterle concluded that the procedure was an option for patients with severe angina who are not suitable for angioplasty or for coronary bypass surgery.

• Michael H. Crawford

Infectious Diseases

The discovery of a genetic "master switch" that allows bacteria to cause infections was reported in May 1999 by molecular biologist Michael J. Mahan and his colleagues at the University of California in Santa Barbara. The researchers said the discovery could lead to new methods of preventing and treating infections.

Mahan's team studied a bacterium called *Salmonella typhimurium*, which causes food poisoning in humans. The 2,500 other known strains of *Salmonella* also cause diseases, including typhoid fever. Each strain carries many *virulence genes,* genes that are switched on when the bacterium finds a host and which help the microbe thrive.

The researchers identified a protein called DNA adenine methylase, or Dam, which switches on more than 20 of the virulence genes. Mahan's team inactivated the gene that produced Dam in *S. typhimurium* and injected the altered bacteria into mice. Consequently, some of the virulence genes were never turned on and the bacteria did not cause disease. In addition, the genetically altered *S. typhimurium* acted as a vaccine against the disease. The mouse immune systems produced antibodies that destroyed the unaltered version of the bacteria. Scientists hoped the *Salmonella* research could also lead to a new family of antibiotics that work by inactivating Dam genes.

AIDS menace. Acquired immune deficiency syndrome (AIDS) became the world's most deadly infectious disease in 1998, overtaking tuberculosis, according to a May 1999 report by the World Health Organization (WHO) in Geneva, Switzerland. Human immunodeficiency virus (HIV), which causes AIDS, killed more than 2.28 million people worldwide in 1998, while tuberculosis killed about 1.5 million people. WHO also noted that AIDS was the leading cause of death in Africa, accounting for about 19 percent of all deaths.

Faced with such statistics, public health workers stepped up efforts to control the epidemic. The first clinical trials in Africa of an HIV vaccine began in February 1999 in Uganda. AIDS has killed about 500,000 of the country's 20 million people and left about 1 million children orphaned. The United States National Institute of Allergy and Infectious Diseases (NIAID) in Bethesda, Maryland, began the vaccine trial with 40 volunteers.

Origin of HIV. An international team of scientists announced in February 1999 that they had traced the origin of HIV to a virus in a chimpanzee species in western equatorial Africa. Scientists had long suspected that the AIDS virus had descended from a strain of simian immunodeficiency virus (SIV), but the virus had been found in only three chimps and their SIV strains seemed only remotely related to HIV.

The research team, led by virologist Beatrice H. Hahn of the University of Alabama at Birmingham, discovered a fourth infected chimp and used sophisticated genetic analysis to study the various SIV strains and their four hosts. The researchers then compared the chimp viruses with various strains of HIV. Putting together many bits of evidence, Hahn's group concluded that HIV originated in a chimp species called *Pan troglo-dytes troglodytes.* They determined that the virus was probably transmitted to humans in three separate occurrences, most likely when hunters butchered infected chimps for meat.

NIAID Director Anthony A. Fauci said the finding may have many applications in AIDS research. Although the chimps are infected with the HIV-like virus, they stay healthy. Fauci noted that understanding how chimps resist the virus may lead to drugs that can protect humans from HIV.

Prion diseases. New discoveries about the structure of protein particles called prions may make it possible to breed sheep and cattle that are resistant to deadly nerve disorders, researchers at the University of California at San Francisco (UCSF) reported in April 1999. Prions are proteins normally found in the brains of all animals. Abnormally shaped or infectious prions, however, can cause brain-deteriorating diseases, such as

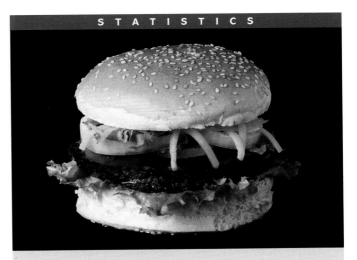

S T A T I S T I C S

Salmonella contamination decreases

The U.S. Department of Agriculture (USDA) reported in March 1999 that a new inspection system at meat-processing plants had reduced the prevalence of the disease-causing *Salmonella* bacteria. USDA officials stated that a comparison of contamination levels in raw meat products before and after the program was implemented in January 1998 revealed the benefits of the new program.

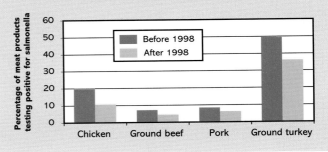

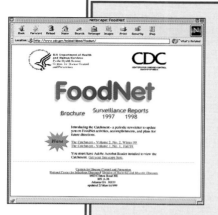

And the surveillance says ...

The United States Centers for Disease Control and Prevention (CDC) in Atlanta, Georgia, coordinates a program called the Foodborne Diseases Active Surveillance Network, or FoodNet. Working with several state and federal agencies, the CDC tracks the cases of foodborne illness in the United States, conducts studies to determine the source of these diseases, and evaluates the success of various food safety programs. Results of FoodNet studies, information about various foodborne illnesses, and copies of the FoodNet newsletter can be found on the Internet at http://www.cdc.gov/ncidod/dbmd/foodnet/.

scrapie in sheep, bovine spongiform encephalopathy (BSE) or "mad cow disease" in cattle, and Creutzfeldt-Jakob disease (CJD) and several other diseases in humans.

Disease occurs when an infectious prion acts as a template for altering the shape of the healthy prions it encounters. Nerve cells with the infectious form of the protein stop working normally. Although much about the origin of infectious prions remained mysterious in the 1990's, researchers had determined that the disease could cross species. In other words, beef infected with BSE could cause a form of CJD, called variant CJD (vCJD).

The UCSF researchers, led by pharmaceutical chemist Thomas L. James, described the three-dimensional structure of prions. In particular, they determined that a region of the prion is susceptible to change and that the kind of change that occurs determines what disease develops. The researchers also found that the prions of some individual animals were resistant to change. They hypothesized that breeding animals with such prions could prevent disease.

Meningitis drug. The first effective drug treatment for viral meningitis, the most common infection of the central nervous system in humans,

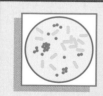

Dangerous dogs

From December 1998 to February 1999, nine meat-processing companies in the United States recalled more than 45 million pounds of hotdogs and lunch meats after an outbreak of food poisoning from the bacterium *Listeria monocytogenes*. The U.S. Centers for Disease Control and Prevention (CDC) in Atlanta, Georgia, attributed 21 deaths to the *Listeria* contamination. CDC officials also made the following warnings:

- All meat products, including such precooked meats as hotdogs, should be cooked thoroughly.

- *Listeria monocytogenes* can survive at refrigerator and freezer temperatures and is usually not killed in microwave ovens.

- Consumers should carefully wash all utensils that have touched uncooked meats.

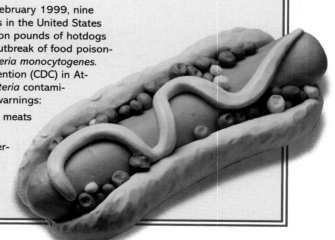

was announced in May by scientists at the University of California at San Diego. Meningitis, an inflammation of the membranes covering the brain and spinal cord, can be caused by viruses, bacteria, and other microbes.

In clinical trials, the drug called pleconaril proved to be effective in stopping the virus in all 221 children receiving the medication. Pediatrician Mark H. Sawyer, who directed the study, said pleconaril would probably reduce the need for extended hospital stays to treat viral meningitis. The drug, developed by ViroPharma Incorporated in Exton, Pennsylvania, was not yet approved by the U.S. Food and Drug Administration in 1999.

Smallpox virus. In March, a panel of scientists at the Institute of Medicine (IOM) concluded that the smallpox virus could have important applications in medical research that would be lost if the last remaining stocks of the virus were destroyed. IOM is an agency of the National Academy of Sciences in Washington, D.C., that advises the government on science.

After smallpox was eradicated as an infectious disease in 1980, scientists debated a plan to destroy stocks of the virus, which are held in secure laboratories in the United States and Russia. In April 1999, the U.S. government announced that it would preserve its stock.   • **Michael Woods**

- Fighting organ-transplant rejection
- Managing anemia in hemodialysis patients

In the June 1999 issue of the journal *Nature Medicine,* researchers at the Naval Medical Research Center in Bethesda, Maryland, reported progress in preventing the immune system from attacking transplanted organs—a phenomenon known as rejection. The researchers sought to prevent rejection by selectively blocking immune cells that are responsible for attacking a transplanted organ.

When a foreign organism infects the body, Killer T lymphocytes, a type of white blood cell, attack it. However, these cells also attack transplanted organs. Modern antirejection drugs, which work primarily by blocking Killer T cells directly, also suppress the body's ability to fight bacteria and viruses and offer only imperfect protection to the transplanted organ. Patients who take antirejection drugs are therefore always more susceptible to infection and, despite antirejection therapy, more than half of the transplants fail within 10 years.

Instead of blocking the Killer T lymphocytes directly, the researchers attempted to prevent rejection by temporarily blocking the signal that causes Killer T cells to attack. This signal comes from related cells called Helper T lymphocytes. When Killer T lymphocytes are activated by something foreign in the body but then fail to receive this "attack" signal, they die. Different Killer T cells are programmed to attack different invaders. Theoretically, therefore, if all of the

Killer T cells that are activated by the transplant are eliminated before they attack, rejection will not occur. To block the "attack" signal, the researchers used hu5C8, a protein that attaches to Helper T cells and prevents them from recognizing a foreign invader. Without this interaction, the Helper T cells send no attack signal.

The researchers gave kidney transplants to a group of rhesus monkeys. Nine of these monkeys were also given huC58 for five months and no medication after that. All of the monkeys who did not receive huC58 rejected the transplants, but none of the huC58-treated monkeys showed any sign of rejection. Furthermore, none of the treated monkeys showed any evidence of illness to suggest that their immune systems had been weakened. At the time of the report, one monkey had been off the hu5C8 for almost a year. Although the monkeys did develop antibodies to the transplants and the transplants had abnormal amounts of white blood cells within them, all of the kidneys still functioned normally.

Managing anemia. In August 1998, American investigators reported on the results of a multicenter clinical trial studying the most effective use of a drug used to treat *anemia* (an abnormally low number of red blood cells) in patients who require *hemodialysis* (mechanical filtration of impurities from the blood). Virtually all

Facts about kidney stones

An estimated 600,000 people in the United States develop kidney stones each year. Kidney stones are created when substances in urine (mainly calcium) crystallize and clump together. Small stones pass unnoticed out of the body by urination, but larger ones sometimes get stuck in the urinary tract, causing excruciating pain. Kidney stones are often removed using an endoscope inserted into the *urethra* (tube that carries urine out of the body). The stone is either pulled out or broken up with ultrasonic waves or a laser beam. Another method, called extracorporeal shock wave lithotripsy, employs powerful sound waves to break up kidney stones from outside the body. Symptoms of a kidney stone include severe abdominal pain radiating to the groin, urgent need to urinate, and blood in the urine.

hemodialysis patients develop anemia. This is due to a lack of *erythropoietin,* a hormone produced by the kidneys that stimulates red blood cell production. Synthetic erythropoietin (sold as Epogen) has been used since 1989 to correct this deficiency, but physicians have questioned whether raising the traditional dosage would produce greater benefits.

The researchers evaluated 1,233 patients with cardiovascular disease who were receiving hemodialysis. Half of the patients received Epogen to maintain a *hematocrit* (the relative volume of blood cells in a given amount of blood) of 30 percent, the standard for dialysis patients. The others received higher doses of Epogen to raise their hematocrit to 42 percent, the normal level for healthy people.

The researchers halted the study when the data indicated that the high hematocrit group had a slightly higher rate of death. Surprisingly, the higher death rate occurred among patients who for some reason had failed to achieve a higher hematocrit despite the higher dosage. Patients who did achieve a higher hematocrit had a lower death rate. Because the researchers were unable to explain this result, they concluded that their strategy should not be used without further study.　　• Jeffrey R. Thompson

Medical Ethics

• Placebos and surgery
• Jack Kevorkian convicted
• Oregon suicide law
• HIV discrimination

The medical community in late 1998 and 1999 debated the use of a *placebos* (inactive substances) in some medical experiments. The debate involved the use of placebo surgical procedures.

In clinical trials, one group of patients may be given an experimental drug while another group is given a placebo. The researchers can then determine whether the new drug has any benefits over the placebo. Most of the controversies involving placebos in the late 1990's focused on whether participants who received placebos were being denied a drug already known to be effective. But by 1998, the debate broadened to include the use of placebo surgery, a practice that had ended in the early 1970's but made a reappearance in some medical research in the 1990's.

In April 1999, a group of researchers from the University of Colorado in Denver reported that they conducted a surgical clinical trial in 1997 using placebo treatment on 40 people who had been diagnosed with Parkinson disease. Parkinson disease is a degenerative disorder characterized by the death of nerve cells in a part of the brain. These cells produce a chemical called dopamine, which controls body movements. As the cells die, the concentration of dopamine in the brain decreases, and the affected person develops tremors, muscle stiffness, and loss of balance.

As part of the 1997 study, neuro-surgeons drilled four tiny holes through the patients' foreheads into their skulls. Half of the patients received injections of fetal cells that researchers theorized might help repair the patients' deteriorated brain cells; the other half of the patients received no treatment.

Officials with the National Institutes of Health, which sponsored the Parkinson trials, argued that placebo surgery is the only way to obtain valid medical research information. Other physicians and medical ethicists also supported such surgery as a legitimate research tool. Studies underway in 1999 that used surgical placebos included additional research on Parkinson disease, cancer research, and the value of knee surgery for certain types of arthritis.

Other ethicists opposed the use of surgical placebos. They reasoned that placebo drugs (usually sugar pills) pose no health risk to patients. But surgical placebos use invasive procedures that may harm a patient.

As surgery is increasingly subjected to the kinds of rigorous evaluation that applied to new medicines in the 1990's, medical ethicists said that this sort of trial will undoubtedly create more controversy in the 2000's.

Jack Kevorkian convicted. A Michigan jury in March 1999 convicted 70-year-old Jack Kevorkian of second-degree murder for the 1998 physician-assisted suicide of a 52-year-old man. Kevorkian, a Michigan pathologist whose medical license had been revoked, claimed to have helped more than 130 people commit suicide since 1990. Kevorkian had been tried five times before the verdict on other charges of physician-assisted suicide. In four cases he was acquitted, and the fifth was declared a mistrial. The 1999 case was the first murder charge against Kevorkian.

In September 1998, Kevorkian videotaped the death of Thomas Youk, a Michigan man who suffered from amyotrophic lateral sclerosis, or Lou Gehrig's disease, after injecting him with a lethal dose of chemicals. In prior cases, Kevorkian had only provided the patients with a "suicide machine," a device containing lethal

doses of medicine that the patients operated themselves. Kevorkian later gave the videotape to the television news program "60 Minutes," which broadcast excerpts.

In April 1999, a Michigan judge sentenced Kevorkian to 10 to 25 years in prison with the possibility of parole after 6 years and 8 months. Kevorkian, who insisted on defending himself during the trial, appealed his conviction. He maintained that he had received poor legal advice.

Opponents of assisted suicide applauded Kevorkian's conviction. Others, including Youk's family, defended Kevorkian's methods and called his actions merciful.

Guilty verdict

A guard escorts Jack Kevorkian, *below,* a former pathologist, from a Michigan courtroom in March 1999 after a jury convicted him of second-degree murder. The jury convicted Kevorkian of the September 1998 physician-assisted suicide death of a man who had been diagnosed with amyotrophic lateral sclerosis, also known as Lou Gehrig's disease.

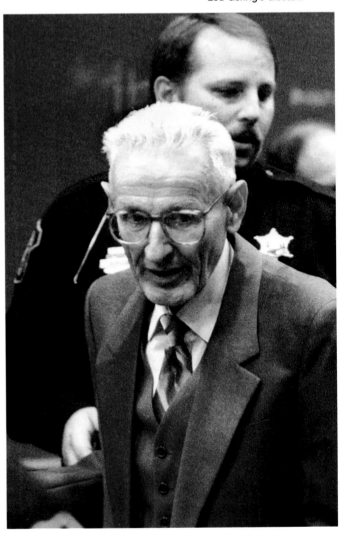

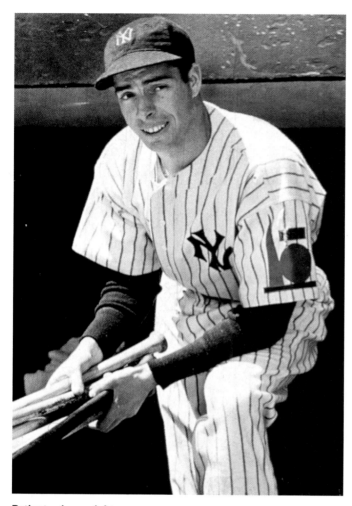

Patient privacy rights

Published reports about the health of baseball Hall-of-Famer Joe DiMaggio, *above,* sparked a debate in 1999 about medical privacy. DiMaggio, who died in March 1999 following a five-month battle with cancer, had criticized physicians for releasing details of his health to the media. Many physicians said that patient confidentiality was more important than the public's "need to know."

Oregon suicide law. Oregon health officials reported in a February 1999 edition of *The New England Journal of Medicine* that during 1998, 15 terminally ill people ended their lives by lethal doses of medication. The first report on Oregon's Death with Dignity Act was issued one year after Oregon became the first state to legalize physician-assisted suicide for terminally ill patients.

The report showed no evidence that any of the patients who died had suffered painful, lingering deaths—as some opponents of the law had feared. Rather, state health officials said that the law had been used by strong-willed patients who wanted to have control over the way in which they died.

According to the Oregon Health Division report, a total of 23 people received prescriptions for drugs to end their lives in 1998, but 6 died from their illnesses before taking the drugs, and 2 were still alive as of Jan. 1, 1999. Thirteen of the 15 patients who died suffered from cancer. The other two patients were suffering from heart or lung diseases, according to the report. The average age of those who died was 69.

The Death with Dignity Act was originally approved by Oregon voters in 1994, making it the first state to enact such a law. Oregon voters in 1997 turned back an effort to repeal the law.

HIV discrimination. The United States Supreme Court voted 5 to 4 on June 25, 1998, that people infected with human immunodeficiency virus (HIV), the virus that causes AIDS, are entitled to protection against discrimination. The case involved a Maine dentist, Randon Bragdon, who refused to treat a patient in 1994 because she was HIV-positive.

The patient filed a lawsuit claiming that she was entitled to treatment under the 1990 Americans with Disabilities Act (ADA), which protects people from discrimination in public accommodations, including medical offices. The dentist countersued, claiming that the woman was not protected under the ADA, since she did not have AIDS, did not have any symptoms, and therefore did not have a disability.

The Supreme Court, however, ruled that HIV is a physical impairment because the infection always impairs the immune system. They also ruled that HIV is a disability because it limits a person's ability to reproduce.

Some health care advocates in 1999 said that the Supreme Court's decision may have an effect far beyond HIV. They said that people with such conditions as diabetes, epilepsy, infertility, alcohol addiction, or some genetic trait that could be transmitted to their children may also be protected against discrimination. Other experts in 1999 predicted that whether such people have a disability under the ADA would be a matter for future court cases. • Carol Levine

Internet use may lead to depression and loneliness, according to a study conducted by researchers at Carnegie Mellon University and published in *The American Psychologist* in September 1998. The two-year study marked the first concentrated examination of the social and psychological effects of Internet use at home.

Researchers interviewed members of nearly 100 families before and after they obtained Internet access. Participants in the study who used the Internet for even a few hours a week experienced higher levels of depression and loneliness than those who used the network less often. Internet use itself appeared to cause a decline in psychological well-being.

In order to rule out the possibility that people who were more depressed and lonely might be more attracted to the Internet, researchers assessed the psychological health of the subjects at the beginning of the study. Participants filled out standard questionnaires used to assess psychological health. They were asked to agree or disagree with statements such as "I felt everything I did was an effort," "I enjoy life," and "I can find companionship when I want it." People who were lonelier and more depressed at the start of the study were no more attracted to the Internet than those who were happier and more socially engaged. But at the

end of the study, researchers found that one hour on the Internet per week led to a slight increase in depression and loneliness. Subjects who used the Internet for one hour per week also lost an average of 2.7 members of their social circle.

The results came as a surprise to the social scientists who designed the study, as well as to the corporations who helped fund it. The $1.5 million project, titled HomeNet, was financed by the National Science Foundation and such technology companies as Apple Computer, AT&T Research, Hewlett Packard, and Intel Corporation.

Some social scientists consider the Internet more stimulating than television and other media. It allows users to choose the information they want and use such active communication options as e-mail, chat rooms, and electronic bulletin board postings. But the HomeNet study suggested that the interactivity of the Internet does not necessarily make it more stimulating than television or other media.

HomeNet participants used social features of the Internet, such as e-mail and chat, rather than passive features such as reading or watching videos. But as people in the study spent more time online, they interacted less with family members and friends. Researchers hypothesized that although the Internet allows

- Internet use and depression
- Aging may bring happiness
- Effectiveness of antidepressants
- Body dysmorphic disorder
- Good news for working moms

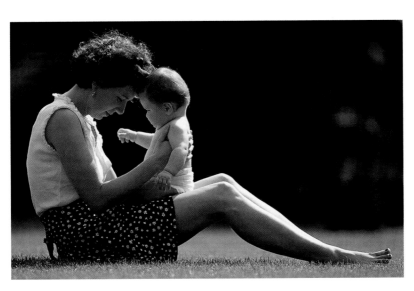

Don't worry, mom

A large, long-term study at the University of Connecticut in Storrs reported that children of working mothers suffer no lasting psychological damage. The research was published in the March 1999 issue of the journal *Developmental Psychology*.

users to get in touch with people from far away, it tends to build shallow relationships. These relationships lead people to feel less connected overall. HomeNet suggested that maintaining social ties with people who are physically nearby could lead to better psychological health. The researchers recommended that the Internet be used to foster more intense development of services that support communities and strong relationships.

Researchers predicted a national debate over how public policy on the Internet should evolve and how the technology might be shaped to enhance social health. Internet use was expanding rapidly in 1999. According to Nielsen Media Research, nearly 70 million adult Americans were online in the fall of 1998. As the use of the Internet continues to grow, it could become the tool that fragments American society—or the one that unifies it—according to researchers.

Aging may bring happiness. In a study of more than 2,700 adults from the ages of 25 to 74, Daniel Mroczek and Christian Kolarz of Fordham University found that older people tend to be happier. Their report appeared in the November 1998 issue of the *Journal of Personality and Social Psychology.*

The researchers asked study participants to respond to questions designed to assess happiness and life satisfaction. The older respondents in the study more frequently reported feeling positive emotions, such as cheerfulness, good spirits, and happiness, within the previous 30 days. Even when other factors that might affect the results—like education, health, marital status, personality, and stress—were taken into account, age had a stronger influence on the happiness level of the participants.

The link between increasing age and happiness was strongest for men. The men showed an increase in positive emotions and a decrease in negative emotions—feeling hopeless, nervous, sad, or worthless—as they grew older. Aging women seemed to have more positive emotions but just as many negative emotions as younger women.

Although the data seem to paint a clear picture of the relationship between happiness and aging, the results were difficult for researchers to interpret. The older participants may have been happier, or they may have been less willing to reveal unhappiness. It was also possible that, for a generation of people who lived through the Great Depression of the 1930's and at least one world war, "happiness" has a broader range of possibilities, said the researchers.

Dr. Laura Carstensen, a Stanford University psychologist, also found a positive relationship between age and well-being. She suggested that older

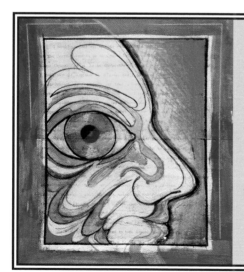

Problems of Internet "addiction"

People who spend an excessive amount of time on the Internet tend to have various psychiatric disorders, psychiatrist Nathan Shapira of the University of Cincinnati College of Medicine reported in May 1999. He studied 14 people whose "addiction" to the Internet resulted in such problems as broken relationships and job loss. Eleven of the people he studied had been diagnosed with manic-depression; seven had experienced an anxiety disorder; six had suffered from an eating disorder; seven had either lost control over their anger or were unable to curb their urge to shop; and eight had abused alcohol or some other substance. Internet addiction is not a recognized disorder. Shapira suggested that it should be. He suggested that it be called "Netomania" and categorized as an impulse control disorder.

people may feel happier because they have survived more of life's ups and downs and are more likely to find satisfaction in the moment.

Effectiveness of antidepressants. Prozac and other antidepressant drugs known together as selective serotonin reuptake inhibitors (SSRIs) are no better, and no worse, at treating people suffering from major depression than the older generation of tricyclic drugs such as Pamelor. These findings were released in March 1999 by the Agency for Health Care Policy and Research of the U.S. Department of Health and Human Services.

The study also found that depressed patients in clinical trials continue taking the older generation of drugs at about the same rate as they continue SSRIs, despite more severe side effects from the older tricyclics.

The number of prescriptions written for all antidepressants has been increasing at an average of about 20 percent annually since 1994. But most of the growth during that time is in the SSRIs, since the number of prescriptions of tricyclics has been relatively stable, rising from 43 million annually to 51 million in 1998.

According to IMS Health of Plymouth Meeting, Pennsylvania, a group that collects data on the pharmaceutical industry, the number of SSRI prescriptions written annually more than doubled between 1994 and 1998, rising from 35 million in 1994 to 77 million in 1998. Prescriptions for Prozac increased from 16 million to almost 25 million annually.

The researchers analyzed 315 clinical trials to evaluate the benefits and drawbacks of each category of antidepressants. They also reviewed the effects of three herbal treatments— kava, St. John's wort (hypericum), and valierina. The researchers found that the newer and older antidepressants were about equally effective in alleviating major depression, but the SSRIs also appeared to help prevent relapse in recovered patients. The researchers did not have enough evidence to draw any conclusions about the effectiveness of the three herbal treatments.

The report's recommendation that

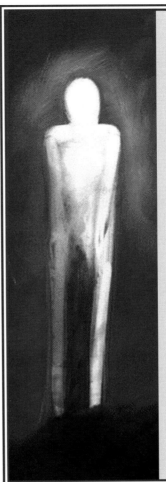

Types of anxiety disorders

Panic disorder—Repeated episodes of intense fear that strike often and without warning.

Obsessive-compulsive disorder—Repeated, unwanted thoughts or compulsive behaviors that seem impossible to stop or control.

Post-traumatic stress disorder—Persistent symptoms, such as nightmares and depression, that occur after experiencing a traumatic event.

Social phobia—An overwhelming and disabling fear of scrutiny, embarrassment, or humiliation in social situations, which leads to avoidance of many potentially pleasurable and meaningful activities.

Generalized anxiety disorder—Constant, exaggerated worrisome thoughts and tension about everyday routine events and activities.

Source: National Institute of Mental Health.

doctors reconsider the use of tricyclics could be significant, especially for primary care physicians who diagnose and treat a growing percentage of depression cases. Experts in depression say these family doctors have grown comfortable prescribing SSRIs in the late 1990's, but generally have shied away from the tricyclics because of their more disruptive side effects. The 1999 study could reduce this reluctance.

The study also has financial implications. The SSRIs generally cost significantly more than tricyclics, which can be purchased as generics since most patents have expired. The annual cost of SSRIs increased from $2.3 billion in 1994 to $5.6 billion in 1998, according to IMS Health.

Body dysmorphic disorder. Many teen-agers obsess about parts of their bodies, whether it be a case of acne or pointed elbows. But those who agonize unduly over appearance may have a mental disorder known as body dysmorphic disorder (BDD), a severe preoccupation with an imagined or slight defect in appearance. BDD was the subject of a report published in the April 1999 issue of the *Journal of the American Academy of Child & Adolescent Psychiatry.*

Researchers at Brown University compiled the report, which documented a study of 33 young people, ages 6 to 17, who had been diagnosed with BDD. The researchers found that almost all of the children had experienced disruption in school, jobs, and social life.

These children were most preoccupied with their skin and hair. Some subjects complained about short legs and gaps between their teeth. Five never left their homes because they were afraid to show the public their "defects"—all of which were either nonexistent or slight. Twenty-two subjects had thought about suicide, and seven had attempted it.

The severe preoccupation with bodily appearance is not just an adolescent disorder. BDD is also common in adults, affecting up to 1 in 50 people. Women in their 30's are most likely to have BDD. Yet, most cases begin before age 18.

Although no one knows what causes BDD, biological, psychological, and sociocultural factors may all play a part, according to the researchers.

Good news for working moms. A large, long-term study at the University of Connecticut in Storrs concluded that children of working mothers suffer no lasting psychological damage. The research was published in the journal *Developmental Psychology* in March 1999.

The researchers evaluated 6,000 children whose mothers worked during the first three years of their lives. They evaluated the youngsters for as long as 12 years, specifically in terms of the effects of their mothers' employment on behavioral problems, academic success, self-esteem, and language development. No significant differences were found among children of working mothers, when compared with children of stay-at-home moms. The researchers reported that certain issues, including the bond between mother and child and the quality of the day-care experience, are critical to the well-being of children of working mothers.

These findings contradicted previous research of the same children at a younger age, which had suggested that children with working mothers experienced social and developmental difficulties.

• Renée Despres

• Fiber and colon cancer

• Tomatoes and cancer prevention

• Mediterranean diet

• Nuts and heart disease

• An apple a day

Dietary fiber plays no role in reducing the risk of colon cancer, according to a January 1999 report by researchers at Brigham and Women's Hospital, Harvard Medical School, and the Harvard School of Public Health in Boston. The finding came as a surprise to many health care professionals. Although research about the role of fiber in preventing colon cancer has been inconclusive, most nutrition specialists had endorsed the high-fiber theory since the 1970's.

The 1999 report was part of an ongoing program called the Nurses' Health Study. In 1980, more than 88,000 female nurses ages 34 to 59 completed a dietary questionnaire. Follow-up research on the partici-

pants continued for 16 years. When the investigators compared women with the highest fiber intake (about 25 grams a day) with those eating the least amount of fiber (about 10 grams a day), they found that fiber had no beneficial effect on reducing the risk of colon cancer.

In an editorial that accompanied the report in the *New England Journal of Medicine,* cancer specialist John Potter of the Fred Hutchinson Cancer Research Center in Seattle discussed why investigating possible links between fiber and colon cancer is a complex task. He noted that measuring food intake by asking people to remember how often they ate a particular food during the past year can

Dietary supplement labels

The U.S. Food and Drug Administration introduced new labels in 1999 for dietary supplements to help consumers make informed decisions about these products. The standard label, *right*, must include the following information:

- Manufacturer's recommended serving size.

- The amount of each ingredient that is present at a significant level and its percentage of the recommended daily allowance.

- Any other ingredient regardless of how little is present.

When a supplement includes an herb, the label must use the common name of the plant and indicate what part of the plant was used. If the manufacturer uses a *proprietary* (patented) blend of herbs, the label can indicate the total amount of the blend rather than the amount of each herb.

Supplement Facts

Serving Size 1 Tablet

Amount Per Serving		% Daily Value for Children Under 4 Years of Age	% Daily Value for Adults and Children 4 or more Years of Age
Calories	5		
Total Carbohydrate	1 g	†	< 1%*
Sugars	1 g	†	†
Vitamin A	2500 IU	100%	50%
(50% as beta-carotene)			
Vitamin C	40 mg	100%	67%
Vitamin D	400 IU	100%	100%
Vitamin E	15 IU	150%	50%
Thiamin	1.1 mg	157%	73%
Riboflavin	1.2 mg	150%	71%
Niacin	14 mg	156%	70%
Vitamin B$_6$	1.1 mg	157%	55%
Folate	300 mcg	150%	75%
Vitamin B$_{12}$	5 mcg	167%	83%

* Percent Daily Values are based on a 2,000 calorie diet.
† Daily Value not established.

Other ingredients: Sucrose, sodium ascorbate, stearic acid, gelatin, maltodextrins, artificial flavors, dl-alpha tocopheryl acetate, niacinamide, magnesium stearate, Yellow 6, artificial colors, stearic acid, palmitic acid, pyridoxine hydrochloride, thiamin mononitrate, vitamin A acetate, beta-carotene, folic acid, cholecalciferol, and cyanocobalamin.

---

produce inaccurate results. He also suggested that scientists should be looking at specific kinds of fiber rather than lumping all fiber into one category. Scientists also speculate, Potter wrote, that the amount of sugar in the diet, rather then the lack of fiber, could be the important factor in colon cancer risk. Potter called for more research on how fiber functions in the body before scientists tried to settle the debate.

Also, in spite of the 1999 report, nutritionists noted that even if fiber plays no protective role in colon cancer, a high-fiber diet rich in fruits, vegetables, and grains is still a source of important vitamins and *phytochemicals* (plant chemicals). Previous studies found that high-fiber diets are linked with a lower risk of high-blood pressure, heart disease, and adult-onset diabetes. High-fiber diets may also help with weight control and improve intestinal health.

Tomatoes and cancer prevention. Eating tomatoes and tomato-based products reduces the chance of developing several kinds of cancers, according to a report in January by nutritionist Edward Giovannucci of the Harvard School of Public Health. After reviewing the findings of 72 studies, Giovannucci found that 35 studies demonstrated that tomato-based products were associated with a significantly reduced cancer risk.

The beneficial substance, according to numerous studies, is lycopene, the substance that creates the red color in tomatoes. Lycopene acts as an *antioxidant,* a compound that blocks the effects of a cellular process called *oxidation,* which occurs when oxygen combines with food molecules to produce energy for the body. A by-product of oxidation is a molecule called a *free radical,* which can cause cellular damage that leads to cancer. Antioxidants can interact with free radicals, rendering them harmless. Lycopene may also control the level of some hormones that can increase the chances of developing cancer.

Lycopene is present in fresh tomatoes, but when tomatoes are cooked, cells release even more of the substance. Nutritionists have noted that other red foods—watermelon, red grapefruit, and guava—are also good sources of lycopene.

Although the benefit of tomato-based products was most strongly associated with a reduced risk of prostate, lung, and stomach cancers, Giovannucci also noted a lower risk of pancreatic, colon, mouth, breast, and cervical cancers.

Mediterranean diet. In February 1999, researchers in France reported on the healthful benefits of a Mediterranean diet on the heart. The Lyon Diet Heart Study evaluated the effect of diet on people who had already suffered a heart attack.

Some of the participants in the study ate a typical Western European diet, with saturated fats from meats and dairy products and substances known as omega-6 polyunsaturated fatty acids, which are found in oils from corn, sunflower, and safflower. Other participants ate a Mediterranean diet, which includes less meat and more bread, root and green vegetables, fruits, beans, and moderate amounts of fish and red wine. Most of the oils used for cooking or seasoning were olive or canola oil. The researchers followed their subjects for 46 months and found that the Mediterranean diet group had a 50 to 70 percent lower risk of suffering a second heart attack.

The Lyon researchers concluded that the Mediterranean diet was healthier because of high levels of alpha-linolenic acid, which belongs to a group of substances known as omega-3 polyunsaturated fatty acids. Alpha-linolenic acid—found in olive oil, numerous seed oils, and nuts—is believed to reduce the irregular heart rhythms that can accompany heart attacks. It may also prevent inflammation in blood vessels, which can lead to *plaque* (fatty deposit) build-up.

The researchers also noted that olive oil is rich in monounsaturated fats, which are less susceptible than other fats to oxidation, a process that may play a role in plaque development. The Mediterranean diet also includes high levels of antioxidant vitamins such as vitamin C.

In an editorial accompanying the Lyon study, Alexander Leaf, a fatty acid specialist at Massachusetts General Hospital in Boston, wrote that an important message of the study is that individuals should lower their intake of omega-6 polyunsaturated fats and eat more foods rich in alpha-linolenic acid. Diets should include only small quantities of meat and be rich in fruits, grains, nuts, beans and vegetables, according to Leaf.

Nuts and heart disease. In November 1998, researchers participating in the Nurses' Health Study reported that women who ate 1 ounce (28 grams) of nuts at least five times a week cut their risk of heart disease by 35 percent compared with those who ate few nuts or none at all. The conclusions were based on the dietary questionnaires given to more than 86,000 women and follow-up research over a 14-year period.

Previous studies had suggested that eating nuts could help keep the heart healthy, and scientists have offered several theories to explain the theory.

Some experts believe the benefits arise because most of the fat in nuts is polyunsaturated or mono-unsaturated, both of which can lower cholesterol when substituted for saturated fat. Others cite the high levels of *arginine,* an amino acid that can help form the chemical nitric oxide, which relaxes blood vessels and may inhibit blood clotting. Nuts also contain heart-healthy minerals, including copper, magnesium, and potassium. Almonds are good sources of vitamin E,

What is a serving?

The United States government recommends daily servings from each of the major food groups for a healthy diet. The following chart clarifies what nutrition specialists consider a single serving of various foods.

Sources: U.S. Department of Agriculture, U.S. Department of Health and Human Services, and National Dairy Council.

Recommended Daily Allowance

Dairy
2–3 servings

Milk
1 cup

Yogurt
1 cup

Cheese
1 ½–2 ounces

Ice cream
½ cup

Meat
2–3 servings

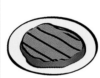
Lean meat
2–3 ounces

Lean poultry or fish
2–3 ounces

Egg
1

Peanut butter
2 tablespoons

Vegetables
3–5 servings

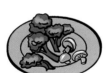
Cooked vegetable
½ cup

Raw vegetables
½ cup

Raw leafy vegetables
1 cup

Potato
1 medium

Fruit
2–4 servings

Juice
¾ cup

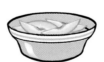
Canned fruit
½ cup

Apple, banana, orange, or pear
1 medium

Grapefruit
½

Grains
6–11 servings

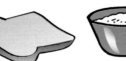
Bread
1 slice

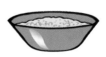
Pasta, rice, cooked cereal
½ cup

Cold cereal
1 ounce

Bagel
¼

Modified Food Pyramid for 70+ Adults

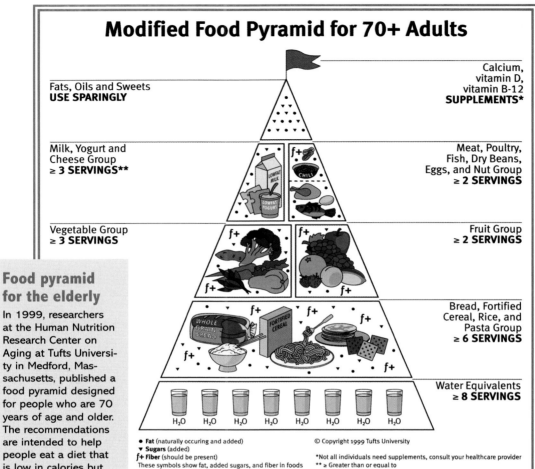

Fats, Oils and Sweets
USE SPARINGLY

Calcium,
vitamin D,
vitamin B-12
SUPPLEMENTS*

Milk, Yogurt and
Cheese Group
≥ 3 SERVINGS**

Meat, Poultry,
Fish, Dry Beans,
Eggs, and Nut Group
≥ 2 SERVINGS

Vegetable Group
≥ 3 SERVINGS

Fruit Group
≥ 2 SERVINGS

Bread, Fortified
Cereal, Rice, and
Pasta Group
≥ 6 SERVINGS

Water Equivalents
≥ 8 SERVINGS

H₂O H₂O H₂O H₂O H₂O H₂O H₂O H₂O

● **Fat** (naturally occuring and added) © Copyright 1999 Tufts University
▼ **Sugars** (added)
f+ **Fiber** (should be present)   *Not all individuals need supplements, consult your healthcare provider
These symbols show fat, added sugars, and fiber in foods   ** ≥ Greater than or equal to

Food pyramid for the elderly

In 1999, researchers at the Human Nutrition Research Center on Aging at Tufts University in Medford, Massachusetts, published a food pyramid designed for people who are 70 years of age and older. The recommendations are intended to help people eat a diet that is low in calories but high in important vitamins and minerals.

The pyramid emphasizes the need to drink plenty of water because older adults often do not feel thirsty even if they are not drinking adequate amounts of water. The flag at the top of the pyramid is a reminder that certain dietary supplements may be necessary and should be taken as recommended by a physician.

and walnuts provide alpha-linolenic acid. Nuts also contain phytochemicals that may act as antioxidants or as cholesterol-lowering agents.

The scientists noted, however, that it was too early to conclude that eating nuts can definitely lower the risk of heart disease. One nutritional drawback is that nuts are extremely high in calories and can easily lead to weight gain.

An apple a day. Scientists may have an explanation for the old adage that an apple a day keeps the doctor away. Researchers at the University of California at Davis reported in April 1999 that apple juice and fresh apples contain significant amounts of antioxidants. In a laboratory study,

they found that oxidation of the low-density lipoprotein (LDL) cholesterol—a process that leads to plaque development in blood vessels—dropped by as much as 34 percent depending on the brand of juice. Apples had a similar effect.

Other researchers had determined that apples and apple juice contain high concentrations of phytochemicals that may reduce the risk of heart disease, cancer, and other diseases. Some of these chemicals may prevent cancer-causing agents from damaging genes. Others boost enzymes that make cancer causing substances easier to excrete. Apples are also a good source of the soluble fiber pectin, which has been linked with a reduction in cholesterol.   ● Jeanine Barone

Both short and long intervals between pregnancies can lead to problems such as preterm birth and small babies according to two separate studies published in 1999. Low birth weight is one of the main causes of infant illnesses and death in the United States.

Researchers at the U.S. Centers for Disease Control and Prevention (CDC) in Atlanta, Georgia, and the School of Public Health at the University of North Carolina in Chapel Hill reported in May on their review of birth certificates in North Carolina from 1988 to 1994. They found an increased risk of preterm birth and small babies when the interval between the birth of one child and the beginning of another pregnancy was less than six months.

They also discovered that shorter intervals between pregnancies were more common among women who were in other high-risk categories —adolescents, unmarried women, those who smoked cigarettes, women who received prenatal care late in the pregnancy or not at all, and those who previously had small or preterm babies. However, even after taking these factors out of the equation, the researchers still observed a slightly increased risk with intervals of less

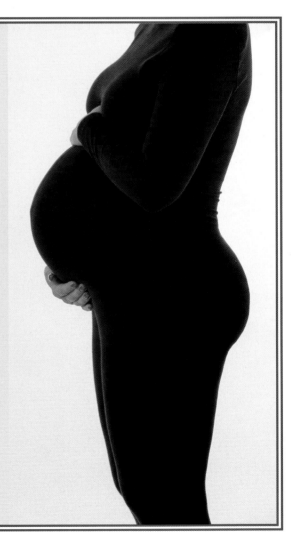

After a Cesarean delivery

The natural and generally safest way for a baby to be delivered is through the mother's vagina. Sometimes, however, a physician must perform a *Cesarean section,* a delivery through an incision in the mother's abdomen and *uterus* (the organ that contains the fetus), when a vaginal delivery is not possible or the life of the mother or baby is in danger. Like all surgical procedures, however, a Cesarean delivery presents risks.

An additional concern for a mother is whether she can deliver another baby vaginally after undergoing a Cesarean delivery. A vaginal birth after Cesarean delivery (VBAC) does have risks, particularly the dangers of rupturing the uterus along the surgical scar.

Several studies about VBAC's have been conducted since the 1970's, and opinions about their safety vary. In July 1999, the American College of Obstetricians and Gynecologists issued guidelines to help physicians decide when VBAC is an appropriate option. For example, the guidelines noted that some kinds of incisions have a greater risk for rupturing than others. The guidelines also directed physicians to counsel women about the benefits and risks of VBAC, a second Cesarean delivery, and an emergency Cesarean delivery after an unsuccessful attempt of VBAC.

than six months. They also noted that as the interval between pregnancies increased, the risks decreased.

The researchers did not determine why short intervals caused problems, but they noted other studies suggesting that during a short interval the mother does not have time to heal or build up nutritional reserves. These conditions may then disrupt the growth of the next baby.

Risks of long intervals. In a related study published in February 1999, researchers at the Utah Department of Health in Salt Lake City and the CDC reported similar findings linking low birth weight, preterm birth, and

small babies to short intervals and to intervals of more than 23 months.

The investigators reviewed information from birth certificates in Utah from 1989 to 1996. After taking into consideration other risk factors, they found problems occurred more often with intervals of less than 6 months and more than 23 months. The pregnancies with the lowest risks began between 18 to 23 months after the birth of a previous baby.

Pregnancy intervals of less than six months occurred more often in young women who were unmarried, used tobacco, did not have prenatal care, and previously had a baby that was small or born prematurely. Long intervals occurred more often in older women who were unmarried and used tobacco and alcohol during pregnancy.

Diabetes and pregnancy

Diabetes is a condition in which the body has trouble making or using *insulin,* the hormone that helps process sugar and starches. During pregnancy, a woman's body produces hormones that can affect how insulin works, causing *gestational* (pregnancy-related) diabetes. It can cause a baby to become overly large, posing problems during delivery as well as physical problems in the baby.

Women who are over 30 years old, overweight, or have a family history of diabetes are especially at risk for gestational diabetes. Physicians can prescribe exercise, diet, and medication to control diabetes during pregnancy.

Women who have diabetes before becoming pregnant are at risk for complications, such as miscarriages, birth defects, and breathing problems in the baby. If diabetes is under control before a pregnancy, the risks are not as great.

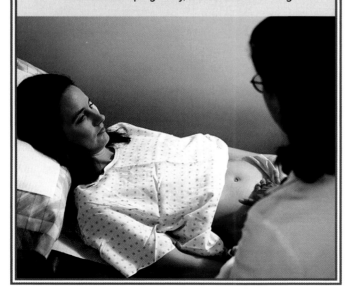

Stopping the spread of HIV. In October 1998, the Institute of Medicine in Washington, D.C., issued a document recommending that all pregnant women be tested for human immunodeficiency virus (HIV) to help reduce HIV infection from mother to baby during pregnancy and birth. The Institute of Medicine, which enlists members of the scientific and medical community to examine public health policies, assembled a panel of 19 experts representing federal agencies, professional organizations, and other groups involved in controlling the spread of HIV, the virus that causes AIDS.

Although there was progress in reducing the spread of HIV in the late 1990's, infected babies continued to be born to mothers who did not know they had HIV. Officials hoped that the new guidelines, "Reducing the Odds: Preventing Perinatal Transmission of HIV in the United States," would have a major impact on the care of pregnant women and the prevention of HIV infection in babies.

HIV can be passed from a mother to her baby during pregnancy or delivery. If HIV infection is detected during the pregnancy, the mother can begin treatment that can prevent the transmission of the virus to the baby. Without treatment, the risk of passing the infection from mother to baby is about 25 percent, but with treatment, the risk drops to 5 to 8 percent.

Previous federal guidelines did not include HIV testing as a routine part of prenatal examinations. Instead, physicians were advised to give patients pretest counseling about the risk of AIDS and the benefits of being tested for HIV. With this approach, many cases of HIV were missed. The counseling took time and special skills that were not necessarily available to women at all health care facilities. And many women chose not to be tested.

The special panel argued that by making HIV tests a part of routine prenatal care, some of the barriers to testing would be broken down. For example, physicians would not have to base a recommendation for tests on the patient's probable risk level for HIV infection. Also, making HIV tests routine may remove some of the stigmas that discourage women from getting tested. Nonetheless, the panel recommended that patients should still be allowed to refuse an HIV test.

The panelists also noted that many women who are infected with HIV do not receive health care unless they are pregnant. Having access to testing and prenatal care, the panel reasoned, would bring these women into the health care system.

Cesarean delivery and HIV. A *Cesarean birth,* the delivery of a baby through a surgical opening in the mother's abdomen, can lower the risk of passing HIV from mother to baby, according to research published in April 1999. The finding was reported by the International Perinatal HIV Group, a panel of experts from the U.S. National Institutes of Health, the CDC, and the American College of Obstetricians and Gynecologists, a medical specialty association based in Washington, D.C., that represents women's health physicians.

The researchers analyzed the results of 15 clinical studies. They found that Cesarean delivery that occurs before labor begins or before a pregnant woman's membranes rupture can lower the risk of passing HIV from mother to child, whether or not the woman received HIV treatment. The rupture of membranes, which usually occurs just before labor begins, is the breaking of the sac of fluid that surrounds the fetus.

The panel also noted that Cesarean delivery does not prevent HIV transmission after labor begins or membranes rupture. Therefore, the group recommended that a Cesarean be planned for week 38 of a pregnancy rather than at the normal time of delivery around week 40. The panel also proposed that women with HIV should still receive treatment to further reduce the risk of infecting the baby and that the mother should be able to decide whether to have a Cesarean delivery.   • Rebecca D. Rinehart

- Pulmonary hypertension
- New lung disease identified
- Loss of lung function due to asthma

In the May 4, 1999, issue of the *Annals of Internal Medicine,* a team of researchers led by cardiologist Vallerie V. McLaughlin of Rush Heart Institute Center for Pulmonary Heart Disease in Chicago reported on the success of a drug called prostacyclin to treat patients with a condition known as secondary pulmonary hypertension. Most people are familiar with general *hypertension* (high blood pressure) and its relationship to heart disease, kidney disease, and stroke. However, the public is less knowledgeable about pulmonary hypertension, which refers to the elevation of blood pressure in the *pulmonary arteries* (arteries that route blood through the lungs). Pulmonary hypertension is a progressive condition with a high mortality rate. In severe cases, patients may need to undergo a lung transplant. It can be classified as either *primary* (unknown cause) or *secondary* (associated with other factors, such as the use of the weight-loss drug dexfenfluramine).

Studies have shown that continuous infusion of prostacyclin, a *vasodilator* (drug that causes blood vessels to widen), can significantly reduce pulmonary hypertension and improve survival rates of patients with primary pulmonary hypertension. As a result, prostacyclin has become an approved therapy for primary pulmonary hypertension. Because treatments available in the late 1990's for secondary pulmonary hypertension were disappointing, McLaughlin's group set out to determine whether prostacyclin would offer similar benefits to patients with this condition.

The researchers treated 33 patients with secondary pulmonary hypertension with prostacyclin, which was delivered continuously by a portable infusion pump. The patients were followed for an average of about one year. Subsequent tests showed that prostacyclin significantly reduced blood pressure in the pulmonary arteries. The patients also had better *cardiac output* (output of oxygen-rich blood from the heart) and more endurance on a treadmill, and showed an improvement in their overall heart function. This outcome, the investigators said, should encourage further, more complete studies of prostacyclin therapy for patients with certain types of secondary pulmonary hypertension.

New lung disease identified. A new occupational lung disease resulting from exposure to nylon flocking was described in the Aug. 15, 1998, issue of the *Annals of Internal Medicine*. David Kern and colleagues from Memorial Hospital in Rhode Island and the University of Washington named this condition "flock worker's lung." The disorder is a chronic inflammation of the *interstitium* (tissue surrounding the air sacs in the lung) resulting from inhaling nylon flock. This substance is a short, fluffy nylon filament that is

glued onto fabric to make a velvety material often used in upholstery, carpeting, and plush toys.

The report described the diagnosis in 1996 of two workers at a Rhode Island nylon flocking plant who were found to have an unknown type of interstitial lung disease. The researchers evaluated other employees of the same plant and found eight cases of uncategorized lung disease that they classified as flock worker's lung. All of the workers reported coughs and breathing difficulty, and three also reported intermittent chest pain.

The authors suggested that a diagnosis of flock worker's lung depends on finding persistent respiratory symptoms, previous work in the flocking industry, and *histologic evidence* (having to do with the microscopic structure of tissues) of interstitial lung disease, and no better explanation for the abnormalities. The management of this condition includes removal of the patient from the flocking plant and, if necessary, the administration of corticosteroids to reduce inflammation. Doctors had previously not considered nylon to be a cause of lung disease. However, this report suggests that this disorder may be real and underdiagnosed.

Asthma and loss of lung function. In October 1998, researchers in Denmark reported on the long-term effects of asthma. The study used data

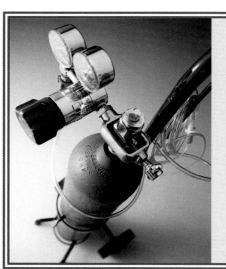

Emphysema facts

Emphysema is a lung disease which destroys the *alveoli* (air sacs) in the lungs. The alveoli lose their ability to release carbon dioxide into the airways so that it can be exhaled. The lungs stretch out and overinflate, resulting in labored breathing and a decrease in overall respiratory function. Although there is no cure for emphysema, physicians can help people with the disease live more comfortably by providing relief of symptoms and prevent the disease from worsening. Common treatment strategies include:

• Quitting smoking.

• Exercise, including breathing exercises to strengthen the muscles used in breathing.

• Drugs that relax and open air passages in the lungs.

• Lung transplant surgery.

from the Copenhagen City Heart Study, which was conducted from 1976 to 1994 to assess the health of adult citizens of Copenhagen, Denmark.

The investigators studied 17,506 subjects, 1,095 of whom had been diagnosed with asthma, over a 15-year period. Each subject completed a survey and underwent pulmonary function testing on three separate occasions over the observation period. Pulmonary function was assessed by measuring the amount of air that a person could forcibly expire in one second, adjusted for the individual's height. The investigators found that people with asthma lost significantly more lung function over the observation period compared with nonasthmatic people. This was true of both males and females, smokers and nonsmokers. In fact, asthmatic and nonasthmatic smokers both exhibited a loss of lung function over time, but the asthmatic smokers lost the most lung function of any group.

From these results the researchers concluded that asthma may lead to a loss of pulmonary function over time, no matter how severe the asthma or how good pulmonary function is at the time of diagnosis. This study also confirmed the harmful effects that cigarette smoking has on pulmonary function.　● Robert A. Balk

---

A national campaign to prevent and treat injuries could save thousands of lives and billions of dollars in health care costs each year, a study by the Institute of Medicine (IOM) concluded in October 1998. The IOM is an agency of the National Academy of Sciences, a nonprofit organization in Washington, D.C., that advises the United States government on science issues. According to the IOM, injuries were the leading cause of death and disability for people under age 35 in the United States in the mid-1990's.

The IOM campaign urged special emphasis on reducing firearm injuries. Gunshots caused about 36,000 deaths in 1995, second only to the 42,000 deaths caused by automobile accidents. But while highway fatalities decreased from the mid-1980's to the mid-1990's, firearm injuries and deaths increased, according to the IOM. The group recommended a national policy for preventing gunshot injuries that incorporates many elements of the successful campaign against motor vehicle injuries. The highway injury reduction effort involved new federal laws, improvements in road and vehicle design, and driver education programs.

The IOM suggested that firearm safety efforts begin with measures to keep guns away from children and adolescents, who account for many firearm injuries. The plan would involve reducing the access of children and teens to guns and ammunition, designing guns with safety features to prevent accidental or unauthorized use, and making community conditions safer for young people.

The study also recommended improvements in trauma care, more research on the most effective kinds of trauma care, and new local and state injury-prevention programs.

Accident trends. The National Safety Council (NSC), a nonprofit organization based in Itasca, Illinois, that works to prevent accidents, reported in September 1998 that the number of deaths from accident injuries decreased in 1997 for the first time since 1993. The 1997 accident death rate was 35 per 100,000 people, the second lowest since the NSC was formed in 1913. (The lowest rate was 34 per 100,000 people in 1992.) Accidents continued to be the fifth leading cause of death, after heart disease, cancer, stroke, and chronic lung disease.

The NSC estimated that 93,800 Americans died in accidents in 1997. About 60.5 million Americans sought medical care for accident injuries or had to limit their activities for at least one day because of an injury. Of those, 37.2 million people sought care in hospital emergency departments and 2.6 million people were hospitalized. The NSC estimated that the total cost of accident injuries in 1997 was $478.3 billion—$1,800 for each person in the country.

Fire deaths. Despite a decline in the number of people who die annually in fires in the United States, the fire-related death rate remains one of the highest of any industrialized country. The U.S. Fire Administration (USFA), part of the Federal Emergency Management Agency, reported that finding in December 1998. A study of 14 industrialized countries showed that only Hungary has a higher number of fire-related deaths per person than the United States.

The agency estimated, however, that about 3,400 Americans will die of fire-related causes in 1999, down from 6,215 in 1988. Experts credited the decline to greater use of home smoke detectors and sprinkler systems, the development of child-proof cigarette lighters, and a reduction in cigarette smoking, which is a major cause of home fires. These factors also contributed to a decline in the number of people injured in fires, as did the trend toward eating in restaurants. As fewer people cook at home, according to the USFA, fewer are injured in cooking-related fires.

Highway accidents. The number of Americans killed in motor vehicle accidents decreased in 1998 to its lowest level in four years, the National Highway Traffic Safety Administration (NHTSA) reported in May 1999. Traffic deaths fell to 41,480 in 1998, compared with 42,103 in 1997. Alcohol-related traffic deaths fell to a record low of 15,936, down from 16,189 in 1997.

The National Transportation Safety Board (NTSB) recommended new regulations in May 1999 to reduce fatigue among truck and bus drivers, railroad engineers, pilots, and ship captains. The NTSB said fatigue among people who operate powered vehicles causes thousands of accidents each year. Companies that operate trucking lines, for instance, should adopt new work rules that limit the number of hours truckers can drive without taking a sleep break.

The NTSB also urged that commercial motor vehicles install accident recorders similar to those required on commercial air planes. The recorders would keep track of a vehicle's speed, steering, and braking so that crash investigators could better determine the cause of fatal crashes.

Seat belt progress. The U. S. Department of Transportation (DOT) announced in February 1999 that about 70 percent of motor vehicle drivers and passengers used seat belts in November 1998, an increase from 65 percent in May 1998. The new figure reflected the highest percentage of seat belt use ever recorded in the United States. Based on the 1998 figure, DOT Secretary Rodney E. Slater predicted that 1,500 deaths and tens of thousands

A study reported by the U.S. National Highway Traffic Safety Administration in 1998 showed that older drivers—particularly men—are more likely to be involved in deadly auto accidents than teen-age drivers. However, driving is important for many elderly people to maintain their independence and self-sufficiency. Highway safety experts noted that new methods for assessing driving skills, education programs for older drivers, and the development of safer cars and better roads may help to bring down the fatality rate for older drivers.

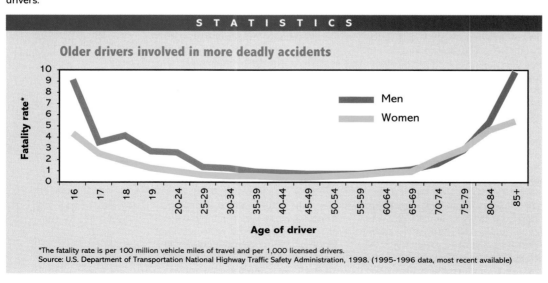

STATISTICS

Older drivers involved in more deadly accidents

*The fatality rate is per 100 million vehicle miles of travel and per 1,000 licensed drivers.
Source: U.S. Department of Transportation National Highway Traffic Safety Administration, 1998. (1995-1996 data, most recent available)

of injuries from motor vehicle accidents would be prevented in 1999. DOT further estimated that if 90 percent of U.S. drivers used seat belts, more than 5,500 deaths and 132,000 injuries would be prevented each year.

Slater reported that several factors had led to the record-high seat belt usage. They included stricter laws requiring drivers and occupants to use seat belts, tougher enforcement of seat belt laws by police, and public education campaigns that made people more aware that seat belts save lives. One such campaign, begun in March 1998, encouraged parents to act as seat belt role models for their children. Slater cited evidence that children often do not buckle their own seat belts when the driver in a vehicle rides unbuckled. The program placed a message to parents on more than 8,500 billboards along roads throughout the United States.

In addition, in February 1999, DOT announced new regulations that would make it easier for parents to properly anchor safety seats in cars and other motor vehicles. Under the new ruling, the rear seats of all cars beginning with the 2000 model year would be required to have standard anchoring points for child safety seats. Every new child seat would have attachment points that easily fit into the anchors. The system would reduce the risk of a child safety seat coming loose during an accident or emergency stop. DOT estimated that the new requirement could prevent up to 3,000 injuries each year.

Trunk release levers. Ford Motor Company announced in March 1999 that it would become the first automaker to install emergency trunk release levers as standard equipment in the trunks of its automobiles starting with the 2000 model year. Other car makers offered emergency release levers as an option at added cost.

The step came amid increased concern about children dying of heat exhaustion after being trapped in locked trunks. Eleven children died in such incidents in the summer of 1998. Many of the deaths occurred during hide-and-seek games in which children climbed into automobile

trunks without a parent's knowledge and locked the lid. Safety experts also urged parents to prevent trunk locking incidents by teaching children not to play inside or around cars.

Ford's trunk-release system consists of a T-shaped handle attached to a cable that controls the luggage compartment latch. The fluorescent handle glows in the dark, making it visible to individuals trapped in a trunk. Pulling the handle in any direction unlatches the trunk. Safety experts noted that the emergency levers would also allow victims of carjackings and other crimes to escape.

Falling TV's. Televisions placed on wobbly furniture pose a threat of serious injury or death to children, a

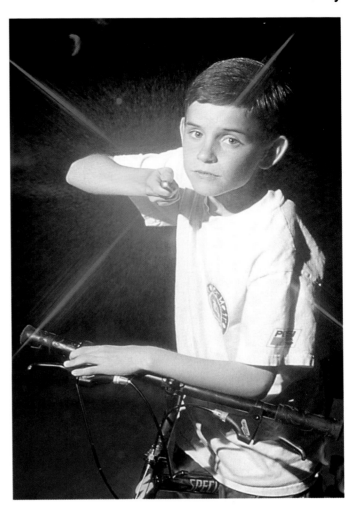

Laser pointer hazards
Laser pointers pose a wide range of hazards, according to a statement issued by the American Optometric Association in April 1999. Eye care specialists warned that flashing the pointer at someone's eye could cause temporary visual impairment. Prolonged contact could result in permanent eye damage.

study at the University of Alabama in Birmingham reported in September 1998. Researchers analyzed 73 reports of children, aged newborn to 11 years, injured or killed by falling television sets.

The researchers found that big-screen television sets placed on wobbly stands, tables, or dressers were the most dangerous. The large, top-heavy TV's were liable to tip over and cause a severe head injury to young children. Children were usually injured while trying to reach and adjust television controls. Three-year-old toddlers were at greatest risk. The researchers recommended that big-screen TV's be placed on secure supports in a child-safe location.

Biking accidents. About half of all bicycle riders wore helmets regularly in 1998, an increase from only 18 percent in 1991, according to a U.S. Consumer Product Safety Commission (CPSC) study released in April 1999. But the CPSC also found that 43 percent of the estimated 80.6 million bike riders never wear helmets and 7 percent wear them less than half the time.

CPSC chairman Ann Brown said biking accidents kill 900 people each year and cause 567,000 injuries serious enough to require treatment in a hospital emergency department. Wearing a bike helmet can reduce the

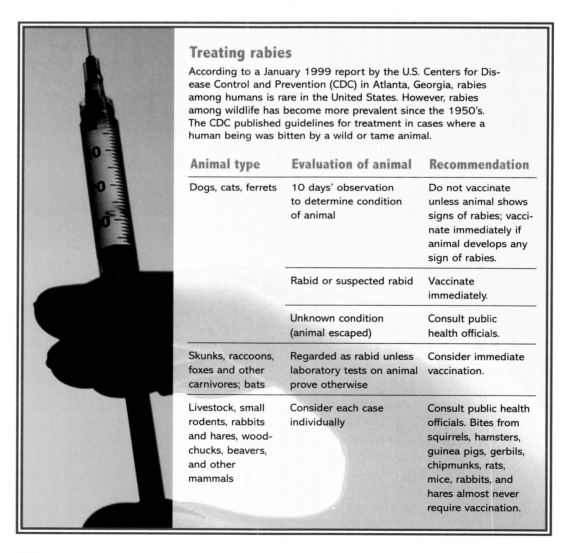

Treating rabies

According to a January 1999 report by the U.S. Centers for Disease Control and Prevention (CDC) in Atlanta, Georgia, rabies among humans is rare in the United States. However, rabies among wildlife has become more prevalent since the 1950's. The CDC published guidelines for treatment in cases where a human being was bitten by a wild or tame animal.

Animal type	Evaluation of animal	Recommendation
Dogs, cats, ferrets	10 days' observation to determine condition of animal	Do not vaccinate unless animal shows signs of rabies; vaccinate immediately if animal develops any sign of rabies.
	Rabid or suspected rabid	Vaccinate immediately.
	Unknown condition (animal escaped)	Consult public health officials.
Skunks, raccoons, foxes and other carnivores; bats	Regarded as rabid unless laboratory tests on animal prove otherwise	Consider immediate vaccination.
Livestock, small rodents, rabbits and hares, woodchucks, beavers, and other mammals	Consider each case individually	Consult public health officials. Bites from squirrels, hamsters, guinea pigs, gerbils, chipmunks, rats, mice, rabbits, and hares almost never require vaccination.

risk of a head injury, the most common serious biking injury, by 85 percent, she added.

The study found that 69 percent of children under age 16 wear a helmet regularly while riding a bike, and 38 percent of adult riders do so. About 70 percent of bikers who wore helmets said they did so because a parent or spouse insisted on it, and about 44 percent cited local or state laws as their main reason for using a helmet. Bikers reported several reasons for not wearing a helmet. These included taking a short ride, forgetting to wear or buy one, and feeling that helmets are uncomfortable.

Teen-safe cars. Parents choosing a car for teen-age drivers should be made aware that big, heavy vehicles are the safest, researchers at the Harborview Injury Prevention and Research Center in Seattle reported in November 1998. Safety considerations are especially important for teens, they noted, because young drivers are 4 times more likely than older drivers to be involved in a crash.

Researchers asked 331 parents of teen-agers attending a driver education course to rank the safety value of various automobile features. Only 40 percent of the parents ranked vehicle size and weight as important or very important in deciding which family-owned car the teen-ager would be allowed to drive. Most based the deci-

sion on whether a car had automatic transmission, a good repair record, and low gas mileage.

The researchers said knowledge about the safety advantages of large, heavy vehicles is especially important for the 20 percent of families who buy another vehicle when a teen-ager begins driving. By selecting a big vehicle, parents may reduce the risk of a serious injury or fatality.

Workplace safety. The National Institute for Occupational Safety and Health (NIOSH) recommended in September 1998 that employers take additional steps to protect workers from job-related hearing loss. NIOSH is an agency of the U. S. Department of Health and Human Services that works to prevent workplace illnesses and injuries.

NIOSH estimated that 30 million U.S. workers are exposed to hazardous levels of noise that may damage hearing. The agency suggested that a worker's average noise exposure for an 8-hour day should not exceed 85 decibels—the equivalent level of sound experienced approximately 3 feet (1 meter) from an electric drill as it is going through a piece of wood. NIOSH urged employers to monitor workers more often to prevent excess noise exposure and use better ways of identifying and protecting workers who are experiencing job-related hearing loss. • **Michael Woods**

Gonorrhea and syphilis remain serious problems in several cities in the United States, though they have been nearly wiped out nationwide, according to a study released in December 1998. The U.S. Centers for Disease Control and Prevention (CDC) in Atlanta, Georgia, ranked the 20 cities with the highest rates for both of these sexually transmitted diseases (STD's). Baltimore, Maryland, led the United States in both gonorrhea and syphilis infection rates.

Gonorrhea and syphilis infections have been reduced to all-time lows in the United States. But high rates for both diseases are still found in several cities, the CDC's numbers showed. In Baltimore, 991 of every 100,000

people were infected with gonorrhea in 1997, the CDC said. Nationwide, the rate of infection was 123 per 100,000 people. And though syphilis infects just 3 people per 100,000 nationwide, the rate was 99 per 100,000 in Baltimore.

Fourteen other cities appeared on both lists: Washington, D.C; St. Louis, Missouri; Detroit, Michigan; Richmond, Virginia; Newark, New Jersey; Norfolk, Virginia; New Orleans, Louisiana; Memphis, Tennessee; Oklahoma City, Oklahoma; Birmingham, Alabama; Nashville, Tennessee; and Milwaukee, Wisconsin.

Gonorrhea causes painful, burning urination and a puslike discharge from the urethra or vagina. Syphilis

Sexually Transmitted Diseases

- STD's on the rise in cities
- Chlamydia rates in teens
- Teens more cautious about sex
- Teens underestimate STD risk

Sexually Transmitted Diseases

The number of new sexually transmitted disease cases each year has risen to 15.3 million, 3.3 million more than health experts previously thought, according to a report released by the Kaiser Family Foundation in December 1998. The number is higher because doctors now have better ways of detecting sexually transmitted diseases that cause no noticeable symptoms.

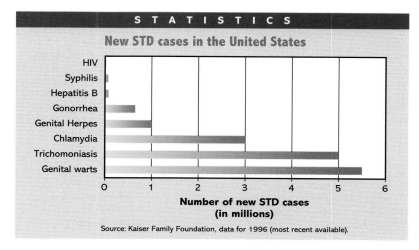

STATISTICS

New STD cases in the United States

Number of new STD cases
(in millions)

Source: Kaiser Family Foundation, data for 1996 (most recent available).

causes rashes and lesions and, if left untreated, can lead to the degeneration of bone, heart, and nerve tissue.

The CDC also listed states that reported the highest levels of chlamydia among young women. Chlamydia, a parasite that can cause infertility and tubal pregnancies, was in 1999 the most widely reported infectious disease. It infects about 4 million Americans each year, the CDC said.

Looking at chlamydia infections among 15- to 24-year-old women tested in family planning clinics, the CDC found that infections reached 11 percent in Alabama, Arkansas, Mississippi, North Carolina, and South Carolina.

Chlamydia rates in teens. The sexually transmitted disease chlamydia has become so common among teenage girls in some parts of the United States that in 1998, doctors began to recommend that sexually active girls be tested for the disease twice a year, instead of once a year, as called for by national medical guidelines.

The call for testing twice a year, by researchers at Johns Hopkins University, was based in part on their study of 3,202 girls ages 12 to 19 in Baltimore who went to clinics for birth control, pregnancy, or sexually transmitted diseases. The highest rate of infection, 27.5 percent, occurred in 14-year-olds, but older girls also had a high rate, about 20 percent.

The study found that among the girls who tested positive and were

treated, more than half became infected again within six to seven months.

According to the CDC, the infection and its complications cost the United States $2.4 billion a year. In October 1998, researchers with the sexually transmitted diseases branch of the National Institute of Allergy and Infectious Diseases reported that the incidence of the disease did not appear to be rising, but that increased testing had revealed disturbingly high rates of infection.

Teens more cautious about sex. The percentage of high school students who reported having engaged in sexual intercourse declined from 1991 to 1997, according to a survey released in September 1998 by the CDC. The findings of the ongoing survey of teen-age risk behavior were in keeping with other studies that suggested U.S. youth were growing more cautious about sex.

A majority of students surveyed said they had not had sexual intercourse, the first time in the 1990's that abstainers were in the majority. The findings further showed that teaching teen-agers about safe sex had not resulted in more promiscuity.

The CDC analyzed data from a sample of high school students every two years from 1991 through 1997. In the 1997 survey, completed by 16,262 students, 48.4 percent said they were sexually experienced compared with 54.1 percent in 1991.

Asked if they had ever had sexual intercourse, 52 percent of those surveyed in 1997 said no, compared with 46 percent in 1991. Asked if they used a condom the last time they had sex, 57 percent of students said yes, compared with 46 percent in 1991. Sixteen percent of students said they had sex with four or more partners, down from 19 percent in 1991.

The trend toward abstinence was in sharp contrast to the 1970's and 1980's, when sexual activity ballooned among teen-agers. Sexual activity among girls 15 to 19 jumped to 57 percent in 1988 from 29 percent in 1970, according to the CDC.

Teens underestimate STD risk.
Sexually active teen-agers in the United States underestimate their chances of getting a sexually transmitted disease other than AIDS, according to a survey released in March 1999. The random telephone survey of 400 teens ages 15 to 17 was conducted by the Henry J. Kaiser Family Foundation.

Fully three-quarters of the teens surveyed underestimated the incidence of sexually transmitted disease. That attitude may put them at greater risk for infection, said the survey authors, who noted that about 4 million teens contract a sexually transmitted disease every year. • Laura Bushie

---

Sunscreen may foster the development of moles, probably by encouraging children to remain longer in the sun, a study released in March 1999 found. The number of moles a person has is a strong predictor of the lifetime risk of melanoma, a deadly form of skin cancer. The incidence of melanoma increased dramatically among white populations around the world in the 1990's.

Researchers from the European Institute of Oncology in Milan, Italy, studied 631 children from four countries with a variety of climates. Doctors examined the children for moles, and parents described the children's history of sun exposure, frequency of sunburns, and their use of sunscreen and protective clothing.

The scientists reported that the children who regularly used sunscreen had the highest risk of developing moles. The data took into account a child's sensitivity to sun, eye color, and other characteristics. Sunburns were not associated with the appearance of moles.

Children who used the most sunscreen, and had the highest number of moles, also had spent the longest time in the sun, according to the researchers. Most of their exposure occurred during vacation.

Skin

- Sunscreen and moles
- Skin cancer risks
- Skin and the psyche
- Depression and cosmetic surgery
- Nickel allergies on the rise

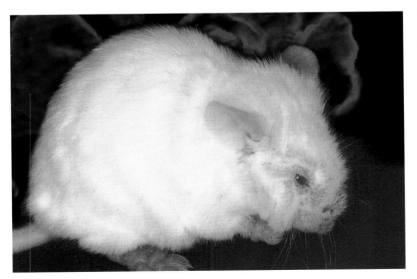

Furry mice advance research on baldness
University of Chicago researchers reported in November 1998 that they had used genetic-engineering techniques to produce mice with extra-furry coats, *left*. The researchers produced the mice by giving them a gene that codes for a protein important to the development of hair follicles. Additional research on the gene might lead to a treatment for baldness or to methods for stopping abnormal hair growth.

Skin cancer risks. A history of non-melanoma skin cancer may raise the risk of dying from another type of cancer, researchers at Emory University and the U.S. Centers for Disease Control and Prevention in Atlanta, Georgia reported. The findings, published in a September 1998 issue of the *Journal of the American Medical Association*, focused on 12-year outcomes of more than 1 million adults.

The authors found that subjects with a history of nonmelanoma skin cancer, which is slow growing and easy to treat, had a 20 percent to 30 percent higher incidence of other cancers than those without such histories. For example, men and women with previous nonmelanoma tumors faced increased risk of lung cancer, non-Hodgkin's lymphoma, and subsequent melanoma. Men showed increased risk for cancer of the testes, prostate, salivary glands, and bladder, and for leukemia. Women had a higher risk for breast cancer.

Skin and the psyche. For people who have chronic skin conditions that are resistant to treatment, the psychological impact of a traumatic event may partly explain the symptoms, according to a study released in November 1998.

Researchers at Kent and Canterbury Hospital in Canterbury, England, studied 64 people with chronic skin problems. They discovered that 44 of these people had experienced a major life event, such as a serious illness or death of a loved one, just before or at about the same time that their skin problems began. The researchers met with each person and encouraged them to discuss the stressful or traumatic episode.

Over the course of the five-year study, symptoms of the skin conditions, including psoriasis and eczema, either improved or disappeared in 40 of the 60 people. The researchers offered a few possible explanations for the improvement. First, having a chance to talk about a traumatic or stressful event may have helped some people deal with their past. In addition, having someone pay attention to their problems also may have provided a boost to the patients.

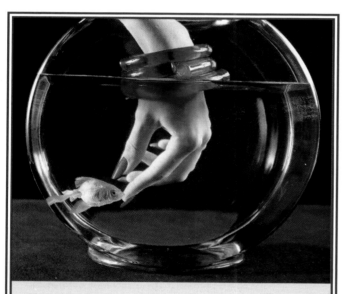

Fish tank-itis

Physicians warn that fish owners should keep their hands out of the fish tank. Fish tank granuloma, an infection caused by bacteria in tank water, can affect tropical fish keepers who have cuts on their arms and hands. The infection can develop into a painful red lesion.

- **Symptoms:** Fish tank granuloma causes swelling and red, raised lumps that form a line on the infected skin. It is often misdiagnosed as warts or an injury.

- **Prevention:** Physicians recommend wearing rubber gloves and using a long-handled tool when cleaning the fish tank.

- **Treatment:** Fish tank granuloma is treated with antibiotics.

Source: Mayo Clinic.

Depression and cosmetic surgery. People who request cosmetic surgery on their faces are more likely to be suffering from mental health disorders, according to a study released in April 1999. The study revealed that half of those individuals seeking cosmetic alterations to their nose suffer from clinical depression and nearly a third have attempted suicide.

The study's author, Henri Gaboriau of the Department of Otolaryngology at Tulane University in New Orleans, Louisiana, said the study was intended to help doctors decide in which cases plastic surgery was appropriate. The finding showed that there was a high level of conflict between

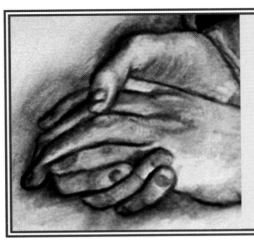

Fingernail facts

- Fingernails form under the cuticle and grow out toward the tip of the finger, so cuticle injuries can change the look of a fingernail. It takes about six months for a nail to grow from cuticle to fingertip.

- Nail ridges are seldom dangerous, but they can be a sign of serious illness. Longitudinal ridges are typically hereditary. Horizontal ridges are usually the result of small injuries or of a harsh manicure.

- Nail growth varies from person to person and from finger to finger. Thumb and pinky nails grow more slowly than those on the middle and index fingers. Men's nails grow a little faster than women's.

surgeons and patients suffering personality disorders after surgery, and that these patients were more likely to seek legal redress.

The researchers reviewed a wide range of studies of patients who had undergone plastic surgery. They found that more than two-thirds of all cosmetic surgery was carried out on the face or neck and that nearly a third of these operations were on the nose. Assessments of the patients prior to their operations showed that 50 percent were clinically depressed, 70 percent suffered from anxiety, 20 percent had problems with substance abuse, and nearly 30 percent had attempted suicide.

Nickel allergies on the rise. Doctors in 1999 announced a steep rise in nickel allergies in the United States. In 1990, 10.5 percent of Americans were sensitive to nickel, but by 1999 the figure rose to 14.3 percent.

Nickel allergies are a form of contact dermatitis, a condition that occurs when a substance to which a person is allergic rubs against the skin. Several medical studies in 1998 and 1999 suggested that the increase in nickel allergies may be linked to body piercing, which has exposed more people's skin to jewelry made of nickel. Newly pierced skin is the most likely to react to nickel.

• Laura Bushie

Smoking

Approximately 64 million people—or about 3 out of every 10 Americans over the age of 12—were tobacco smokers in 1997. That finding was reported in August 1998 as part of the annual National Household Survey on Drug Abuse. The survey was conducted by the United States Health and Human Services Department's Substance Abuse and Mental Health Services Administration (SAMHSA). A person was considered a current smoker if they had smoked in the month prior to the survey.

The SAMHSA report also showed that 6.4 million people—about 3 percent of Americans over age 12—reported using smokeless tobacco. In addition, men had a slightly higher smoking rate than women, and adults who had not completed high school were more likely to smoke than college graduates.

Cigarettes and students. Researchers at the University of Michigan in Ann Arbor reported in December 1998 that smoking rates among students aged 13 to 18 declined for the first time after having increased for several years. That finding was part of the 1998 Monitoring the Future Study, which has tracked drug use by American high school students since 1975 and tracked 8th and 10th grade students since 1991. The study was sponsored by the National Institute on Drug Abuse.

The researchers surveyed approximately 50,000 students in 422 schools nationwide. They reported that the number of 8th graders who had ever smoked declined 1.9 percent, to 19.1 percent, between 1996 and 1998. The survey showed that the number of 10th graders who had ever smoked dropped 2.8 percent, to 27.6 percent, in the same period. Between 1997 and 1998, the number of 12th graders who had smoked fell 1.4 percent, to 35.1 percent.

The researchers theorized that the decline was linked to educational efforts in the 1990's about the adverse health consequences of smoking and numerous lawsuits against the tobacco industry. Despite the decreases in young cigarette smokers, the product's accessibility remained high. According to the study, 73.6 percent of 8th graders and 88.1 percent of 10th graders surveyed in 1998 responded that it was easy to obtain cigarettes, a 2 percent decline from the 1997 survey.

Smoking and college. Cigarette smoking among college students rose between 1993 and 1997, according to a Harvard School of Public Health Study published in November 1998. The researchers in 1997 surveyed 14,521 students in 116 colleges in the United States about their smoking habits. They then compared the results with a survey of 15,103 students conducted in 1993. The researchers found that 22.3 percent of students were current smokers in 1993, compared with 28.5 percent in 1997.

The researchers attributed the increase in part to the general rise in adolescent smoking in the early 1990's. Twenty-eight percent of the smokers surveyed in 1997 reported having started smoking regularly while in college. Half of the smokers reported trying to quit at least once in the past year.

Risks of cigar smoking. Men who regularly smoke cigars may be at a greater risk for heart disease and certain cancers, according to a study published in June 1999 by researchers at Kaiser Permanente Medical Care Program in Oakland, California. Researchers examined the medical histories of 17,774 men—1,546 of whom smoked only cigars on a regular basis—from 1971 to 1995.

According to the study, men who smoked fewer than five cigars each day had a 34 percent higher risk of throat and oral cancers and a 57 percent increased risk of lung cancer than those men who were nonsmokers. Men who smoked five or more cigars daily had a 620 percent greater risk of throat and oral cancers and a 220 percent greater risk of lung cancer. There was also an increased risk—56 percent—of heart disease among men who were cigar smokers.

Cigarette companies reach settlement

In November 1998, the attorneys general of 46 states agreed to settle their lawsuit against the major producers of the tobacco industry—R. J. Reynolds Tobacco, Philip Morris Companies, Lorillard Tobacco Company, and Brown & Williamson Tobacco Corporation. The 46 states had sued the cigarette manufacturers to recover Medicaid money spent treating diseases related to smoking. Under the agreement, the tobacco manufacturers were to pay $206 billion to the states over 25 years. The only states excluded from this settlement were Florida, Minnesota, Mississippi, and Texas, which resolved their individual lawsuits before the comprehensive deal.

In April 1999, cigarette ads were removed from more than 4,100 cigarette billboards across the United States as part of the tobacco settlement. Cigarette makers agreed to pay rent on the billboards until the end of 1999, at a cost of more than $100 million. Antismoking messages were put up on the billboards for the duration of the lease.

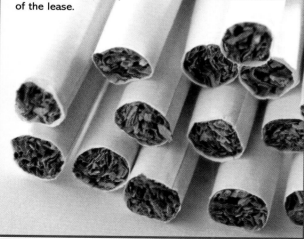

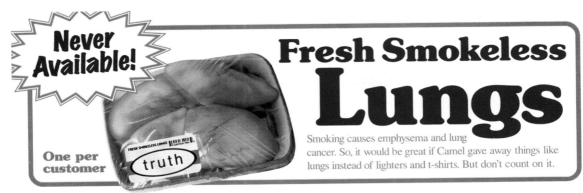

Never Available!

One per customer

truth

Fresh Smokeless Lungs

Smoking causes emphysema and lung cancer. So, it would be great if Camel gave away things like lungs instead of lighters and t-shirts. But don't count on it.

In response to such studies, U.S. Surgeon General David Satcher in 1999 called for greater restrictions on the sale of cigars, an increase of the federal tax on cigars, more warning labels on cigar products and advertisements, and greater information on the harmful effects of secondhand cigar smoke.

A Government Printing Office report on tobacco, published in April 1999, found that cigar sales in the United States increased 50 percent between 1993 and 1998, reversing a decline in cigar usage that had existed since the 1970's. The report stated that 3.75 billion cigars were sold in 1998, a 75 percent increase from 1993. Young and middle-aged men accounted for the greatest number of new cigar smokers, though the number of women and teen-agers also increased.

IRS and insurance coverage. The Internal Revenue Service (IRS) in June 1999 announced that it would allow smokers to claim some out-of-pocket costs of treatment for addiction to nicotine as a tax deduction. The decision would not allow smokers to claim nonprescription medications, such as nicotine patches or nicotine chewing gum, as deductions unless such treatments were obtained with a prescription. Also, only medical expenses reaching at least 7.5 percent of a taxpayer's adjusted gross income will qualify as a deduction. Possible deductions included medical bills, and stop-smoking programs offered by hospitals or other treatment facilities that are not reimbursed by an employer or insurance plan.

The decision to allow tax deductions for smokers trying to quit reversed a 1979 decision that excluded nicotine addiction from deductions that had been allowed for the treatment of alcoholism and drug addiction. The IRS justified its reversal by citing Surgeon General reports issued since 1988 that documented the addictiveness of nicotine and the negative health effects of smoking.

The tax deductions may encourage private insurers to include smoking cessation programs in their coverage. Such insurance coverage is relatively uncommon, though a few studies have shown that comprehensive coverage leads to a greater rate of smoking cessation.

For example, a study published in September 1998 showed that four times as many people would use smoking cessation services—such as nicotine gum or behavior modification techniques—under full coverage than any level of reduced coverage. Furthermore, the study, by researchers at the Group Health Cooperative of Puget Sound and the University of Washington, both in Seattle, found that almost twice as many smokers would quit under a full coverage program than any other coverage plan.

The study also reported that the increase in cost to health plans would be relatively inexpensive—between $2.64 and $4.03 per person annually. Health care professionals said this cost was significantly lower than smoking-related medical expenses for the treatment of hypertension or heart disease.   • David Lewis

Antitobacco campaign Health officials credited an aggressive antismoking advertising campaign, *above,* in Florida with reducing smoking among teen-agers. The U.S. Centers for Disease Control and Prevention, reported in April 1999 that smoking by middle- and high-school students in Florida decreased in 1998. A survey of 21,000 students showed the number of middle-school students who smoked dropped 3.5 percent, while high school smokers decreased by 2 percent.

- More patients can benefit from stroke treatments
- Carotid artery testing
- Potassium lowers stroke risk

The time frame for treating stroke patients with clot-busting drugs can be doubled, from three hours to six hours, without significantly raising the risk of hemorrhage, according to findings from a study of the enzyme prourokinase. The study, carried out by the Cleveland Clinic in Ohio, was presented at the February 1999 American Heart Association stroke conference.

Since 1995, most stroke victims have been eligible for treatment with another clot-dissolving drug, tissue plasminogen activator (TPA). Many physicians thought TPA would revolutionize the field, but its usefulness

proved limited because it is effective only if administered within three hours of the stroke's onset.

Stroke victims sometimes wait days instead of hours to report symptoms. The Cleveland Clinic researchers found that only 19 percent of patients reach hospitals within three hours, and they estimated that only 5 percent of stroke victims in the United States were receiving treatment.

The Cleveland Clinic studied only patients with one of the most serious forms of stroke, blockage of the middle cerebral artery. Unlike TPA, which is administered intravenously, prourokinase is injected directly into

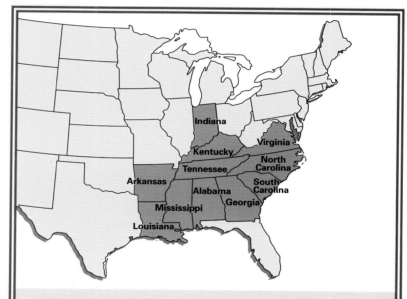

Mapping stroke risk

What do the southeastern states stretching from Louisiana to North Carolina have in common? They are part of the "stroke belt." Residents of this area are more likely to have a fatal stroke than other Americans. Some medical experts place 8 states in the stroke belt, while others identify 11 at-risk states. Most experts exclude Florida. An area covering the coastal plains of North Carolina, South Carolina, and Georgia is called the "stroke buckle" because the stroke death rate there is about twice as high as in the rest of the country.

The high stroke rates in the stroke belt appear to have multiple causes. A stroke belt resident is more likely than the average American to be overweight. Obesity also increases the risk of diabetes, which increases the risk of stroke. Diet is another factor. Southerners as a group tend to eat more fried food and less fruit than other Americans.

Source: The American Heart Association.

the artery in the brain close to the site of the clot. The presence of the clot causes the prourokinase to break down into the enzyme urokinase, which dissolves the obstruction.

The study showed that 67 percent of the blocked arteries were cleared by the prourokinase. Furthermore, 40 percent of those treated were judged to have little or no impairment three months after their stroke compared with 25 percent of the patients who did not receive the treatment. The results suggested that more patients could benefit from treatments that could reduce or reverse the effects of strokes as they are happening.

Carotid artery testing. Thickening of the carotid artery walls in the neck is a more powerful predictor of heart attack or stroke in elderly people than even high cholesterol or high blood pressure, according to a study released in January 1999 took ultrasound measurements of the two carotid arteries in people over age 65 with no history of heart disease or stroke-related illness. The two carotid arteries carry blood from the heart to the brain. Ultrasound can detect cumulative damage to the blood vessels before the patient experiences any symptoms, according to researchers from Tufts-New England Medical Center in Boston.

The study looked at 4,476 Medicare beneficiaries with an average

age of 72. None had a history of heart attacks or stroke. An average of six years later, the 20 percent with the thickest artery walls had more than three times the risk of a heart attack or stroke than the 20 percent with the thinnest artery walls, even after risk factors such as high cholesterol were taken into account.

Potassium lowers stroke risk. A study released in September 1998 that tracked nearly 44,000 men over eight years found that those whose diets included large amounts of potassium had one-third fewer strokes than those whose diets did not. The benefits were greatest for men with high blood pressure.

The study, conducted by the Harvard School of Public Health in Cambridge, Massachusetts, also found that the rate of strokes was lower for men who consumed higher levels of magnesium and cereal fiber.

The major finding was that men in the top 20 percent for potassium consumption (eating an average of nine potassium-rich servings a day) had 38 percent fewer strokes than those in the bottom 20 percent, who consumed less than four servings. Men without high blood pressure who had high intakes of magnesium had a 30 percent lower risk of stroke. Men who ate large amounts of cereal fiber had a 40 percent lower risk than those who did not.　● Laura Bushie

---

Researchers published two studies in October 1998 on new techniques for bone marrow transplants that improve patient-donor matching and expand the pool of suitable donors. Bone marrow is the tissue within bones that produces blood cells. In a bone marrow transplant, physicians replace a patient's defective or destroyed bone marrow with healthy marrow from another person. This is often done for patients who suffer from *leukemia* (a type of cancer characterized by abnormal white blood cells).

For a transplant to succeed, the donor and recipient must have similar types of HLA (human leukocyte antigen) genes, which control the body's immune system. A simple blood test

is usually used to determine this match. However, the blood test is unable to detect subtle genetic differences that could result in the patient's body rejecting the transplant.

A research team led by geneticists at Kyushu University in Japan reported that survival rates for transplant recipients could be doubled by using a matching system that relies on an analysis of deoxyribonucleic acid (DNA), the molecule that makes up genes. After analyzing the DNA in the HLA genes of 880 unrelated donors and recipients, the scientists determined that a perfect match of three HLA genetic factors (HLA-A, HLA-B, and HLA-C) was best for reducing a patient's risk of rejecting a transplant.

Surgery

- Better bone marrow transplants
- Hand transplants
- Prophylactic mastectomies
- New circumcision policy

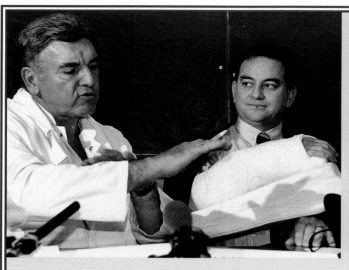

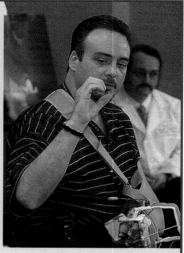

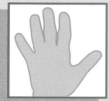

World's first hand transplants

Physician Jean-Michel Dubernard, *left,* describes the hand transplant operation that he and other surgeons performed on Clint Hallam, holding up his new hand in a cast. The operation, performed in September 1998 at Edouard Herriot Hospital in Lyons, France, was the first successful hand transplant in history. In January 1999, Matthew Scott, *right,* became the second person to successfully receive a hand transplant.

His surgery was performed at Louisville Jewish Hospital in Kentucky. Both procedures involved removing a hand from a deceased donor and attaching it to an arm of the patient. Hallam received a right hand, and Scott a left. Each man had lost his hand in an accident several years before. To prevent their immune systems from rejecting the hands, Hallam and Scott need to take potent antirejection drugs for the rest of their lives. As of mid-1999, both men had limited use of their new hands and could do such tasks as picking up a glass and writing with a pen. However, their doctors said it would take at least a year to determine if nerves would regenerate enough to give the hands normal sensation.

In the other bone marrow study, scientists at the University of Perugia in Italy and the Weizmann Institute in Israel reported on a technique that allows bone marrow mismatches to be used in transplants if the marrow is specially treated prior to the surgery. The technique involves using drugs to boost the marrow's production of *hematopoietic stem cells* (cells that give rise to blood cells), and removing most of the marrow's *T-lymphocytes* (cells that help destroy foreign substances).

The researchers reported that 41 of 43 bone marrows so treated were accepted by leukemia patients. However, only 12 of the patients were alive and free of disease 1 ½ years after treatment. The researchers hoped that additional studies into this technique would boost the survival rate of patients.

Hand transplants. Clint Hallam, a 48-year-old from Australia, became the first person in history to successfully receive a hand transplant in September 1998. The operation, using a hand from a deceased, anonymous donor, was performed at Edouard Herriot Hospital in Lyons, France, by a team of physicians led by microsurgeon Earl Owen. Hallam had lost his right hand in a circular saw accident in 1984.

Surgeons at Louisville Jewish Hospital in Louisville, Kentucky, performed a second hand transplant in January 1999. The surgeons attached the left hand of a donor to the arm of Matthew Scott, a 37-year-old American who had his hand blown off by a firecracker in 1985.

Surgeons first attempted a hand transplant in 1964 in Ecuador, but the patient's immune system immediately rejected the new hand. By 1998, advances in microsurgery and antirejection drugs made it more likely that limb transplants would succeed. Both Hallam and Scott reported limited use of their new limbs within a few weeks of the surgery. However, their physicians said it would be at least a year before they could determine if sensory nerves would regenerate enough to allow the men to have normal sensations in the hands.

While many physicians said the success of the hand transplants might lead to transplants of other body parts, critics called the procedures unnecessary and dangerous. Of greatest concern to these observers was the fact that the transplant recipients would need to take potent antirejection drugs for the rest of their lives to prevent their immune systems from rejecting the hands. Critics noted that these drugs increased vulnerability to life-threatening infections and cancer.

Prophylactic mastectomies. Women who undergo *bilateral prophylactic mastectomy* (surgical removal of both breasts while healthy) reduce their risk of getting breast cancer by at least 90 percent, according to a January 1999 report by researchers at the Mayo Clinic in Rochester, Minnesota. The study was the first detailed analysis of this radical procedure, which is sometimes chosen by women with a family history of breast cancer who want to reduce their risk of getting the disease.

The team of Mayo physicians reviewed the cases of 639 women who had both breasts removed between 1960 and 1993. The researchers classified the women into two categories—high risk (if they had a family history of multiple cancers) and moderate risk (if they had a personal history of multiple breast lumps).

For the high-risk group, the researchers compared the women with their own sisters, who were pre-

sumed to be at a similar risk level. Based on the number of breast cancers that developed in the sisters who had not had mastectomies, the physicians calculated that between 37 and 53 cancers would have developed among the mastectomy patients if they had not had their breasts removed. The researchers also concluded that at least 10 of these women would have died.

However, only three cancers and two deaths actually occurred among the women who underwent early breast removal. These figures represented a 90 to 94 percent risk reduction for cancer and an 81 to 94 percent risk reduction for death.

For the moderate-risk group, investigators used computer *models* (simulations) of how breast cancer develops. Based on these models, the researchers concluded that 37 women who had the breast surgery would have otherwise developed cancer, and that 10 of them would have died from the disease. In reality, only 4 of the women developed cancer (a 90 percent risk reduction), and none of them died.

Despite these findings, the researchers stressed that women have far less invasive options for preventing breast cancer than mastectomy. These options include self-examination of the breasts, *mammograms* (X rays of the breast), and tamoxifen, a drug approved for preventing breast cancer by the U.S. Food and Drug Administration in October 1998.

New circumcision policy. In March 1999, the American Academy of Pediatrics (AAP) acknowledged the potential health benefits of infant *circumcision* (the removal of the foreskin of the penis), but concluded that the benefits "are not significant enough" to recommend the routine performance of the procedure. The statement revised the AAP's previous policy, which referred only to the potential benefits of routine circumcision.

The AAP said it changed its policy partly because of recent studies, including some showing there is much less difference in the risk for urinary tract infections between circumcised and uncircumcised infants than previously believed.   • Suzanne Baker

- Fluid intake reduces bladder cancer risk
- Viagra ineffective in women?
- Home cancer test approved

In May 1999, a study led by Dominique S. Michaud of the Harvard School of Public Health in Boston, Massachusetts, reported that drinking large quantities of fluids can reduce the risk of developing bladder cancer. Cancer of the urinary bladder is the fourth most common type of cancer among American men. Some experts believe that bladder cancer can result when *carcinogens* (cancer-causing agents) in the urine come in contact with the lining of the bladder. For this reason, frequent urination may decrease the risk of bladder cancer by reducing the time that carcinogens in the urine are in contact with the bladder lining. Investigations designed to assess the association of specific fluids, such as coffee and alcohol, with the development of bladder cancer have been largely inconclusive.

The study, which was initiated in 1986, included more than 48,000 male health professionals who responded to a detailed questionnaire on diet and medical history. Among the study group, 252 cases of bladder cancer were diagnosed during the study period. Patients who drank more than 2.5 liters (85 fluid ounces, or about 10 cups) of beverages per day had the lowest risk, while those who drank less than 1.3 liters (44 fluid ounces, or about 5½ cups) had the greatest risk of developing bladder cancer.

An editorial accompanying the study pointed out that the survey did not assess the sources of the water consumed by the subjects. This missing element may be important, since in some areas of the world drinking large amounts of well water contaminated with carcinogens may increase the risk of bladder cancer. The editorial concluded with the statement, "The quality of what you drink may therefore be as important as how much (or little) you imbibe."

Viagra ineffective in women? A study published in March 1999 reported that Viagra, the impotence drug that has helped millions of men with sexual dysfunction, does not offer similar benefits to women. The study was led by urologist Steven Kaplan of Columbia Presbyterian Center of New York Presbyterian Hospital.

Viagra, known generically as sildenafil, increases the effects of nitric oxide in the body. This improves sexual function by helping to boost blood flow to the genitals. Theoretically, it should work the same way in women as it does in men.

Kaplan's team studied 33 postmenopausal women with self-described sexual dysfunction for at least the previous six months. The most common symptoms of sexual dysfunction included decreased arousal, inadequate vaginal lubrication, and inability to achieve orgasm. After 12 weeks, 25 percent of the women had some

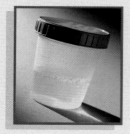

Hematuria: A common warning sign

Hematuria is the clinical term for the presence of red blood cells in the urine. Hematuria can be either *microscopic* (consisting of a higher-than-normal amount of red-blood cells in a urine sample) or *macroscopic* (with visible blood—as pink or red coloration or blood clots in the urine). The source of the bleeding can be anywhere along the urinary tract, which includes the kidneys, the urinary bladder, the *ureters* (tubes connecting the kidneys and urinary bladder), the prostate gland (in men), or the *urethra* (tube that carries urine from the bladder out of the body).

It is important that a physician evaluate all cases of hematuria to rule out a serious problem causing the condition. Fortunately, however, hematuria usually does not indicate a serious problem. Some of the most common causes include kidney or bladder stones and urinary tract infections. In men 50 years of age or older, the most common reason for hematuria is benign prostate enlargement. Other causes of hematuria include:

- Trauma, such as a strong blow to the kidneys
- Urinary tract blockages
- Viral infections of the urinary tract and certain sexually transmitted diseases, particularly in women
- Urinary tract tumors (cancerous or noncancerous)
- Various kidney diseases and disorders

Any amount of blood in the urine is potentially serious, whether or not it is accompanied by pain, so it should never be ignored. People who notice hematuria should see their physician or urologist as soon as possible.

improvement in sexual function. However, this percentage was statistically too small to prove that the drug was responsible for the effect.

The authors pointed out that the study had several limitations—it comprised only a small number of women and the trial period was relatively short. In addition, the cases of sexual dysfunction were self-described, not clinically diagnosed. Several larger, controlled clinical trials of Viagra's effect on sexual dysfunction in women were being conducted in 1999.

Home cancer test approved. An in-home urine test for bladder cancer received U.S. Food and Drug Admin-

istration approval in December 1998. The test, available by prescription only, was intended for use by bladder-cancer patients being monitored for a recurrence of the disease.

The BTA Stat Test, developed by Bion Diagnostic Sciences, Inc., of Redmond, Washington, uses *monoclonal antibodies* (artificial proteins designed to attack a specific substance in the body) to detect BTA (bladder tumor-associated antigen), a protein associated with bladder cancer tumors that can be found in urine. The test gives results within five minutes and reportedly detected bladder cancer with an accuracy of 90 percent. • Glenn S. Gerber

Public health authorities and veterinarians in the Southern United States were on the lookout for domestic animals infested with the screwworm in 1998 and 1999. The surveillance for the insect pest was prompted by the discovery of a small number of screwworm cases in Texas and by the return of U.S. military personnel and their pets through southern airports from closed bases in Panama, where the screwworm was common.

The screwworm is the *larvae* (immature form) of *Cochliomyia hominivorax,* a fly that lays its eggs in the skin of livestock and other animals. The larvae feed on an animal's body

tissue and infect the animal with harmful bacteria. The infected animal may die within just a few days.

The U.S. Department of Agriculture (USDA) led a project that eliminated the screwworm within U.S. borders by 1982. This project involved the release of large numbers of sterilized male flies, which produced no offspring when they mated with female flies. The pest was also eliminated in Mexico and most countries in Central America, but it remained a problem in Costa Rica and Panama.

The USDA was working with the U.S. Army in 1999 to verify that every pet entering the United States

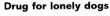

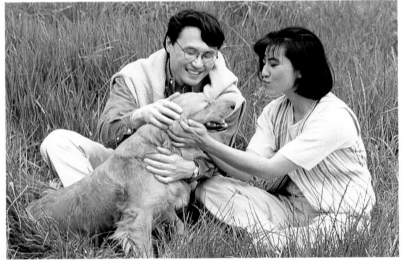

Drug for lonely dogs
The drug Clomicalm was approved by the U.S. Food and Drug Administration in December 1998 to treat separation anxiety in dogs. This condition is characterized by such behavior as constant barking and the destruction of house furnishings when a dog is left home alone. However, veterinarians warned that for the drug to be effective, owners must also work to modify their dog's behavior through proper training.

from Panama was screwworm free. In addition, the Texas Animal Health Commission was monitoring the situation and was prepared to release sterile male flies if any more screwworms were found.

Contaminated reptiles. Most, if not all, iguanas sold as pets carry internal populations of *Salmonella* bacteria, which are shed in their feces. The bacteria usually wind up on the iguana's skin, where they can pose a serious threat to human health. Those conclusions were announced in July 1998 by a team of biologists led by Bruce Burnham of the U.S. Air Force Academy near Colorado Springs, Colorado.

Green iguanas have been implicated as the source of many cases of the human disease salmonellosis. The disease, which occurs when humans ingest the microbes, causes diarrhea, abdominal pain, and fever in most people. In some cases, it causes a massive infection and is fatal.

The researchers purchased 12 green iguanas from different pet dealers in the Colorado Springs and Denver areas. The iguanas were isolated and fed diets free from *Salmonella* to prevent the spread of the bacteria. Despite these precautions, all of the animals were found to have the microorganism in their intestinal tracts.

The researchers said that the disease-causing microbes are probably in the bodies of all iguanas, as well as in most other reptile pets, including turtles and snakes. To reduce the risk of *Salmonella* transmission to people, the researchers advised individuals to always wash their hands after touching a reptile and to keep reptiles out of kitchens.

Preventable pet problems. A nationwide survey of 52 veterinary clinics, released in May 1999, confirmed that most health problems of dogs and cats can be prevented with proper pet care. The survey, led by veterinarian Elizabeth Lund of the University of Minnesota at St. Paul, found that the most common problem requiring medical treatment in the 46,710 cases examined was dental and gum disease. About 40 percent of the dogs and cats in the survey had this condition, which can be prevented by periodic teeth cleanings.

Among dogs, other common medical problems, in descending order of occurrence, were ear infections, skin problems, flea infestation, allergies, lumps, and lameness. Besides flea infestations, cats were usually seen by veterinarians for different reasons than dogs, including ear mites, abscesses, respiratory tract infections, injuries from the bites of other cats, and tapeworm infections.

• Philip H. Kass

In the Consumer Health section, see CONTROLLING THE COST OF PET CARE.

Weight Control

- Weight control and diabetes
- Heart damage and fen-phen
- Energy-regulating gene identified
- FDA approves orlistat
- Overfed babies and obesity

A study reported in May 1999 suggested that young, overweight men might be at an increased risk for developing adult onset diabetes, also known as Type II diabetes. In Type II diabetes, the pancreas produces insulin, the hormone that regulates *glucose* (blood sugar) levels, but not enough to meet the body's needs, especially when the person is overweight. Type II diabetes occurs mainly in people over age 40. The study was conducted by researchers at Johns Hopkins University in Baltimore.

The team of researchers, led by Frederick L. Brancati, an associate professor of medicine and epidemiology at Johns Hopkins, tracked 916 former medical students who graduated between 1948 and 1964. The researchers discovered that 35 of the men had Type II diabetes. The men in the study who were overweight at age 25, and those who became overweight between 35 and 45, were more than three times more likely to develop diabetes than those participants who were not overweight. The researchers concluded that weight control in early adulthood may prevent occurrences of Type II diabetes.

Heart damage and fen-phen. A study presented in March 1999 at a meeting of the American College of Cardiology in New Orleans confirmed that people who had taken two popular weight-loss drugs—fenfluramine and phentermine, commonly known as "fen-phen"—for more than six months showed unusually high rates of heart valve disease. People who reported taking the drugs for less than six months did not suffer from heart valve damage.

The study, conducted by Duke University Medical Center cardiologist Thomas Ryan, tracked 1,163 former fen-phen users. Patients who took the combination for less than six months had a 4.5 percent incidence rate of heart valve disease. Patients who had never taken fen-phen had a 3.6 percent incidence rate of heart valve disease. Those who used fen-phen for more than six months had a 7 per-

cent incidence rate of heart valve disease. The rate of heart valve disease increased to 13.6 percent for those people who had taken fen-phen for one to two years and it jumped to 17.4 percent for people who had used fen-phen for more than two years. Those patients who took fen-phen and had heart valve disease experienced only minor symptoms. However, researchers in 1999 did not know whether those health problems would worsen over time.

Fenfluramine was voluntarily removed from markets in the United States in 1997 by its manufacturer. Although the United States Food and Drug Administration (FDA) never ap-

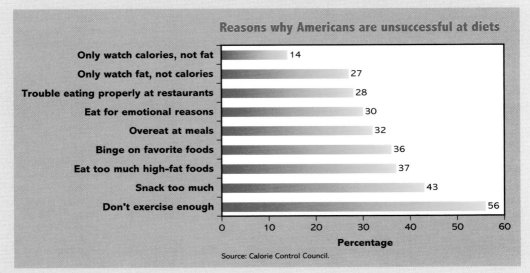

STATISTICS

Losing weight

A survey published in 1998 by the Calorie Control Council, an international association of low-calorie and re-duced-fat food and beverage manufacturers, revealed that the number of American adults on a diet had decreased since the mid-1980's. The council surveyed 1,163 adults and projected that 27 percent of all Americans—about 54 million people—were on a diet in 1998. More than half of those surveyed reported failing at their diets because of a lack of exercise.

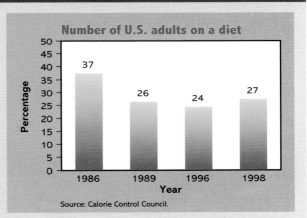

Number of U.S. adults on a diet

Year	Percentage
1986	37
1989	26
1996	24
1998	27

Source: Calorie Control Council.

Reasons why Americans are unsuccessful at diets

	Percentage
Only watch calories, not fat	14
Only watch fat, not calories	27
Trouble eating properly at restaurants	28
Eat for emotional reasons	30
Overeat at meals	32
Binge on favorite foods	36
Eat too much high-fat foods	37
Snack too much	43
Don't exercise enough	56

Source: Calorie Control Council.

proved combining the two drugs, about 25 million prescriptions for fen-phen were written by doctors in the mid-1990's in hopes that the drug would help obese patients control their weight.

The Duke University study was the largest of its kind to examine the connection between heart valve disease and fenfluramine. Researchers in 1999 did not know why fenfluramine caused heart valve disease.

Energy-regulating gene identified. In March 1999, scientists at Millennium Pharmaceuticals in Cambridge, Massachusetts, announced the discovery of a gene thought to regulate metabolism and the expenditure of energy. The gene, known as "Mahogany" (a reference to the brown fur of the mice used as test subjects), or the MG gene, was believed to suppress obesity and regulate the way the body burns calories.

The Millennium researchers fed mice diets that included various amounts of fat. Those mice with a mutated MG gene did not gain weight regardless of the amount of fat in their diet. Mice with the normal MG genes gained weight when they were given a high-fat diet. The researchers were optimistic that similar results would be found in humans. They hoped that their findings would lead to the development of a safe and effective weight-loss drug.

FDA approves orlistat. The FDA in April 1999 approved the use of orlistat, sold as Xenical, as a treatment for obesity. In clinical trials, orlistat blocked an enzyme that absorbs dietary fat in the gastrointestinal tract. As a result, orlistat cuts absorption of dietary fat by about 30 percent.

Researchers from Hoffman-LaRoche Laboratories, Inc., of Nutley, New Jersey—the company that manufactures orlistat—announced in May that a two-year study of 247 obese women over the age of 45 showed that 56.1 percent of patients taking orlistat had lost more than 5 percent of their initial body weight compared with 39.4 percent of patients who had received a *placebo* (inactive substance). All of the women in the study had followed a low-calorie diet

in the first year of treatment and a weight-maintenance diet prescribed to them in the second year.

Researchers recommended the drug for patients who were at least 20 percent overweight and had conditions aggravated by obesity, such as diabetes, high cholesterol, or high blood pressure. Experts said that orlistat should be used in conjunction with a well-balanced diet and regular exercise program.

Researchers said that the drug also carried some side effects. For example, orlistat reduces the absorption into the body of fat-soluble vitamins, including vitamins A, D, E and K, and beta carotene. Other effects included gas and frequent bowel movements.

Overfed babies and obesity. Researchers at the Children's Hospital in Cincinnati, Ohio, reported in October 1998 that mothers who overfeed their young children may promote obesity later in life. The researchers studied three groups of 14 mothers with children ranging in age from 1 year to 3 years.

The mothers who participated in the study reported a belief that high infant weight meant that their children were healthy. They also expressed concerns that their children were not eating enough. Therefore, many of the mothers surveyed fed rice, cereal, and other solid food to their children before the recommended ages.

They also used food to reward their infant's good behavior or to calm them when they were fussy. Many of the mothers told the researchers that they were aware that introducing solid food and using food to control their children's behavior went against the advice of their nutritionists and physicians. Many said that they followed the advice of their mothers in caring for their infants.

The Ohio researchers advised health professionals to avoid implying that infant weight is a good way to measure a child's health. They said that parents who reward their children with food or meet the child's emotional needs by feeding them may be unintentionally promoting obesity in their children. The children may later have difficulty regulating their own food intake. • Lauren Love

1999-2000 DIRECTORY OF HEALTH INFORMATION

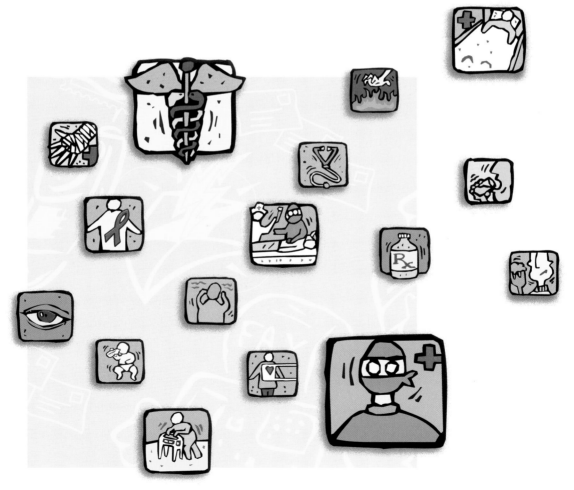

ADDICTIONS

Alcoholics Anonymous provides support and counseling to alcoholics, their families, and their friends.
Phone: 212-870-3312
Mailing address: A.A. World Services, P.O. Box 459, Grand Central Station, New York, NY 10163
Web site: http://www.moscow.com/Resources/SelfHelp/AA/

HabitSmart web site offers an electronic magazine on addictive behaviors that features articles, practical guides, interactive self-help tests, and links to other sites dealing with addiction.
Web site: http://www.cts.com:80/~habtsmrt

National Clearinghouse for Alcohol and Drug Information offers statistics, brochures, educational programs, and the most recent information on drugs and drug abuse.
Phone: 410-225-6910
Mailing address: Office of the Director, Center for Substance Abuse Prevention, Substance Abuse and Mental Health Services Administration, 5600 Fishers Lane, Rockwall II Building, Rockville, MD 20857
Web site: http://www.health.org

Recovery Homepage offers a comprehensive listing of 12-step recovery programs and provides information and support for people suffering from a variety of addictions.
Web site: http://www.shore.net/~tcfraser/recovery.htm
E-mail: tcfraser@shore.net

Web of Addictions web site provides information on addiction and treatment.
Web site: http://www.well.com/user/woa/
E-mail: Razer@ix.netcom.com

ADDISON'S DISEASE

National Adrenal Diseases Foundation provides information and support to individuals suffering from adrenal diseases, especially Addison's disease, which results from insufficient production of several vital hormones by the adrenal gland.
Phone: 516-487-4992
Mailing address: 505 Northern Boulevard, Suite 200, Great Neck, NY 11021

AGING

Children of Aging Parents offers education, support, guidance, and development of coping skills to caregivers of the elderly and provides a referral service.
Phone: 800-227-7294

Eldercare Locator answers questions, provides written information, and makes referrals to local support groups and sources of assistance for the elderly.
Phone: 800-677-1116

Elder Watch web site offers articles, summaries of articles, and links to other health-care sites.
Web site: http://www.wellweb.com/seniors/eldership.htm

Eldercare web site offers Internet resources for seniors and caregivers.
Web site: http://www.ice.net/~kstevens/elderweb.html

National Institute on Aging Information Center provides written information and referrals on various issues affecting aging.
Phone: 800-222-2225; hearing-impaired people can call 800-222-4225.
Web site: http://www.aoa.dhhs.gov/aoa/resource.html

Older Women's League makes referrals to support groups and local chapters.
Phone: 800-825-3695

AIDS

The Body: A Multimedia AIDS and HIV Information Resource web site offers educational information.
Web site: http://www.thebody.com

The Centers for Disease Control AIDS Clearinghouse offers information on HIV/AIDS and provides a referral service.
Phone: 800-458-5231
Web site: http://cdcnac.aspensys.com:86

HIV/AIDS Clinical Trials Information Service answers questions and sends written materials on trials for drugs and experimental therapies.
Phone: 800-874-2572
Web site: http://www.actis.org

HIV/AIDS Treatment Information Service web site, operated by the National Library of Medicine, features discussions on scientific issues and research.
Web site:
http://test.nim.nih.gov/atis/list.html

HIV/AIDS Treatment Service provides information on treatment options.
Phone: 800-448-0440
Web site: http://www.hivatis.org

National AIDS Hotline provides information and referrals.
Phone: 800-342-AIDS; Spanish-language information is available at 800-344-7432; people who are hearing impaired can call 800-243-7889
Web site: http://sunsite.unc.edu/ASHA/

Pediatric AIDS Foundation offers support networks and programs for children with AIDS.
Phone: 800-828-3280

Project Inform National HIV/AIDS Treatment Hot Line answers questions about treatment of HIV and AIDS.
Phone: 800-822-7422
Web site: http://www.projinf.org/

ALZHEIMER'S DISEASE

Alzheimer's Association provides information and referrals to local chapters.
Phone: 800-272-3900
Web site: http://www.alz.org/

Alzheimer's Disease Education and Referral Center answers questions and makes referrals to research centers.
Phone: 800-438-4380
Web site: http://www.alzheimers.org/adear

AMYOTROPHIC LATERAL SCLEROSIS

Amyotrophic Lateral Sclerosis (ALS) Association National Office answers questions and provides referrals to support groups and local chapters.
Phone: 800-782-4747
Web site: http://www.alsa.org

ALS web site provides information on cause and treatment of the disease.
Web site: http://www.pslgroup.com/als.htm

ANIMAL WELFARE

American Humane Education Society provides information on animals.
Web site: http://www.mspcu.org

American Society for the Prevention of Cruelty to Animals provides educational information on animals.
Web site: http://www.aspca.org

Electronic Zoo web site provides a listing of animal-health sites on the Internet.
Web site: http://netvet.wustl.edu/e-zoo.htm

ANXIETY DISORDERS

Council on Anxiety Disorders provides information and referrals.
Phone: 910-722-7760
Mailing address: P.O. Box 17011, Winston-Salem, NC 27116

APHASIA

Academy of Aphasia provides research and educational information about aphasia, a speech disorder that often affects victims of stroke.
Phone: 310-206-3206
Mailing address: UCLA, Department of Linguistics, Los Angeles, CA 90024

APLASTIC ANEMIA

Aplastic Anemia Foundation of America serves as an information source for individuals with aplastic anemia, an often fatal disease in which bone marrow fails to produce new blood cells.
Phone: 800-747-2820
Mailing address: P.O. Box 22689, Baltimore, MD 21203

ARTHRITIS

Arthritis Foundation provides information on treatment and local chapters
Phone: 800-283-7800
Web site: http://www.arthritis.org
E-mail: help@arthritis.org

The American Lupus Society sends written information to those who leave their names and addresses on its answering machine.
Phone: 800-331-1802

Lupus Foundation of America provides written information on the cause and treatment of lupus.
Phone: 800-558-0121
Mailing address: 4 Research Place, Suite 180, Rockville, MD 20850-3226

ASTHMA AND LUNG DISORDERS

Allergy and Asthma Network/Mothers of Asthmatics Inc. provides referrals and publishes a monthly newsletter.
Web site:
http://www.podi.com/health/aanma

Allergy, Asthma, and Immunology Online web site, operated by the American College of Allergy, Asthma, and Immunology, provides information on these disorders.
Web site: http://allergy.mcg.edu/

American Lung Association provides information and educational material.
Web site: http//www.lungusa.org

Asthma and Allergy Foundation of America provides written information on asthma and allergies.
Phone: 800-7-ASTHMA

Lungline provides written information on respiratory and immunological problems and an opportunity to speak with a nurse.
Phone: 800-222-LUNG
Web site: http://www.hjc.org

National Asthma Education and Prevention Program Information Center provides fact sheets and articles.
Web site:
http://www.nhlbi.nih.gov/nhibi/nhibi.htm

National Institute of Allergy and Infectious Diseases web site contains information about these disorders.
Web site: http://web.fie.com/web/fed/nih/

ATTENTION-DEFICIT DISORDER

Attention Deficit Disorder Archive web site provides resources on attention deficit disorder to people with this disability.
Web site: http://www.seas.upenn.edu/~mengwong/add/

Children and Adults with Attention Deficit Disorder (CHADD) Online delivers information about attention deficit disorder.
Web site: http://www.chadd.org

National Attention-Deficit Disorder Association Hotline provides information, including referrals to support groups.
Phone: 800-487-2282

AUTISM

Autism Resources web site provides information on the treatment of autism.
Web site:
http://web.syr.edu/~jmwobus/autism/

Autism Society of America offers information on the symptoms and problems of children and adults with autism.
Phone: 800-3-AUTISM

BEHCET'S SYNDROME

American Behcet's Disease Association offers educational and research information on Behcet's syndrome, a disease characterized by painful oral ulcers.
Phone: 800-723-4238

BIRTH DEFECTS

Association of Birth Defect Children Hotline provides information on birth defects and offers help in adjusting to the problems faced by people with physical malformations.
Phone: 800-313-ABDC

Cornelia De Lange Syndrome Foundation seeks to ensure early and accurate diagnosis of the syndrome (a birth defect resulting in babies who develop at a slower rate).
Phone: 800-223-8355

March of Dimes Birth Defects Foundation promotes the prevention of birth defects by focusing on child health issues.
Web site: http://www.modimes.org

BLADDER DISORDERS

Bladder Health Council provides written materials on bladder cancer and other bladder disorders.
Phone: 800-242-2383
Web site:http://www.access.digex.net~afud

BLOOD

National Rare Blood Club offers information to people with rare blood types.
Phone: 212-889-8245

BRAIN INJURY

Brain Injury Association Family Help Line (formerly National Head Injury Foundation) answers questions, provides written information, and makes referrals to local resources.
Phone: 800-444-6443

Traumatic Brain Injury web site provides information and links to other web sites.
Web site:
http://canddwilson.com/tbi/tbiepil.htm

BREAST DISEASE

American Society of Breast Disease provides information on breast diseases.
Phone: 214-368-6836

Breast Cancer Information Clearinghouse provides information and free publications and brochures on breast cancer detection and treatment.
Phone: 800-4-CANCER
Web site: http://nysernet.org/bcic/

A Patient's Guide to Breast Cancer Treatment web site provides information on breast cancer and its treatment.
Web site: gopher://nysernet.org:70/00/bcic/sources/strang-

BURNS

American Burn Association offers information on the treatment of burns.
Phone: 800-548-2876
Web site: http://www.ameriburn.org

National Burn Victim Foundation provides information on treatment. Maintains 24-hour emergency burn referral.
Phone: 800-803-5879

Phoenix Society for Burn Survivors offers a self-help service for burn survivors and their families.
Phone: 800-888-BURN

CANCER

American Brain Tumor Association provides information on brain tumors and brain tumor research.
Phone: 800-886-2282
Mailing address: 2720 River Road, Suite 146, Des Plaines, IL 60018

American Cancer Society provides special services to cancer patients.
Phone: 800-ACS-2345
Mailing address: 1599 Clifton Road NE, Atlanta, GA 30329
Web site: http://www.cancer.org

Association for Research of Childhood Cancer offers information on various pediatric cancers.
Phone: 716-681-4433
Mailing address: P.O. Box 251, Buffalo, NY 14225-0251

Cancer Information Service of the National Cancer Institute answers questions and provides written information and referrals to treatment centers, mammography facilities, and support groups. The web site offers an online library.
Phone: 800-4-CANCER; hearing-impaired people can reach the service by TDD at 800-332-8615
Web site: http://www.icic.nci.nih.gov

Cancer Pain Education for Patients and Families web site, operated by the University of Iowa, provides information about pain control.
Web site: http://coninfo.nursing.uiowa.edu/www/nursing/apn/cncrpain/toc.htm

Cancer Response System of the American Cancer Society provides written information and referrals to local ACS programs and resources.
Phone: 800-ACS-2345
Web site: http://www.cancer.org

Cansearch: A Guide to Cancer Resources web site features step-by-step instructions on how to access resources.
Web site: http://access.dignex.net/~mkragen/cansearch.html

International Myeloma Foundation provides research information on myeloma, a blood cancer.
Phone: 800-452-CURE
Web site: http://www.comed.com/Aboutccihf.spml

Leukemia Society of America provides information and financial aid for patients and sponsors support groups.
Phone: 800-955-4LSA

OncoLink web site offers information guides on the nature of cancer, its causes, and screening and prevention, information on clinical trials, financial guides, and a feature about childhood cancer.
Web site: http://cancer.med.upenn.edu/

Prostate Cancer Infolink web site provides information and resources for patients with prostate cancer.
Web site: http://www.comed.com/prostate/

Prostate Cancer Support Network sends written information and provides referrals to local support groups.
Phone: 800-828-7866
Web site: http://www.access.digex.net~afud

Quick Information About Cancer for Patients and Their Families web site provides information on causes of cancer, treatment, and support.
Web site: http://asa.ugl.lib.umich.edu/chdocs/cancer/

Skin Cancer Foundation offers information on the prevention and early recognition of skin cancer.
Phone: 800-SKIN-490

Y-ME National Breast Cancer Organization allows callers to speak to counselors who have survived breast cancer; offers a men's hotline staffed by male counselors; and supplies wigs and prostheses to women who cannot afford them.
Phone: 800-221-2141; Spanish speakers may call 800-986-9505
Web site: http://www.y-me.org

CELIAC DISEASE

Celiac Disease Foundation provides information to individuals with celiac disease (the small intestine is damaged by ingestion of certain foods).
Phone: 818-990-2354
Mailing address: 13251 Ventura Boulevard, Suite 3, Studio City, CA 91604-1838

CEREBRAL PALSY

United Cerebral Palsy Associations provides information and referral services.
Phone: 800-USA-5UCP
Mailing address: 1522 K Street NW, Suite 1112, Washington, DC 20005
Web site: http://www.ucpa.org
E-mail: uspnatl@ucpa.org

CHILD ABUSE AND NEGLECT

Childhelp/IOF Foresters National Child Abuse Hotline provides trained professional counselors for crisis intervention 24 hours a day, 7 days a week.
Phone: 800-4ACHILD; hearing-impaired people can reach the hotline at 800-2ACHILD

Child Quest International offers referrals for abused and exploited children.
Phone: 800-248-8020

National Clearinghouse on Child Abuse and Neglect Information provides information on child abuse and neglect.
Phone: 800-394-3366

National Committee to Prevent Child Abuse provides resources on child maltreatment and prevention.
Phone: 800-CHILDREN
Mailing address: 332 South Michigan Avenue, Suite 1600, Chicago, IL 60609

CHILDHOOD DISEASES

American Pediatric Gastroesophageal Reflux Association provides information to parents of children who suffer from gastroesophageal reflux.
Phone: 617-926-3586
Mailing address: 23 Acton Street, Watertown, MA 02172

Children's Blood Foundation provides information on diseases of the blood in children, such as leukemia, hemophilia, and diseases of the immune system.
Phone: 212-297-4336
Mailing address: 333 East 38th, 8th Floor, New York, NY 10016

Children's Medical Center web site, sponsored by the University of Virginia Health Sciences Center, provides information on childhood diseases.
Web site: http://galen.med.virginia.edu/~smb4v/cmchome.html

Cyclic Vomiting Syndrome Association provides support and information to individuals suffering from cyclic vomiting syndrome, a disorder that usually affects children aged 3 to 7 and is characterized by recurrent attacks of nausea and vomiting.
Phone: 414-784-6842
Mailing address: 13180 Caroline Court, Elm Grove, WI 53122

National Vaccine Information Center provides information about childhood vaccines.
Phone: 800-909-SHOT
Mailing address: 512 Maple Avenue West, Suite 206, Vienna, VA 22180

Pedinfo web site provides information on childhood diseases, on-line publications, support groups, and links to dozens of other sites.
Web site:
http://www.lhl.uab.edu:80/pedinfo/

CHRONIC FATIGUE SYNDROME

Chronic Fatigue and Immune Dysfunction Syndrome Association of America provides free information to callers who leave a message on its answering machine.
Phone: 800-442-3437

Chronic Fatigue Syndrome web site offers information and resources.
Web site: http://www.cais.com/cfs-news/

National Chronic Fatigue Syndrome and Fibromyalgia Association provides educational material about the illnesses.
Phone: 816-931-4777
Mailing address: 3521 Broadway, Suite 222, Kansas City, MO 64111

CHRONIC PAIN

American Academy of Head, Neck, and Facial Pain serves as a referral service for patients suffering from head, facial, and neck pain.
Phone: 800-322-8651
Mailing address: 520 West Pipeline Road, Hurst, TX 76053-4924

American Chronic Pain Association offers support and information to individuals suffering from chronic pain.
Phone: 916-632-0922
Mailing address: P.O. Box 850, Rocklin, CA 95677

The National Chronic Pain Outreach Association Hotline provides information and referrals.
Phone: 540-997-5004

The Worldwide Congress on Pain web site offers information and educational material on chronic pain.
Web site: http://www.pain.com

CLEFT PALATE

Children's Craniofacial Association provides financial assistance and a referral service to craniofacially deformed individuals.
Phone: 800-535-3643

Cleft Lip and Palate web page provides a collection of Internet resources on the disorders.
Web site:
http://www.samizdat.com/pp3.html

Cleft Palate Foundation offers information about cleft lip and palate and provides research programs and children's services.
Phone: 800-24-CLEFT
Mailing address: 1218 Grandview Avenue, Pittsburgh, PA 15211

Forward Face provides medical, psychological, and financial support services.
Phone: 800-FWD-FACE
Mailing address: 317 East 34th Street, New York, NY 10016

COMA

Coma Recovery Association provides support to coma survivors.
Phone: 516-355-0951

COSMETIC SURGERY

National Foundation for Facial Reconstruction sponsors programs for patients with facial disfigurements.
Phone: 800-422-FACE

CROHN'S DISEASE AND COLITIS

Crohn's and Colitis Foundation of America, Inc. provides information and referrals.
Phone: 800-932-2423

Crohn's Disease, Ulcerative Colitis, and Inflammatory Bowel Disease web site provides information on the treatments of various bowel disorders.
Web site: http://qurlyjoe.bu.edu/

CYSTIC FIBROSIS

Cystic Fibrosis Foundation provides written information and referrals to accredited cystic fibrosis care centers.
Phone: 800-FIGHT CF
Web site: http://www.cff.org

The Cystic Fibrosis web site provides online information about the disease.
Web site:
hppt:www.ai.mit.edu/people/mernst/cf/

A Family Guide to Cystic Fibrosis Testing web site provides information about the disease and testing procedures.
Web site:
http://www.phd.msu.edu/cf/fam.html

DEATH AND DYING

GriefNet web site provides resources to help people cope with loss and grief.
Web site: http://rivendell.org/

DEGENERATIVE DISEASES

Independent Citizens Research Foundation for the Study of Degenerative Diseases provides information on the causes of degenerative diseases.
Phone: 914-478-1862

DENTISTRY

American Academy of Oral Medicine provides information on the cause, prevention, and the control of diseases of the teeth.
Phone: 703-684-6649
Mailing address: 631 29th Street South, Arlington, VA 22202-2312

American Dental Association provides news and information on dental health.
Phone: 312-440-2500
Mailing address: 211 East Chicago Avenue, Chicago, IL 60611
Web site: http://www.ada.org

Dental-Related Internet Resources web site, operated by New York University College of Dentistry, provides a listing of dental information on the Internet.
Web site: http://www.nyu.edu/dental/

DERMATOLOGY

American Dermatological Association provides educational and research information.
Phone: 706-721-6496
Mailing address: Medical College of Georgia, Department of Dermatology, Augusta, GA 30912-2900

American Hair Loss Council provides information regarding treatments for hair loss in both men and women.
Phone: 800-274-8717
Mailing address: 401 North Michigan Avenue, 22nd Floor, Chicago, IL 60611-4212

Dystrophic Epidermolysis Bullosa Research Association of America offers information on the cause and treatment of dystrophic epidermolysis bullosa, a group of inherited disorders of the skin characterized by formation of blisters.
Phone: 212-693-6610
Mailing address: 40 Rector Street, New York, NY 10006

Eczema Association for Science and Education provides research and educational information on eczema.
Phone: 503-228-4430
Mailing address: 1221 Southwest Yamhill, No. 303, Portland, OR 97205

Foundation for Ichthyosis and Related Skin Types provides information and support to people suffering from ichthyosis, a hereditary disease that causes the skin to be thick, dry, taut, and scaly.
Phone: 800-545-3286
Mailing address: P.O. Box 20921, Raleigh, NC 27619

International Livedo Reticularis Network provides information on livedo reticularis, a condition characterized by a reddish-blue mottling of the skin.
Phone: 512-353-7451
Mailing address: 215 Lazy Lane, San Marcos, TX 78666

National Association for Pseudoxanthoma Elasticum provides support and information on pseudoxanthoma elasticum, a disease marked by an exaggeration of the normal creases and folds of the skin.
Phone: 303-832-5055
Mailing address: 1420 Ogden Street, Denver, CO 80218

National Psoriasis Foundation provides information and support to people suffering from psoriasis (a chronic skin disease characterized by red patches covered with white scales) or psoriatic arthritis.
Phone: 800-723-9166
Mailing address: 6600 Southwest 92nd, Suite 300, Portland, OR 97223-7195
Web site: http://www.psoriasis.org/

DIABETES

American Diabetes Association answers questions and provides written information. The web site offers information on diabetes and how to cope with it.
Phone: 800-ADA-DISC
Web site: http://www.diabetes.org

The Diabetic Foot web site, operated by the Foot and Ankle Institute of St. George, Utah, provides information on foot problems associated with diabetes.
Web site: http://www.infowest.com/doctor/index.html

Diabetes Home Page offers information on support groups and organizations, research, and sources of insulin pumps, sugar-free chocolates, and diet plans.
Web site: http://www.nd.edu/~hhowisen/diabetes.html

Diabetes Research Institute Foundation serves as an information clearinghouse and offers a referral service.
Phone: 800-321-3437
Mailing address: 3440 Hollywood Boulevard, Suite 100, Hollywood, FL 33021

International Diabetic Athletes Association provides a network and support group for athletes with diabetes.
Phone: 800-898-IDAA
Mailing address: 1647 West Bethany Home Road, No. B, Phoenix, AZ 85015

Juvenile Diabetes Foundation International Hotline answers general questions and supplies written information.
Phone: 800-223-1138
Web site: http://www.jdfcure.com
E-mail: info@jdfcure.com

Managing Your Diabetes web site features a diabetes reference manual and provides information on the disease.
Web site: http://www.Lilly.com/diabetes

The National Institute of Diabetes and Digestive and Kidney Disease of the National Institutes of Health web site offers educational materials and information on several disorders.
Web site: http://www.niddk.nih.gov/
E-mail: kranzfeldk@hq.niddk.nih.gov

DIGESTIVE DISEASE

Digestive Disease National Coalition offers information on digestive diseases and related nutrition.
Phone: 202-544-7497
Mailing address: 711 2nd Street Northeast, Suite 200, Washington, DC 20002

Intestinal Digestive Diseases Information Clearinghouse serves as a central information resource on the prevention and management of digestive diseases.
Phone: 301-654-3810
Mailing address: 2 Information Way, Bethesda, MD 20892-3570

North American Society for Pediatric Gastroenterology and Nutrition provides information on gastrointestinal disorders.
Phone: 216-844-1767

DISABILITY AND REHABILITATION

Accent on Information provides a computerized retrieval system that offers access to information on products and serv-ices available to the disabled.
Phone: 309-378-2961
Mailing address: P.O. Box 700, Bloomington, IL 61702

American Amputee Foundation offers counseling to new amputees and their families, legal assistance, and referral concerning prosthetics.
Phone: 501-666-2523
Mailing address: P.O. Box 250218, Hillcrest Station, Little Rock, AR 72225

American Disability Association provides information on disability issues, children's services, and support services.
Phone: 205-323-3030
Mailing address: 2121 8th Avenue North, Suite 1623, Birmingham, AL 35203

Americans with Disabilities Act (ADA) Document Center web site contains infor-mation on ADA implementation, the rights of the disabled, and instructions on how to file a complaint.
Web site:
http://janweb.icdi.wvu.edu/kinder/

Amputee Shoe and Glove Exchange facilitates swaps of unneeded shoes and gloves by amputees.
Mailing address: P.O. Box 27067, Houston, TX 77227

The Association of Retarded Citizens provides information on legislation, support services, and publications.
Phone: 202-467-4179
Mailing address: Department of Government Affairs, 1522 K Street Northwest, S-516, Washington, DC 20005-1247
Web site: http://TheArc.org/welcome.html

Canine Companions for Independence offers information on obtaining specially trained dogs for the disabled.
Phone: 800-767-2275
Mailing address: P.O. Box 446, Santa Rosa, CA 95402

Center for Information Technology Accommodation web site provides a list of accessibility resources, a handbook on in-formation technology issues, a section on legislative issues, and links to other sites.
Web site: http://www.gsa.gov/coca/
E-mail: Susan.Brummel@gsa.gov

Clearinghouse of Disability Information provides information on federally funded programs serving the disabled.
Phone: 202-205-8241
Mailing address: U.S. Department of Education, Office of Special Education and Rehabilitative Services, Switzer Building, Room 3132, Washington, DC 20202-2524

Direct Link for the Disabled serves as an information resource and referral service linking local, state, and national resources for all disabilities, health conditions, and rare disorders.
Phone: 805-688-1603
Mailing address: P.O. Box 1036 Solvang, CA 93464

Federation for Children with Special Needs is a coalition of parents' organiza-tions acting on behalf of children and adults with disabilities that offers educa-tional material and referrals.
Phone: 800-331-0688
Mailing address: 95 Berkley Street, Suite 104, Boston, MA 02116

Job Accommodation Network provides international information and referral services for people with disabilities.
Electronic bulletin board: 800-DIALJAN
Phone: 800-526-7234; hearing-impaired people can call 800-526-7234

National Information Center for Children and Youth with Disabilities provides infor-mation and referrals to other organizations, prepares information packets, and assists parents.
Phone: 800-695-0285
Mailing address: P.O. Box 1492, Washington, DC 20013

National Information Clearinghouse for Infants with Disabilities and Life-Threatening Conditions provides informa-tion, assistance, and referrals to caregivers.
Phone: 800-922-9234

National Institute for Rehabilitation Engineering is a service organization of electronic engineers, physicists, psychologists, and optometrists who offer advice to disabled people regarding custom-designed and custom-made tools and devices and training.
Phone: 800-736-2216
Mailing address: P.O. Box T, Hewitt, NJ 07421

National Rehabilitation Information Center acts as a library on topics relating to disability and rehabilitation by searching databases and providing written information. The center also answers questions and provides referrals.
Phone: 800-346-2742
Web site: http://www.naric.com/naric

Rehabilitation Learning Center web site features a slide show that explains how spinal-cord-injury patients can master tasks such as getting in and out of a car, bed, shower, or wheelchair. Anatomic drawings allow patients to access diagrams of the spinal cord and spot the location of an injury.
Web site:
http://weber.u.washington.edu/~rlc/
E-mail: rlc@washington.edu/~rlc

DOWN SYNDROME

Down Syndrome Web Page includes Internet resources on Down syndrome and basic scientific information.
Web site: http://www.nas.com/downsyn/
E-mail: trace@nas.com

Mental Retardation Association of America provides information, referrals, and educational material.
Phone: 801-328-1575
Mailing address: 211 East 300 South, Suite 212, Salt Lake City, UT 84111

National Down Syndrome Society Hotline answers questions, supplies written information, and provides referrals to local support groups of parents of children with Down syndrome.
Phone: 800-221-4602
Web site: http://www.pcsltd.com/ndss/

DRINKING WATER

Safe Drinking Water Hotline, operated under contract for the Environmental Protection Agency, answers questions and provides written information about federal regulation of public water.
Phone: 800-426-4791

DYSLEXIA

Dyslexia Archive web site provides a collection of material covering all aspects of dyslexia.
Web site: http://www.hensa.ac.uk/dyslexia/www/homepage.html

The Orton Dyslexia Society sends written information to callers who leave their names and addresses on its answering machine.
Phone: 800-222-3123—answering machine; staff members answer questions at 410-296-0232.

EATING DISORDERS

American Anorexia/Bulimia Association serves as an information and referral service.
Phone: 800-924-2643
Mailing address: 293 Central Park West, Suite 1R, New York, NY 10024

Anorexia Nervosa and Related Disorders provides support groups, medical referrals, and counseling for anorectics, bulimics, and their families.
Phone: 541-344-1144
Mailing address: P.O. Box 5102, Eugene, OR 97405

National Association of Anorexia Nervosa provides information on eating disorders.
Phone: 847-831-3438

EPILEPSY

Epilepsy Foundation of America answers questions; provides information; and makes referrals.
Phone: 800-EFA-1000
Mailing address: 4351 Garden City Drive, Landover, MD 20785
Web site: http://www.efa.org

Epilepsy Support Organizations Guide
web site provides addresses and phone numbers organizations providing support and education for people with epilepsy.
Web site: http://neurosurgery.mgn.harvard.edu/ep-resrc.htm

Washington University Epilepsy Links
web site provides a comprehensive list of epilepsy-related resources.
Web site:
http://www.neuro.wustl.edu/epilepsy/

EYES AND VISION

American Council of the Blind makes referrals, provides information on consumer items for blind people, and provides updates on legislation affecting the blind.
Phone: 800-424-8666
Mailing address: 1155 15th Street Northwest, Suite 720, Washington, DC 20005
Web site: http://www.acb.org

American Foundation for the Blind
provides information to individuals who are blind or visually impaired.
Phone: 800-AFB-LINE
Mailing address: 11 Penn Plaza, Suite 300, New York, NY 10001

Association for Macular Diseases provides information on the causes, treatment, and prevention of macular diseases, which include inflammations, tumors, retinal growths, and degenerative problems.
Phone: 212-605-3719
Mailing address: 210 East 64th Street, New York, NY 10021

Council of Citizens With Low Vision provides information and referral to people who are partially sighted and to people with low vision.
Phone: 800-733-2258
Mailing address: 1400 North Drake Road, No. 218, Kalamazoo, MI 49006

Eyenet web site, operated by the American Academy of Ophthalmology, features a forum where ophthalmologists answer frequently asked questions about eye disorders, eye care news, and a detailed illustration of the human eye.
Web site: http://www.eyenet.org

Glaucoma Research Foundation provides information about glaucoma and offers referrals and support services.
Phone: 800-826-6693
Mailing address: 490 Post Street, Suite 830, San Francisco, California 94102

Glaucoma 2001 provides information for people suffering from glaucoma.
Phone: 800-391-EYES
Mailing address: Foundation of the American Academy of Ophthalmology, 655 Beach Street, P.O. Box 7424, San Francisco, California 94120-7424

Guide Dog Foundation for the Blind, Inc. provides guide dogs free of charge to qualified people who are legally blind. The toll-free line has information specialists who answer questions.
Phone: 800-548-4337
Web site: http://www.guidedog.org

National Association for Parents of the Visually Impaired provides referrals to support groups.
Phone: 800-562-6265

National Eye Care Project provides referrals to physicians who treat on a volunteer basis people 65 years and older who are unable to afford eye care.
Phone: 800-222-EYES

National Eye Research Foundation
answers questions, sends out written information, and provides referrals.
Phone: 800-621-2258
E-mail: nerf1955@aol.com

Prevent Blindness America answers general questions and provides written information on vision, eye health, care, and safety.
Phone: 800-331-2020
Web site: http://www.prevent-blindness.org
E-mail: 74777.100@compuserve.com

FEET

American Academy of Orthopedic Surgeons provides written information about problems that affect the feet.
Phone: 800-346-AAOS
Mailing address: 6300 North River Road, Rosemont, IL 60018-4226

American Orthopedic Foot and Ankle Society provides information about problems that affect the feet and offers professional referrals.
Phone: 800-235-4855
Mailing address: 701 16th Avenue, Seattle, WA 98122

Foot Care Information Center Hotline, operated by the American Podiatric Medical Association, provides written materials and referrals to callers who leave their names and addresses on its voice mail.
Phone: 800-FOOT CARE

FERTILITY

National Infertility Network Exchange provides referrals and support for individuals and couples suffering from infertility.
Phone: 516-794-5772
Mailing address: P.O. Box 204, East Meadow, NY 11554

Resolve, Inc. offers information, referral, and support to people with problems of infertility.
Phone: 617-623-0744
Mailing address: 1310 Broadway, Somerville, MA 12144-1731
Web site: http://www.resolve.org/

FOOD AND NUTRITION

Ask the Dietitian web site provides an interactive forum on nutrition.
Web site:
http://www.hoptechno.com/rdindex.htm
E-mail: jlarsen@skypoint.com

Center for Food Safety and Nutrition web site, operated by the Food and Drug Administration, contains information about food safety, cosmetics, product labeling, and proper nutrition.
Web site: http://vm.cfsan.fda.gov/list.html
E-mail: lrd@vm.cfsan.fda.gov

Consumer Nutrition Hotline of the American Dietetic Association's National Center for Nutrition and Dietetics answers questions on food and nutrition and offer referrals to local dietitians. Callers can listen to taped messages on food and nutrition.
Phone: 800-366-1655
Web site: http://www.eatright.org

Food and Nutrition Information Center provides publications on nutrition. The web site, operated by the U.S. Department of Agriculture, offers information on the USDA research service and library.
Phone: 301-504-5719
Web site: //www.nalusda.gov/fnic/

Meat and Poultry Hotline, operated by the United States Department of Agriculture, provides an opportunity to speak to a food safety specialist weekdays from 10 a.m. to 4 p.m. Eastern time.
Phone: 800-535-4555
Web site: http://www.usda.gov/agency/fsis/homepage.htm

North American Vegetarian Society web site provides information on vegetarian events, conferences, and nutrition.
Web site: http://mars.superlink.com/user/dupre/navs/index.html
E-mail: dupre@mars:superlink.com

Seafood Hotline, operated by the United States Food and Drug Administration, provides information on seafood.
Phone: 800-FDA-4010
Web site: http://www.fda.gov/

GENERAL HEALTH INFORMATION

American Medical Association offers information about research materials to consumers and medical professionals. The web site provides information about the activities and policies of the AMA, access to abstracts of its journals and publications, and other resources.
Phone: 312-464-5000
Mailing address: 515 North State Street, Chicago, IL 60610
Web site: http://www.ama-assn.org
E-mail: webAdmin@web.ama-assn.org

The American Red Cross web site provides information on current relief efforts, Red Cross services, locating the Red Cross chapter near you, and volunteering.
Web site: http://www.crossnet.org/

CenterWatch web site provides information about clinical trials and new drug therapies recently approved by the Food and Drug Administration.
Web site: http://www.CenterWatch.com

Department of Health and Human Services provides consumer-oriented health-care information. This federal government web site provides information on health concerns and issues, financial assistance, legal documents, and educational materials.
Mailing address: Hubert H. Humphrey Building, 200 Independence Avenue, SW, Washington, DC 20201
Web site: http://www.os.dhhs.gov/
E-mail: tthomso@os.dhhs.gov

Global Health Network web site, sponsored by the University of Pittsburgh, offers thousands of Internet links to schools and organizations.
Web site:
http:www.pitt.edu/home/ghnet/ghnet.html
E-mail: rlaporte@vms.cis.pitt.edu

The Good Health web site offers a database of more than 1,000 health organizations, an interactive forum, and health-related newsgroups.
Web site:
http://www.social.com/health/index.html
E-mail: webmaster@social.com

Health Information Resources web site, operated by the National Information Center, lists toll-free numbers of medical organizations that provide health-related information.
Web site: http://nhic-nt.health.org/

HealthNet web site offers information on hospitals, government, and private medical practices, and provides links to hundreds of other web sites.
Web site:
http://debra.dgbt.doc.ca/~mike/healthnet/
E-mail: x-man@mgcheo.med.uottawa.ca

MedAccess web site offers a consumer's guide to health insurance, health-care professionals, and facilities.
Web site: http://www.medaccess.com

Med Help International web site offers up-to-date information on most known illnesses and diseases.
Web site:
http://medhlp.netusa.net/index.html
E-mail: staff@medhlp.netusa.net

Medical Source web site offers articles, tips, guides on health care, and more than 1,000 links to other health-related sites.
Web site: http://www.medsource.com

National Health Information Center provides referrals to national health organizations and support groups.
Phone: 800-336-4797
Web site: http://nhic-nt.health.org
E-mail: nhicinfo@health.org

The Patient's Network web site, created by caregivers and patients, offers patient education materials, interactive areas, and links to resources.
Web site: http://www.pond.com/wellness/

GENETIC DISEASES

Alliance of Genetic Support Groups provides callers with information on how to contact genetic services and national support groups for various genetic disorders.
Phone: 800-336-GENE
Web site:
http://medhelp.org/www/agsg.htm
E-mail: alliance@capaccess.org

HEADACHE

National Headache Foundation answers questions and provides referrals to support groups.
Phone: 800-843-2256
Web site: http://www.headaches.org

HEARING

American Hearing Research Foundation provides information on hearing disorders.
Phone: 312-726-9670

American Speech-Language-Hearing Information Resource Center provides information on speech, language, and hearing disorders as well as referrals.
Phone: 800-638-8255
Web site: http://www.asha.org

Deaf World web site provides deaf resources organized by country, pen pals for deaf children, and a discussion forum.
Web site:
http://deafworldweb.org/deafworld/
E-Mail: dww@deafworldweb.org

Dial a Hearing Screening Test answers questions, sends written information, and makes referrals to local physicians, audiologists, and hearing-aid specialists. The organization also puts callers in touch with regional centers that give free hearing screening tests over the phone.
Phone: 800-222-EARS
E-Mail: dabiddle@aol.com

Hearing Aid Helpline, operated by the International Hearing Society, answers questions, sends written information on hearing aids and hearing loss, and makes referrals to local hearing-aid specialists.
Phone: 800-521-5247

Hearing Helpline provides written information to the hearing impaired.
Phone: 800-EAR-WELL

HEART DISEASE

American Heart Association provides information on cholesterol and all aspects of heart disease as well as referrals to local heart association chapters weekdays during local business hours. The web site provides resources related to the prevention and treatment of heart disease and stroke.
Phone: 800-AHA-USA-1
Web site: http://www.amhrt.org
E-mail: inquire@amhrt.org

Cardiology Compass web site, operated by the Washington University School of Medicine and Medical Center, provides a list of cardiovascular information resources.
Web site: http://osler.wustl.edu/~murphy/cardiology/compass.html
E-mail: murphy@osler.wustl.edu

The Heart: An Online Exploration web site, operated by the Franklin Institute Science Museum, features a multimedia tour of the heart.
Web site: http://sln.fi.edu/biosci/heart.html
E-Mail: webteam@sln.fi.edu

HEMOPHILIA

Hemophilia Home Page provides information on hemophilia, a hereditary disease in which blood clotting is delayed.
Web site: http://www.web-depot.com/hemophilia/autosite/autosite.cgi

National Hemophilia Foundation operates an information center on hemophilia and provides information on the disorder.
Phone: 212-219-8180
Mailing address: 110 Greene Street, Suite 303, New York, NY 10012

World Federation of Hemophilia provides information about the disorder to individuals suffering from hemophilia.
Web site: http://www.wfh.org/

HEPATITIS

Hepatitis/Liver Disease Hotline, operated by the American Liver Foundation, answers questions, provides information, and makes referrals to individuals with hepatitis or other diseases of the liver.
Phone: 800-223-HEPABC
Web site: http://sadieo.ucsf.edu/alf/alffinal/homepagealt.html

HOSPICE CARE

National Hospice Organization provides written information and answers general questions on hospice and makes referrals to local hospices.
Phone: 800-658-8898
Web site: http://www.nho.org
E-mail: drsnho@cais.com

HUNTINGTON'S DISEASE

Huntington's Disease Society of America provides written information to callers who leave their names and addresses on its answering machine 24 hours a day, 7 days a week.
Phone: 800-345-4372
Web site: http://neuro-www2.mgh.harvard.edu/hdsa/hdsamain.nclk

HYPERTENSION

National Heart, Lung, and Blood Institute's Information Line mails written information on high blood pressure and high blood cholesterol to callers who leave their names and addresses on its answering machine.
Phone: 800-575-WELL

National Hypertension Association provides information on hypertension and conducts hypertension and hypercholesterol detection programs.
Phone: 212-889-3557

HYPOGLYCEMIA

Hypoglycemia Association provides information and support to people with hypoglycemia, a deficiency in the blood sugar that deprives the central nervous system of glucose needed to function.
Phone: 202-544-4044
Mailing address: 18008 New Hampshire Avenue, Box 165, Ashton, MD 20861-0165

IMMUNIZATION

National Immunization Campaign sends information to people who leave a message on their answering machine.
Phone: 800-525-6789

INCONTINENCE

The Simon Foundation for Continence provides free written information and sample products 24 hours a day, 7 days a week.
Phone: 800-237-4666

INJURY CONTROL

Car Accident web site provides information on accidents and injuries related to car accidents.
Web site: http://www.stresspress.com/car/

Injury Control Resource Information Network web site, operated by the University of Pittsburgh Center for Injury Research and Control, provides a list of resources for treating injuries, and links to data bases and organizations.
Web site: http://info.pitt.edu/~hweiss/injury

KIDNEY DISEASE

American Kidney Fund works to alleviate the financial burdens caused by kidney disease.
Phone: 800-638-8299

National Kidney Foundation answers questions and provides written information on various types of kidney disease, research, dialysis, transplants, and diet.
Phone: 800-622-9010

Renal Net web site provides information to patients with renal disorders.
Web site:
http://ns.gamewood.net/renalnet/html

LARYNGECTOMEES

International Association of Laryngectomees offers information and referral for people who have had their larynx removed.
Phone: 404-320-3333
Mailing address: c/o American Cancer Society, 1599 Clifton Road NE, Atlanta, GA 30329

LEAD POISONING

National Lead Information Hotline provides written information on preventing lead poisoning and referrals to agencies that can provide further information to callers who leave their addresses and phone numbers on its answering machine.
Phone: 800-LEAD-FYI

LEARNING DISABILITIES

National Center for Learning Disabilities provides resources and referrals for volunteers, parents, and professionals working with the learning disabled and offers services for children.
Phone: 212-545-7510
Mailing address: 381 Park Avenue South, Suite 1420, New York, NY 10016

LIVER

American Liver Foundation provides information on liver diseases, liver functions, and disease prevention.
Phone: 800-223-0179
Mailing address: 1425 Pompton Avenue, Cedar Grove, NJ 07009

LIVING WILLS

Choice in Dying provides free legal, medical, mental health counseling, and crisis intervention.
Phone: 800-989-9455
Web site: http://www.choices.org

LYME DISEASE

Lyme Disease Foundation assists in the formation of support groups, offers referral service, and provides information on Lyme disease, which is spread to humans by ticks. Symptoms include rashes, joint swelling and pain, fever, severe headaches, and heart arrhythmia.
Phone: 800-886-LYME
Mailing address: 1 Financial Plaza, 18th Floor, Hartford, CT 06103

Lyme Disease Information Network web site provides information on the prevention and treatment of the disease.
Web site:
http://www.sky.net/~dporter/lyme1.html

MARFAN SYNDROME

National Marfan Foundation answers questions, sends written information, and makes referrals to local support groups.
Phone: 800-8-MARFAN
Web site: http://www.marfan.org

MENTAL HEALTH

Internet Mental Health web site offers an online encyclopedia of mental health information, such as information on common mood disorders and common psychiatric medications, and it features an online magazine.
Web site: http://www.mentalhealth.com/

Mental Health Net web site offers a guide to mental health issues by providing links to more than 3,000 resources.
Web site: http://www.cmhc.com/

National Alliance for the Mentally Ill provides information and makes referrals to support groups.
Phone: 800-950-6264
Web site: http://www.cais.com/vikings/nami/index.html

MULTIPLE BIRTH

Center for Study of Multiple Birth provides information on the medical risks of multiple birth.
Phone: 312-266-9093

MULTIPLE SCLEROSIS

Multiple Sclerosis Association of America hotline provides an opportunity for people to speak with counselors.
Phone: 800-833-4672

Multiple Sclerosis Information Source web site provides information on the disorder.
Web site: http://ils.unc.edu/multiplesclerosis/hopk/mspage.html

National Multiple Sclerosis Society provides educational information about MS, counseling, family and social support, equipment assistance, clinical trials, and employment programs.
Phone: 800-FIGHT-MS
Web site: http://www.nmss.org
E-mail: info@nmss.org

MYASTHENIA GRAVIS

Myasthenia Gravis Foundation of America, Inc. answers questions and provides written information.
Phone: 800-541-5454
Web site: http://www.med.unc.edu/mgfa/
E-mail: mgfa@aol.com

NEUROLOGICAL DISORDERS

Cure Paralysis Now web site provides information on research and technology.
Web site: http://www.cureparalysis.org.

National Institute of Neurological Disorders and Stroke answers questions, provides written information, and makes referrals to local agencies.
Phone: 800-352-9424
Web site: http://www.nih.gov/ninds/

Neurosciences on the Internet web site offers a searchable index with resources on neurobiology, neurology, neurosurgery, psychiatry, psychology, and the cognitive sciences.
Web site: http://ivory.lm.com/~nab/

NEWS SERVICES ON THE INTERNET

Medical Reporter, a monthly health-care magazine available only on the Internet, provides articles on diseases, treatments, and public policy issues.
Web site: http://www.dash.com/netro/nex/tmr/tmr.html

NewsFile web site offers newsletters that spotlight health-care issues.
Web site: http://www.newsfile.com

ORTHOPEDICS

Ortho Home Page offers an interactive patient's guide on orthopedics.
Web site: http://www.cyberport.net/ortho/ortho.html

OSTEOPOROSIS

National Osteoporosis Foundation provides written information on the bone disorder.
Phone: 800-223-9994
Web site: http://www.nof.org

PARENTING AND CHILDBIRTH

American Academy of Child and Adolescent Psychiatry web site provides access to more than 45 information sheets published by the AACAP.
Phone: 202-966-7300
Web site: http://www.psych.med.umich.edu/web/AACAP/factsfam/

Ask NOAH web site provides information on topics of interest to parents.
Web site: http://www.noah.cuny.edu

Child Safety Forum web site provides information related to child safety.
Web site: http://www.xmission.com:80/~gastown/safe

La Leche League Helpline answers questions and provides written information on breastfeeding.
Phone: 800-LA LECHE

National Parent Information Network provides information on raising and educating children. The organization's web site offers a monthly online newsletter, a parenting discussion group, and resources on child care, health and nutrition, and education.
Phone: 800-583-4135
Web site: http://ericps.ed.uiuc.edu/npin/npinhome.html

PARKINSON DISEASE

American Parkinson Disease Association, Inc. provides information and makes referrals.
Phone: 800-223-2732
Web site: http://neuro-chief-e.mgh.harvard.edu/parkinsonsweb/main/pdmain.html

Parkinson Disease Information Center web site provides information on the disease and its treatment.
Web site:
http://www.efn.org/~jskaye/pd/index.html

PHARMACEUTICALS

Drug Info Net, Inc. web site offers information on drugs.
Web site: http://www.druginfonet.com

PharmInfoNet web site offers information on thousands of drugs' trade names, generic names, and characteristics.
Web site: http://pharminfo.com

RxList web site offers information on more than 4,000 drug products.
Web site: http://www.rxlist.com/

PITUITARY DISORDERS

Human Growth Foundation provides information to families of children with physical growth problems.
Phone: 800-451-6434

PREMENSTRUAL SYNDROME

PMS Access provides recorded information on PMS.
Phone: 800-222-4767

RARE DISORDERS

National Organization for Rare Disorders provides information on more than 1,000 rare disorders.
Phone: 800-999-6673
Web site: http://www.nord-rdb.com/~orphan

REYE'S SYNDROME

National Reye's Syndrome Foundation answers questions and provides written information.
Phone: 800-233-7393

SAFETY

Consumer Product Safety Commission Hot Line provides taped information on product recalls, corrective actions, and other product safety questions.
Phone: 800-638-2772

The National Highway Traffic Safety Administration Auto Safety Hotline provides information on recalls, crash-test results, tire quality, and other automotive safety topics. Callers can also obtain written information and report auto safety problems.
Phone: 800-424-9393
Web site: http://www.nhtsa.dot.gov/index.

Occupational Safety and Health Administration (OSHA) web site provides information on OSHA regulations and documents, advisories, legislation, and a list of frequently asked questions about OSHA.
Web site: http://www.osha.gov/

SCLERODERMA

United Scleroderma Foundation answers questions; provides written information; and makes referrals to physicians, local chapters, and support groups.
Phone: 800-722-HOPE
Web site: http://www.scleroderma.com

SCOLIOSIS

National Scoliosis Foundation provides information on the disorder.
Phone: 617-926-0397
Mailing address: 72 Mt. Auburn Street, Watertown, MA 02172

Scoliosis Association offers information about spinal deviations.
Phone: 800-800-0669

SEXUALLY TRANSMITTED DISEASES

Centers for Disease Control National STD Hotline answers questions and provides written information and referrals.
Phone: 800-227-8922
Web site: http://sunsite.unc.edu/ASHA/

SHINGLES

The VZV Research Foundation provides information on the treatment of shingles.
Phone: 800-472-8478

SICKLE CELL ANEMIA

Sickle Cell Disease Association of America Inc. makes referrals to physicians and local chapters.
Phone: 800-421-8453

SLEEP DISORDERS

Sleep Medicine Home Page provides information on resources, sleep disorder centers, and educational material.
Web site:
http://www.cloud9.net80/~thropy/

SPINA BIFIDA

Spina Bifida Information and Referral Hotline provides information on the disorder.
Phone: 800-621-3141

SPINAL CORD INJURY OR DISORDER

National Spinal Cord Injury Association provides information and makes referrals.
Phone: 800-962-9629

National Spinal Cord Injury Hotline answers questions and makes referrals.
Phone: 800-526-3456
Web site: http://users.aol.com/scihotline
E-mail: scihotline@aol.com

STROKE

American Heart Association Stroke Connection makes referrals to agencies and support groups and provides written information. An answering service operates outside regular hours.
Phone: 800-553-6321
Web site: http://www.amhrt.org/stroke

National Stroke Association answers questions and provides written information about stroke and stroke prevention.
Phone: 800-STROKES
Web site: http://www.stroke.org
E-mail: info@stroke.org

STUTTERING

National Center for Stuttering answers questions, offers suggestions for parents of children who have begun to stutter, makes referrals, and provides written information.
Phone: 800-221-2483
Web site: http://www.stuttering.com

SUDDEN INFANT DEATH SYNDROME

American SIDS Institute provides the opportunity to talk with a doctor or social worker. Also sends written information and makes referrals to local support groups. After regular hours, an answering service at the same number will page a doctor or social worker.
Phone: 800-232-7437; 800-847-7437 within Georgia
Web site: http://www.sids.org

Sudden Infant Death Syndrome Net-work web site provides articles on SIDS, information on reducing the risk for SIDS, recent research, and legislative updates.
Web site: http://q.continuum.net/~sidsnet/

SUICIDE

American Suicide Foundation provides information on the causes and prevention of suicide.
Phone: 800-ASF-4042
Mailing address: 1045 Park Avenue, New York, NY 10028-1030

Suicide Awareness Voices of Education web site provides information about common misconceptions about suicide, what to do if a loved one is suicidal, questions and answers on depression, and a list of books on suicide.
Web site: http://www.save.org/

Suicide Information and Resources web site provides information on suicide and links to other suicide resources.
Web site: http://www.paranoia.com/~real/suicide/

THYROID DISORDERS

Thyroid Foundation of America Hotline provides written information and referrals to physicians.
Phone: 800-832-8321

TINNITUS

American Tinnitus Association provides information about tinnitus.
Phone: 503-248-9985

TOURETTE SYNDROME

Tourette Syndrome Association sends written information to callers who write to the address given on the answering machine.
Phone: 800-237-0717

TRANSPLANTATION and ORGAN DONATION

American Association of Tissue Banks provides research and educational information on transplantation.
Phone: 703-827-9582
Mailing address: 1350 Beverly Road, Suite 220-A, McLean, VA 22101

Lifebanc provides information regarding organ donation.
Phone: 800-558-5433

The Living Bank helps people who, upon their deaths, wish to donate a part or parts of their bodies for the purposes of transplantation, therapy, or medical research.
Phone: 800-528-2971
Mailing address: P.O. Box 6725, Houston, TX 77265

National Bone Marrow Donor Program
provides a registry of bone marrow
donors, searches and matches donor
recipients, and provides educational and
research information.
Phone: 800-627-7692

TRAUMA DISORDERS

**Patient's Guide to Cumulative Trauma
Disorders** web site provides discussions
of trauma disorder, a series of symptoms
and syndromes that come about through
a repetition of stressful activities, such
as overuse of specific muscles, incorrect
posture, or excessive muscle tension.
Web site: http://www.cyberport.net/mmg/
ctd/stuff.html
E-mail: mmg@cyberport.net

TRAVEL HEALTH

**Centers for Disease Control Home
Travel Information Web Page** offers a regional breakdown on risks in 16 parts of
the world, reference materials for the international traveler, information on countries infected with cholera, yellow fever,
and plague and other diseases and epi-
demics.
Web site: http://www.cdc.gov/travel/
travel.html
E-mail: netinfo@cdc1.cdc.gov

Travel Health Information web site,
operated by the Medical College of
Wisconsin, provides information on diseases and immunizations, environmental
hazards, and other travel-related topics.
Web site:
http://www.intmed.mcw.edu/itc/health.html

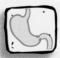

ULCER

National Ulcer Foundation offers infor-
mation on peptic ulcer disease.
Phone: 617-665-6210
Mailing address: 675 Main Street,
Melrose, MA 02176

VICTIMS OF VIOLENCE

National Center for Assault Prevention
provides information on causes and pre-
vention of domestic violence.
Phone: 800-258-3189
Mailing address: 606 Delsea Drive,
Sewell, NJ 08080

National Victim Center answers questions, sends written materials, and makes
referrals to local support groups and organizations for victims of violence.
Phone: 800-FYI CALL
E-mail: nvc@mail.nvc.org
Web site: http://www.nvc.org

WOMEN'S HEALTH

Guide to Women's Health Issues web
site, operated by University of Michigan
School of Information and Library Studies,
serves as a clearinghouse of information
related to women's health.
Web site: http://asa.ugl.lib.umich.edu/
chdocs/womenhealth/womens_health.html

**Institute for Research on Women's
Health** provides information on women's
physical and mental health.
Phone: 202-483-8643

National Council on Women's Health
provides medical information on women's
health.
Phone: 212-535-0031

**National Women's Health Resource
Center** serves as a clearinghouse for
women's health information.
Phone: 202-293-6045
Mailing address: 2440 M Street NW, Suite
325, Washington, DC 20037

Women's Health Resources web site, operated by University of Arizona School of
Information Resources, provides access to
information published by U.S. government
agencies.
Web site: http://timon.sir.arizona.edu/gov-
docs/whealth/agency.htm

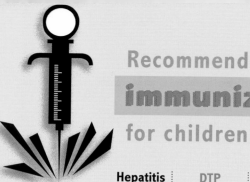

Recommended immunization schedule
for children

	Hepatitis B	DTP (diphtheria, tetanus, pertussis)	Polio	Hib (haemophilis influenza type b)	MMR (measles, mumps, rubella)	Td (tetanus, diphtheria)	Chickenpox
Birth–2 months	X						
1–4 months	X						
2 months		X	X	X			
4 months		X	X	X			
6 months		X		X			
6–18 months	X						
12 months							
12–15 months				X	X		
12–18 months			X				X
15 months							
15–18 months		X					
18 months							
4–6 years		X	X		X		
11–12 years	X					X	
14–16 years							

Source: The Centers for Disease Control and Prevention.

INDEX

How to use the index
This index covers the contents of the 1998, 1999, and 2000 editions.

Each entry gives the last two digits of the edition year and the page number or numbers. For example, this entry means that information on stuttering may be found on page 334 of the 2000 edition.

When there are many references to a topic, some of them are grouped alphabetically by clue words under the main topic. For example, the clue words under Suicide group the major references under several subtopics.

An entry in all capital letters indicates that there is a Health Update with that name in at least one of the three volumes covered by this index. Page numbers for these updates appear after these capitalized headings.

The "see" and "see also" cross-references indicate that references to the topic are listed under another entry in the index.

An entry that only begins with a capital letter indicates that there are no Health Update articles with that title but that information on this topic may be found in the edition and on the pages listed.

The indication (il.) after a page number means that the reference is to an illustration only.

A

G

Garlic, 98: 108, 113
Gasoline fires, 98: 278
Gastroesophageal reflux disease, 00: 249
Gaucher's disease, 00: 41, 43
Gene probe, 00: 41
Gene therapy, 00: 44, 46-47, **99:** 220, 258, **98:** 245
Generalized anxiety disorder, 00: 285
Genes, 00: 40
  aging, **00:** 54
  AIDS, **99:** 257-258, **98:** 197
  Alzheimer's disease, **98:** 213, 246
  anxiety, **98:** 216
  attention deficit disorder, **99:** 108
  blood disorder, **98:** 208-209
  cell death process, **99:** 220
  childhood obesity, **00:** 120
  cystic fibrosis, **98:** 273
  deafness, **99:** 248
  dementia, **99:** 228
  depression, **00:** 187
  Down syndrome, **98:** 243-244
  energy-regulating, **00:** 314
  eye problems, **99:** 256-257, **98:** 241-242
  hair loss, **99:** 296
  heart, **00:** 265
  human behavior, **98:** 222
  inflammatory bowel disease, **98:** 135-136
  intelligence, **99:** 258-260
  lupus, **98:** 204
  multiple sclerosis, **98:** 214
  mutation, **00:** 225
  obesity, **99:** 308 (il.), **98:** 292-293
  orthodontics, **00:** 110
  Parkinson disease, **98:** 214-215
  research, **00:** 39
  speech/language disorder, **99:** 260
  ulcer bacteria, **99:** 242-243
  virulence, **00:** 276
  see also **Cancer; Gene therapy; Genetic engineering; Genetic medicine; Mutations**
Genetic disorders, 99: 259
  correcting, **00:** 45
  Huntington's disease, **00:** 234-235
  information sources, **00:** 328
Genetic engineering, 99: 222, 271-272, **98:** 209, 213, 225
GENETIC MEDICINE, 00: 38-47, 263-266, **99:** 257-260, **98:** 243-246
  advances, **00:** 36-37
  see also **Cloning; Gene therapy; Genes; Genetic engineering**
Genetic screening, 00: 40-42, 43, **98:** 273
Genetically engineered drugs, 00: 42
Genome, 00: 40
Germ theory, 00: 23-24
Germander (herb), **98:** 106
Germanium (element), **98:** 107
Geron Corporation, 00: 59
Gestational diabetes, 00: 292
Gibbon, John, 00: 35
Ginger (herb), **98:** 113
Ginkgo biloba (herb), **99:** 206, 280, **98:** 113
GLANDS AND HORMONES, 00: 28, 266-268, **99:** 260-262, **98:** 247-248

  breast cancer, **98:** 238
  dietary supplements, **98:** 102, 109-111
  reproduction, **99:** 136-144, **98:** 51
  see also **Hormone replacement therapy; and specific glands and hormones**
Glaucoma, 98: 241-242
Glenn, John H., Jr., 00: 212 (il.)
Glucose, 00: 55, 246-247, 312, **99:** 241-242, **98:** 226, 227
  see also **Diabetes**
Gonadotropin releasing hormone, 99: 137, 138 (il.), 144
Gonorrhea, 00: 299-300, **99:** 294, **98:** 279, 280
Gross, Robert E., 00: 33
Guinea worm disease, 98: 258
Gum disease, 00: 245-246
  see also **Periodontal disease**
Gymnastics, 99: 175
Gynecology, 99: 81

H

Haemophilus influenzae type b vaccine, 00: 29
Hair loss, 00: 301(il.), **99:** 296-297
Hand transplants, 00: 308-309
Handwashing, 99: 120-131, **98:** 222 (il.)
Harvey, William, 00: 20
HDL. See High-density lipoprotein
Head injuries, 99: 170
Headache, 00: 328, **99:** 47, 245 (il.), 252-253, 327, **98:** 318
Health care information, 99: 309-336, **98:** 295-336
HEALTH CARE ISSUES, 00: 268-272, **99:** 262-266, **98:** 249-253
  costs, **00:** 50
  pet care costs, **00:** 156-169
  see also **Health care system; Health insurance; Medical ethics**
Health care online, 00: 232
Health care system, 98: 14, 212
  reform, **98:** 251, 316-318
  see also **Managed care**
Health insurance, 00: 264-265, **98:** 13-17, 19, 21, 39-41, 63, 87-90, 95, 263
  mental health coverage, **99:** 278-279
  pet coverage, **00:** 161
  smoking cessation coverage, **00:** 305
  State Children's Health Insurance Program, **00:** 272
  substance abuse coverage, **00:** 220
  see also **Managed care; Medicaid; Medicare**
Health maintenance organizations, 99: 265-266, **98:** 14-19, 31
Hearing. See Ear and hearing
Hearing aids, 98: 234 (il.)
HEART AND BLOOD VESSELS, 00: 272-276, **99:** 267-271, **98:** 253-257
  cardiac arrhythmia, **98:** 232
  erythropoietin, **00:** 226
  fen-phen dangers, **00:** 312-314
  genes, **00:** 265
  laser therapy for pain, **00:** 275-276
  risk of heart attack, **00:** 225-226
  sudden infant death syndrome, **99:** 234-235
  surgical advances, **00:** 33, 35

  thrombotic thrombocytopenic purpura, **00:** 226-227
  valve defects, **99:** 244, 246, 306-307
  varicose veins, **99:** 64-75
  see also **Transplants**
Heart attacks
  aspirin, **99:** 27
  cholesterol level, **99:** 268, **98:** 256
  defibrillators, **99:** 269-270, 290 (il.), **98:** 253
  diagnosis, **99:** 268
  diet, **98:** 256 (il.)
  drug therapy, **99:** 269-270, **98:** 254-255
  ephedra, **98:** 112
  leeches, **00:** 274-275
  risks, **00:** 225-226
  smoking, **98:** 236
Heart disease, 00: 228
  aspirin, **99:** 28
  childhood obesity, **00:** 121
  dental health, **99:** 238-239, 267 (il.)
  DHEA, **98:** 111
  diet, **00:** 288, 290, **98:** 256 (il.)
  diet pills, **98:** 294
  drugs, **98:** 254-256
  exercise, **99:** 270, **98:** 238-239
  growing new vessels, **99:** 270-271
  headache symptom, **99:** 252-253
  hormone replacement therapy, **99:** 58
  information sources, **00:** 329, **99:** 327, **98:** 212, 213, 319-320
  pets, **00:** 158
  sclerotherapy, **99:** 71
  smoking, **98:** 236, 284
  snoring, **98:** 72-73, 75
  surgery, **98:** 254-255
  see also **Atherosclerosis; Cholesterol; Coronary angioplasty; Coronary artery bypass surgery; Heart attacks**
Heartburn, 00: 249
Heart-lung machine, 00: 35
Heartworms, 99: 192
Heat, as pain reliever, 99: 39-43
Heating, and safety, 99: 292
Heel problems, 99: 173, 177
Helicobacter pylori (bacteria), **00:** 249-250, **99:** 242, **98:** 228-229
Helmet, for bicycling, 99: 171, 178
Hematocrit, 00: 280
Hematopoietic stem cells, 00: 308
Hematuria, 00: 310
Hemochromatosis, 98: 208-209
Hemodialysis, 00: 279-280
  see also **Dialysis**
Hemoglobin, 98: 208
Hemophilia, 00: 39, 41, 42, 329, **99:** 222, 328, **98:** 320
Hemorrhoids, 99: 66, 75
Heparin (drug), **99:** 56
Hepatitis
  blood transfusions, **99:** 266, 272
  drugs, **99:** 246
  food safety, **98:** 109, 177, 183, 235, 257 (il.), 276
  information sources, **00:** 329, **99:** 328, **98:** 320
  liver cancer, **00:** 238
  symptoms, **99:** 271 (il.)
  transmission, **99:** 122
  vaccine, **98:** 61-62, 224
  vitamin E, **98:** 269

ACKNOWLEDGMENTS

The publishers gratefully acknowledge the courtesy of the following artists, photographers, publishers, institutions, agencies, and corporations for the illustrations in this volume. Credits should read from top to bottom, left to right on their respective pages. All entries marked with an asterisk (*) denote illustrations created exclusively for this edition. All maps, charts, and diagrams were prepared by the staff unless otherwise noted.

2   Salk Institute; Yerkes Primate Research Center
3   © Reuters/Archive Photos; © PhotoDisc, Inc.; AP/Wide World
4   © Alfred Pasieka/SPL from Photo Researchers; © Laurence Dutton, Tony Stone Images; John Manders*
5   © Craig Hammell, The Stock Market; © Mike Timo, Tony Stone Images; © Oscar Burriel/SPL from Photo Researchers
10   © Alfred Pasieka/SPL from Photo Researchers; Illumination (about 1050) from a Byzantine manuscript by an unknown artist (Granger Collection); © PhotoDisc, Inc.; © Sam Ogden/SPL from Photo Researchers
11   © PhotoDisc, Inc.; © Mehau Kulyk/SPL from Photo Researchers
12   Wellcome Institute Library, London
14   Granger Collection
15   Detail from *The Temptation of St. Anthony* from the Isenheim Altar (about 1515) oil on panel by Matthias Grunewald, Unterlinden Museum, Colmar, France (Eric Lessing from Art Resource)
16   Illumination (about 1050) from a Byzantine manuscript by an unknown artist (Granger Collection)
17   Illumination (about 1440) from a Hebrew edition of *Avicenna's Canon of Medicine* (Granger Collection)
18   © AAA Collection Ltd.
20   Granger Collection
21   Granger Collection; National Library of Medicine; *The First Use of Ether in Dental Surgery* (1846) oil on canvas by W. T. G. Morton, Wellcome Institute Library, London

22   Corbis/Hulton
23   National Library of Medicine
24–25   © PhotoDisc, Inc.
27   Corbis; © PhotoDisc, Inc.
28   © PhotoDisc, Inc.
29   © PhotoDisc, Inc.; Corbis/Bettmann; © PhotoDisc, Inc.
30   Royal Society of Medicine; © PhotoDisc, Inc.
31   Everett Collection
32   © PhotoDisc, Inc.; *The Gross Clinic* (1875) oil on canvas by Thomas Eakins, Jefferson Medical College of Thomas Jefferson University, Philadelphia, PA; © PhotoDisc, Inc.
33   © Ray Ellis, Photo Researchers; © PhotoDisc, Inc.
34–35   © PhotoDisc, Inc.
36   © Alfred Pasieka/SPL from Photo Researchers; © PhotoDisc, Inc.
38   © PhotoDisc, Inc.
40   National Human Genome Research Institute
41   Barbara Cousins*
45   Barbara Cousins*; Ted Thai, *Time* Magazine © Time Inc.
46   Ted Thai, *Time* Magazine © Time Inc.
47   © Sam Ogden/SPL from Photo Researchers
48   © PhotoDisc, Inc.
51   © Mehau Kulyk/SPL from Photo Researchers
53–56   © PhotoDisc, Inc.
57   Barbara Cousins*
58   © PhotoDisc, Inc.
60   © Jon Riley, Tony Stone Images; © Oliver Meckes, Photo Researchers; © John Durham/SPL from Photo Researchers; © Laurence Dutton, Tony Stone Images
61   © Superstock; Beltone Electronics
63   © Laurence Dutton, Tony Stone Images
65–67   Barbara Cousins*

69   © Jon Riley, Tony Stone Images; © Sheila Terry/SPL from Photo Researchers
70   © PhotoDisc, Inc.
71–73   Barbara Cousins*
76   © Markova, The Stock Market
79   Barbara Cousins*
80   © Blair Seitz, Photo Researchers
81   Ann Tomasic*
84–85   © Superstock
86   Beltone Electronics; © Chris Priest/SPL from Photo Researchers; © Uniphoto
88   © John Durham/SPL from Photo Researchers
92   © Oliver Meckes, Photo Researchers
93   Barbara Cousins*
94–95   © Mark Clarke/SPL from Photo Researchers
97   © James King-Holmes/SPL from Custom Medical
99   © PhotoDisc, Inc.
100   Estelle Carol*
102   © David Young Wolff, Tony Stone Images
104   © Donna Day, Tony Stone Images; © Frank Siteman, Index Stock; © PhotoDisc, Inc.; John Manders*
105   © Jim Whitmer, FPG; John Manders*
106   Masel Industries
109   American Association of Orthodontics
110   © PhotoDisc, Inc.
112   WORLD BOOK illustration by Charles Wellek; © 3M Unitek Corporation. All rights reserved
113   American Association of Orthodontics
114   © Frank Siteman, Index Stock
119   © Donna Day, Tony Stone Images
124   © Mark Richards, PhotoEdit; © Robert Ginn, PhotoEdit; © Michael Newman, PhotoEdit;
125   © Jim Whitmer, FPG
126   © Will Hart, PhotoEdit
128   © Keff Zaruba, The Stock Market; © Myrleen Ferguson, PhotoEdit

130–142 © John Manders*
144 © C/B Productions from The Stock Market; © David Madison, Tony Stone Images; © Kathi Lamm, Tony Stone Images; ICON Health & Fitness
145 © Dann Tardif, The Stock Market; © Tom McCarthy, PhotoEdit
149 Life Fitness
150 © Steve Prezant, The Stock Market
151 © Tom McCarthy, PhotoEdit
152 ICON Health & Fitness
154 © C/B Productions from The Stock Market
155 Life Fitness
156 © David Madison, Tony Stone Images
159 © Susan Kuklin, Photo Researchers
160 © Dann Tardif, The Stock Market
162 © David Young-Wolff, PhotoEdit
163 © Marion H. Levy, Photo Researchers
165 © Blair Seitz, Photo Researchers
167 © Kathi Lamm, Tony Stone Images
168 © Craig Hammell, The Stock Market
170 © Richard Nowitz, Photo Researchers; © C/B Productions from The Stock Market; © Bruce Ayres, Tony Stone Images; © Lori Adamski-Peek, Tony Stone Images
171 © Kindra Clineff, Tony Stone Images; © Bill Aron, PhotoEdit
172 © Kindra Clineff, Tony Stone Images
175 © Mug Shots from The Stock Market
176 © Andy Sacks, Tony Stone Images
178 © David Young-Wolff, PhotoEdit

179 © C/B Productions from The Stock Market
182 © Andy Sacks, Tony Stone Images
184 © PhotoDisc, Inc.
189 © Frank Siteman, Tony Stone Images
190 © Richard Nowitz, Photo Researchers
193 © Bob Llewellyn, Uniphoto
194 © Bruce Ayres, Tony Stone Images
196 © Mike Timo, Tony Stone Images
199 © Myrleen Ferguson, PhotoEdit
200–201 © Joe Atlas, Artville
202 © Renee Lynn, Photo Researchers
203 © Lori Adamski-Peek, Tony Stone Images
204 © Ariel Skelley, The Stock Market
207 © Townsend P. Dickinson, The Image Works; © Dion Ogust, The Image Works; © Bill Aron, PhotoEdit
210 © Jon Riley, Tony Stone Images; © PhotoDisc, Inc.; © David R. Frazier
211 © Oscar Burriel/SPL from Photo Researchers
212 AP/Wide World
213 © Oscar Burriel/SPL from Photo Researchers
215 Yerkes Primate Research Center
219 © PhotoDisc, Inc.
221 © Mike Mazzaschi, Stock, Boston
222 © Linda Ziemianski, International Medical News Group
225 Gynetics
226 Biomedical Disposal Inc.
228 © PhotoDisc, Inc.
229 Lunar Corporation
230 © PhotoDisc, Inc.
233 Linda R. Kitabayashi, Salk Institute

235 AP/Wide World; Barbara Cousins*
239 © Simon Fraser/SPL from Photo Researchers
240 © PhotoDisc, Inc.
241 Sara M. O'Hara, Duke University Medical Center
243 Barbara Cousins*; Jeff Guerrant*
245 © Robert Essel, The Stock Market
246 © Paul Barton, The Stock Market
247 © PhotoDisc, Inc.
248 Biocontrol Technology, Inc.
255 © PhotoDisc, Inc.
258 Eric Under*
259 © PhotoDisc, Inc.
260 © James Schnepf, Liaison Agency
261 VISX, Inc.
262 Keravision
263–267 © PhotoDisc, Inc.
269 AP/Wide World
273 Thermo Cardiosystems Inc.
274 © PhotoDisc, Inc.
275 © Eclipse Surgical Technologies
281 © Reuters/Archive Photos
282 © New York Times Company/Archive Photos
283–287 © PhotoDisc, Inc.
290 Tufts University
291–294 © PhotoDisc, Inc.
297 © David R. Frazier
298 © PhotoDisc, Inc.
301 Linda Degenstein and Chuck Wellek, Howard Hughes Medical Center
304 © PhotoDisc, Inc.
305 Chrispin, Porter and Bogusky
308 © Reuters/Archive Photos; AP/Wide World
310 © PhotoDisc, Inc.
311 © Jon Riley, Tony Stone Images
313 © PhotoDisc, Inc.